Prematurity: Art and Science

Guest Editors

ALAN R. FLEISCHMAN, MD
JAY D. IAMS, MD

CLINICS IN PERINATOLOGY

www.perinatology.theclinics.com

Consulting Editor

LUCKY JAIN, MD, MBA

September 2011 • Volume 38 • Number 3

SAUNDERS an imprint of ELSEVIER, Inc.

W.B. SAUNDERS COMPANY
A Division of Elsevier Inc.

Elsevier, Inc. • 1600 John F. Kennedy Blvd. • Suite 1800 • Philadelphia, PA 19103-2899

http://www.theclinics.com

CLINICS IN PERINATOLOGY Volume 38, Number 3
September 2011 ISSN 0095-5108, ISBN-13: 978-1-4557-1118-5

Editor: Kerry Holland
Developmental Editor: Teia Stone

Clinics in Perinatology (ISSN 0095-5108) is published quarterly by Elsevier Inc., 360 Park Avenue South, New York, NY 10010-1710. Months of issue are March, June, September, and December. Business and Editorial Offices: 1600 John F. Kennedy Blvd., Ste. 1800, Philadelphia, PA 19103-2899. Customer Service Office: 3251 Riverport Lane, Maryland Heights, MO 63043. Periodicals postage paid at New York, NY and additional mailing offices. Subscription prices are $256.00 per year (US individuals), $382.00 per year (US institutions), $306.00 per year (Canadian individuals), $485.00 per year (Canadian institutions), $376.00 per year (foreign individuals), $485.00 per year (foreign institutions) $122.00 per year (US students), and $176.00 per year (Canadian and foreign students). Foreign air speed delivery is included in all Clinics subscription prices. All prices are subject to change without notice. **POSTMASTER:** Send address changes to *Clinics in Perinatology,* Elsevier Health Sciences Division, Subscription Customer Service, 3251 Riverport Lane, Maryland Heights, MO 63043. **Customer Service: Telephone: 1-800-654-2452** (U.S. and Canada); **1-314-447-8871** (outside U.S. and Canada). **Fax: 1-314-447-8029. E-mail: journalscustomerservice-usa@elsevier. com** (for print support); **journalsonlinesupport-usa@elsevier.com** (for online support).

Reprints. For copies of 100 or more, of articles in this publication, please contact the Commercial Reprints Department, Elsevier Inc., 360 Park Avenue South, New York, NY 10010-1710. Tel. (212) 633-3812; Fax: (212) 482-1935; email: reprints@elsevier.com.

Clinics in Perinatology is also pubilshed in Spanish by McGraw-Hill Interamericana Editores S.A., P.O. Box 5-237, 06500 Mexico D.F., Mexico.

Clinics in Perinatology is covered in *MEDLINE/PubMed (Index Medicus) Current Contents, Excepta Medica, BIOSIS and ISI/BIOMED.*

Printed and bound by CPI Group (UK) Ltd, Croydon, CR0 4YY

Transferred to Digital Print 2011

Contributors

CONSULTING EDITOR

LUCKY JAIN, MD, MBA
Richard Blumberg Professor and Executive Vice Chairman, Department of Pediatrics,
Emory University School of Medicine, Atlanta, Georgia

GUEST EDITORS

ALAN R. FLEISCHMAN, MD
Senior Vice President and Medical Director, March of Dimes; Clinical Professor of
Pediatrics and Clinical Professor of Epidemiology and Population Health, Albert Einstein
College of Medicine, White Plains, New York

JAY D. IAMS, MD
Frederick P. Zuspan Professor and Endowed Chair, Division of Maternal Fetal Medicine;
Vice Chair, Department of Obstetrics and Gynecology; Co-Chair, Executive Committee,
Ohio Perinatal Quality Collaborative, The Ohio State University Medical Center, Columbus,
Ohio

AUTHORS

MARILEE C. ALLEN, MD
Professor of Pediatrics and Co-Director of the NICU Developmental Followup Clinic,
Kennedy Krieger Institute; The Johns Hopkins School of Medicine, Baltimore, Maryland

JAMIE A. BASTEK, MD
Maternal and Child Health Research Program; Department of Obstetrics and Gynecology,
Center for Research on Reproduction and Women's Health, University of Pennsylvania;
Department of Maternal-Fetal Medicine, Hospital of the University of Pennsylvania,
Philadelphia, Pennsylvania

SCOTT D. BERNS, MD, MPH
March of Dimes National Office, White Plains, New York; Clinical Professor, Pediatrics,
Warren Alpert Medical School of Brown University, Providence, Rhode Island

CLAUDIA BUSS, PhD
Assistant Professor of Pediatrics, University of California Irvine Development, Health and
Disease Research Program, School of Medicine, University of California, Irvine, Orange,
California

DEBORAH E. CAMPBELL, MD
Professor of Clinical Pediatrics, Associate Professor of Clinical Obstetrics and Gynecology
and Women's Health; Director, Division of Neonatology, Albert Einstein College of
Medicine, Children's Hospital at Montefiore, Bronx, New York

LINA F. CHALAK, MD, MSCS
Assistant Professor and Dwight J. Rouse Professor, Division of Neonatal-Perinatal Medicine, Department of Pediatrics, The University of Texas Southwestern Medical Center at Dallas, Dallas, Texas

STEVEN L. CLARK, MD
Medical Director, Women's and Children's Clinical Services Group, Hospital Corporation of America, Twin Bridges, Montana

ELIZABETH A. CRISTOFALO, MD
Assistant Professor of Pediatrics, The Johns Hopkins School of Medicine, Baltimore, Maryland

EDWARD F. DONOVAN, MD
Co-Chair, Executive Committee, Ohio Perinatal Quality Collaborative, Cincinnati Children's Hospital Medical Center, Cincinnati, Ohio

MICHAL A. ELOVITZ, MD
Maternal and Child Health Research Program; Department of Obstetrics and Gynecology, Center for Research on Reproduction and Women's Health, University of Pennsylvania, Philadelphia, Pennsylvania

WILLIAM A. ENGLE, MD
Professor of Pediatrics, Section of Neonatal-Perinatal Medicine, Indiana University School of Medicine, Indianapolis, Indiana

SONJA ENTRINGER, PhD
Assistant Professor of Pediatrics, University of California Irvine Development, Health and Disease Research Program, School of Medicine, University of California, Irvine, Orange, California

ALAN R. FLEISCHMAN, MD
Senior Vice President and Medical Director, March of Dimes; Clinical Professor of Pediatrics and Clinical Professor of Epidemiology and Population Health, Albert Einstein College of Medicine, White Plains, New York

LUIS M. GÓMEZ, MD
Maternal and Child Health Research Program; Department of Obstetrics and Gynecology, Center for Research on Reproduction and Women's Health, University of Pennsylvania; Department of Maternal-Fetal Medicine, Hospital of the University of Pennsylvania, Philadelphia, Pennsylvania

WILLIAM A. GROBMAN, MD, MBA
Associate Professor, Division of Maternal-Fetal Medicine, Department of Obstetrics and Gynecology, Feinberg School of Medicine, Northwestern University, Chicago, Illinois

CHRISTINA S. HAN, MD
Assistant Professor, Department of Obstetrics, Gynecology and Reproductive Sciences, Yale University School of Medicine, New Haven, Connecticut

MARLYSE F. HAWARD, MD
Assistant Professor of Pediatrics, Division of Neonatology, Albert Einstein College of Medicine, Children's Hospital at Montefiore, Bronx, New York

JAY D. IAMS, MD
Frederick P. Zuspan Professor and Endowed Chair, Division of Maternal Fetal Medicine, Vice Chair, Department of Obstetrics and Gynecology; Co-Chair, Executive Committee, Ohio Perinatal Quality Collaborative, The Ohio State University Medical Center, Columbus, Ohio

LUCKY JAIN, MD, MBA
Richard Blumberg Professor and Executive Vice Chairman, Department of Pediatrics, Emory University School of Medicine, Atlanta, Georgia

ALAN H. JOBE, MD, PhD
Division of Pulmonary Biology, Cincinnati Children's Hospital Medical Center, The University of Cincinnati, Cincinnati, Ohio

SARAH A. KEIM, PhD, MA, MS
Assistant Professor of Pediatrics, The Ohio State University College of Medicine, The Research Institute at Nationwide Children's Hospital, Columbus, Ohio

CHRISTINA KIM
The Johns Hopkins School of Medicine, Baltimore, Maryland

NANCY W. KIRSHENBAUM, MD
Assistant Professor of Obstetrics and Gynecology and Women's Health, Department of Obstetrics and Gynecology, Albert Einstein College of Medicine; Director, Westchester Division, Maternal Fetal Medicine Services, Montefiore Medical Center, Bronx, New York

MARK A. KLEBANOFF, MD, MPH
Professor of Pediatrics, The Ohio State University College of Medicine; The Research Institute at Nationwide Children's Hospital, Columbus, Ohio

CHARLES J. LOCKWOOD, MD
The Anita O'Keeffe Young Professor of Women's Health, and Chair, Department of Obstetrics, Gynecology and Reproductive Sciences, Yale University School of Medicine, New Haven, Connecticut

MICHAEL C. LU, MD, MPH
Associate Professor, Department of Obstetrics and Gynecology, Department of Obstetrics and Gynecology, David Geffen School of Medicine, University of California, Los Angeles, Los Angeles, California

SOWMYA S. MOHAN, MD
Assistant Professor, Department of Pediatrics, Emory University School of Medicine, Atlanta, Georgia

BRYAN T. OSHIRO, MD
Associate Professor, Department of Obstetrics and Gynecology, Loma Linda University School of Medicine, Loma Linda, California

MONA PRASAD, DO, MPH
Division of Maternal Fetal Medicine, The Ohio State University Medical Center, Columbus, Ohio

BARBARA ROSE, RN, MPH
Program Director, Ohio Perinatal Quality Collaborative, Cincinnati Children's Hospital
Medical Center, Cincinnati, Ohio

DWIGHT J. ROUSE, MD
Division of Maternal-Fetal Medicine, Department of Obstetrics and Gynecology, Women
and Infants Hospital of Rhode Island; The Warren G. Alpert School of Medicine of Brown
University, Providence, Rhode Island

FREDERICK SCHATZ, PhD
Research Scientist, Department of Obstetrics, Gynecology and Reproductive Sciences,
Yale University School of Medicine, New Haven, Connecticut

PATHIK D. WADHWA, MD, PhD
Professor of Psychiatry and Human Behavior, Obstetrics and Gynecology, Pediatrics, and
Epidemiology, University of California Irvine Development, Health and Disease Research
Program, University of California, Irvine, School of Medicine, Irvine, California

RONALD WAPNER, MD
Department of Obstetrics and Gynecology, Columbia University Medical Center,
New York, New York

AMY E. WONG, MD
Fellow, Division of Maternal-Fetal Medicine, Department of Obstetrics and Gynecology,
Feinberg School of Medicine, Northwestern University, Chicago, Illinois

Contents

Epidemiology

> Preterm birth, defined as a pregnancy ending at less than 37 completed weeks of gestation, is the leading cause of infant mortality in the United States. The occurrence of preterm births rose steadily from 9.4% of all pregnancies in the United States in 1981 to 12.8% in 2006, before declining to 12.7% in 2007 and 12.3% in 2008. Most of the increase was attributable to increases in multiple gestations. Recent research has sought to understand this condition by evaluating its familial occurrence and both clinical and pathologic information to derive an etiologically homogeneous categorization.

Causes

> Preterm birth represents the most significant problem in maternal–child health, with maternal stress identified as a variable of interest. The effects of maternal stress on risk of preterm birth may vary as a function of context. This article focuses on select key issues and questions highlighting the need to develop a better understanding of which particular subgroups of pregnant women may be especially vulnerable to the potentially detrimental effects of maternal stress, and under what circumstances and at which stages of gestation. Issues related to the characterization and assessment of maternal stress and candidate biologic mechanisms are addressed.

> Much emphasis in recent decades has been devoted to inflammation and infection as a premier causal mechanism of preterm birth. This article explores the epidemiologic, clinical, and animal data that exist to support this conceptual paradigm as well as proposed mechanisms through which to potentially mitigate the adversity of prematurity. Truly successful interventions are not likely to occur until the pathogenesis of preterm birth and the

role of inflammation in causing not only parturition but also fetal and neonatal injury is fully elucidated.

Chronic, subacute decidual hemorrhage (ie, abruptio placenta and retrochorionic hematoma formation) is an important contributor to preterm parturition. Such hemorrhage induces thrombin from decidual tissue factor, which plays a pivotal role in the development of preterm premature rupture of membranes and preterm delivery by acting through protease-activated receptors to promote the production of pro-inflammatory cytokines, and matrix-degrading metalloproteinases. Severe, acute abruption can lead to maternal and fetal mortality. Current management of abruption is individualized based on severity of disease, underlying etiology, and gestational age.

Premature delivery of an infant is occasionally performed because of complications of pregnancy. This article reviews common medical indications for preterm delivery and the available evidence supporting delivery before 37 weeks of gestation. In many conditions, few data exist to guide optimal timing of delivery and management is guided by expert opinion. Ultimately, an individual assessment must be made in each case to weigh the risks that pregnancy continuation poses to the mother and/or fetus with the risks of prematurity and its associated morbidities.

Outcomes of Preterm Infants

Over the last 50 years in the United States a rising preterm birth rate, a progressive decrease in preterm mortality, and a lowering of the limit of viability have made preterm birth a significant public health problem. Neuromaturation, the functional development of the central nervous system (CNS), is a dynamic process that promotes and shapes CNS structural development. This article reviews preterm outcomes, recognizing that multiple factors influence neuromaturation and lead to a range of neurodevelopmental disabilities, dysfunctions, and altered CNS processing. Ways to protect preterm infants and support their growth and development in and beyond intensive care are examined.

Infants born preterm are especially vulnerable to cerebral palsy, the risk of which is inversely proportional to gestational age at birth. The contribution of prematurity to the overall burden of cerebral palsy is substantial. This article reviews and discusses potential antenatal and postnatal neuroprotective approaches targeted at the numerous risk factors associated with cerebral palsy among preterm infants, including magnesium sulfate.

Decision-making for extremely immature preterm infants at the margins of viability is ethically, professionally, and emotionally complicated. A standard for prenatal consultation should be developed incorporating assessment of parental decision-making preferences and styles, a communication process involving a reciprocal exchange of information, and effective strategies for decisional deliberation, guided by and consistent with parental moral framework. Professional caregivers providing perinatal consultations or end-of-life counseling for extremely preterm infants should be sensitive to these issues and be taught flexibility in counseling techniques adhering to consistent guidelines. Emphasis must shift away from physician beliefs and behaviors about the boundaries of viability.

Late preterm and early term infants are at higher risk for short-term and long-term morbidities and mortality than term infants. Such outcomes are influenced by many factors, the strongest of which is gestational age. Counseling and educating women and families about risks of late preterm and early term births is helpful for timing and route of delivery, managing the pregnancy and infant, and prognosticating outcomes for infants.

Controversies

Obstetricians and pediatricians share the common goal of a healthy beginning for every baby, mother, and family. This article asserts that miscommunication between the specialties, fostered by separate definitions, metrics, and outcomes, is an impediment to optimal care. Solutions are suggested for improving communication and outcomes.

There is no controversy that women at risk of preterm delivery before 32 to 34 weeks' gestational age should be treated with antenatal steroids. Three recent meta-analyses by the Cochrane Collaboration on the benefits of antenatal steroids, the choice of steroid and dosing, and repeat doses of corticosteroids comprehensively summarize the available clinical information to about 2007. However, there are many unanswered questions about which steroid and dose to use and about their use in selected populations. This review focuses on those areas of uncertainty.

GOAL STATEMENT

The goal of *Clinics in Perinatology* is to keep practicing neonatologists and maternal-fetal medicine specialists up to date with current clinical practice in perinatology by providing timely articles reviewing the state of the art in patient care.

ACCREDITATION

The *Clinics in Perinatology* is planned and implemented in accordance with the Essential Areas and Policies of the Accreditation Council for Continuing Medical Education (ACCME) through the joint sponsorship of the University of Virginia School of Medicine and Elsevier. The University of Virginia School of Medicine is accredited by the ACCME to provide continuing medical education for physicians.

The University of Virginia School of Medicine designates this enduring material activity for a maximum of 15 *AMA PRA Category 1 Credits*™ for each issue, 60 credits per year. Physicians should only claim credit commensurate with the extent of their participation in the activity.

The American Medical Association has determined that physicians not licensed in the US who participate in this CME activity are eligible for a maximum of 15 *AMA PRA Category 1 Credits*™ for each issue, 60 credits per year.

Credit can be earned by reading the text material, taking the CME examination online at http://www.theclinics.com/home/cme, and completing the evaluation. After taking the test, you will be required to review any and all incorrect answers. Following completion of the test and evaluation, your credit will be awarded and you may print your certificate.

FACULTY DISCLOSURE/CONFLICT OF INTEREST

The University of Virginia School of Medicine, as an ACCME accredited provider, endorses and strives to comply with the Accreditation Council for Continuing Medical Education (ACCME) Standards of Commercial Support, Commonwealth of Virginia statutes, University of Virginia policies and procedures, and associated federal and private regulations and guidelines on the need for disclosure and monitoring of proprietary and financial interests that may affect the scientific integrity and balance of content delivered in continuing medical education activities under our auspices.

The University of Virginia School of Medicine requires that all CME activities accredited through this institution be developed independently and be scientifically rigorous, balanced and objective in the presentation/discussion of its content, theories and practices.

All authors/editors participating in an accredited CME activity are expected to disclose to the readers relevant financial relationships with commercial entities occurring within the past 12 months (such as grants or research support, employee, consultant, stock holder, member of speakers bureau, etc.). The University of Virginia School of Medicine will employ appropriate mechanisms to resolve potential conflicts of interest to maintain the standards of fair and balanced education to the reader. Questions about specific strategies can be directed to the Office of Continuing Medical Education, University of Virginia School of Medicine, Charlottesville, Virginia.

The faculty and staff of the University of Virginia Office of Continuing Medical Education have no financial affiliations to disclose.

The authors/editors listed below have identified no professional or financial affiliations for themselves or their spouse/partner:

Marilee C. Allen, MD; Jamie A. Bastek, MD; Scott D. Berns, MD, MPH; Robert Boyle, MD (Test Author); Claudia Buss, PhD; Deborah Campbell, MD; Lina F. Chalak, MD, MSCS; Elizabeth A. Cristofalo, MD; Edward F. Donovan, MD; William A. Engle, MD; Sonja Entringer, PhD; Alan R. Fleischman, MD (Guest Editor); Luis M. Gomez, MD; William A. Grobman, MD, MBA; Christina S. Han, MD; Marlyse F. Haward, MD; Kerry Holland, (Acquisitions Editor); Jay D. Iams, MD (Guest Editor); Lucky Jain, MD, MBA (Consulting Editor); Christina Kim; Nancy W. Kirshenbaum, MD; Michael C. Lu, MD, MPH; Sowmya Mohan, MD; Bryan T. Oshiro, MD; Mona Prasad, DO, MPH; Barbara Rose, RN, MPH; Dwight J. Rouse, MD; Fredrick Schatz, PhD; Pathik D. Wadhwa, MD, PhD; Ronald Wapner, MD; Amy E. Wong, MD.

The authors/editors listed below identified the following professional or financial affiliations for themselves or their spouse/partner:

Steven L. Clark, MD is employed by Hospital Corporation of America.

Michal A. Elovitz, MD is a consultant for KV Pharmaceutical company.

Alan H. Jobe, MD, PhD receives grant support from Fisher and Paykeo, New Zealand, and provides surfactant for sheep research for Cheisi, Parma, Italy.

Sarah A. Keim, PhD, MA, MS owns stock in Abbott Labs, Colgate Palmolive, DuPont, Humana, J&J, Merck, Nestle, Novartis, Sanofi Aventis sponsored Adr., Siemens, and Teva Pharmaceuticals.

Mark Klebanoff, MD, MPH owns stock in Abbott Labs, Colgate Palmolive, DuPont, Humana, J&J, Merck, Nestle, Novartis, Sanofi Aventis sponsored Adr., Siemens, and Teva Pharmaceuticals.

Charles J. Lockwood, MD is on the Advisory Committee/Board for Up-To-Date online journal and Contemporary OB/GYN Journal.

Disclosure of Discussion of Non-FDA Approved Uses for Pharmaceutical Products and/or Medical Devices

The University of Virginia School of Medicine, as an ACCME provider, requires that all faculty presenters identify and disclose any off-label uses for pharmaceutical and medical device products. The University of Virginia School of Medicine recommends that each physician fully review all the available data on new products or procedures prior to clinical use.

TO ENROLL

To enroll in the Clinics in Perinatology Continuing Medical Education program, call customer service at 1-800-654-2452 or visit us online at www.theclinics.com/home/cme. The CME program is available to subscribers for an additional fee of $196.00.

THE CLINICS ARE NOW AVAILABLE ONLINE!

Access your subscription at:
www.theclinics.com

Foreword

Prematurity Viewed Through the Social Ecological Framework

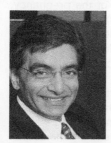

Lucky Jain, MD, MBA
Consulting Editor

Why humans triumphed 45,000 years ago, emerging as the dominant ape of that age, but without any clear biologic underpinnings to help explain this leap, helps put into context the social-ecological framework for advancement of the human race. Scientists believe that the gains came from the emergence of *collective intelligence* nested in communities, rather than individuals, and through rapid interaction and collective behavior, which accelerated the pace of progress.[1] This idea holds hope for health promotion as well, which has become a victim of an excessive focus on the individual and his/her disease management, ignoring the importance of the environment and collective behavior. Proponents of the social ecological framework feel an urgent need to integrate these two seemingly divergent approaches, lifestyle modification and environmental enhancement, to generate the greatest and most enduring impact on health and well-being.

What relevance does this framework have for preterm birth? The dominant causes of death, disease, and suffering globally are directly linked to behavioral factors.[2] Smoking, diet (obesity), sexual behavior, and avoidable injuries are all examples of public health problems that require not only a thorough understanding of relevant theories of behavior change but also interventions that use this knowledge to effectively modify behavior. Research focused on elucidation of pathophysiology and causative mechanisms is important, but has not created the much needed urgency among individuals and communities to embrace preventive methods.

More specifically, the unresolved problem of rising preterm births begs the following questions. First, as Fleishman and colleagues[3] point out in a recent article, has the manmade definition of prematurity (gestational age <37 weeks) perpetuated a false belief that 37-week gestational age fetuses are "term" and therefore safe to deliver? When spontaneous labor and delivery were the norm, the definition was relevant for

Clin Perinatol 38 (2011) xiii–xv
doi:10.1016/j.clp.2011.08.001

data collection and monitoring. However, in situations where nearly 50% of all births follow either induction of labor or cesarean section, one wonders how many 37- to 38-week births could have been prevented if babies <39 weeks gestational age were considered preterm! Second, the widespread belief that fetuses at or beyond 34 weeks achieve sufficient maturity and are at risk for minimal morbidity may have created a feeling that it is safe to deliver when there are maternal or other "soft" indications, even when the risk-benefit analysis would suggest continuation of the pregnancy. Recent attempts at reducing iatrogenic early-term (37-38 weeks) and late preterm (34-37 weeks) births have yielded noteworthy results. Third, one is struck by the glaring racial disparities in prematurity rates, particularly among blacks living in the United States.[4] Is the environment stressful enough to impact pregnancy outcome? If so, what can be done to relieve the stress?

There is strength in the social ecological framework for reproductive health. Indeed, health is determined not just by personal attributes, but by the interaction of these attributes with the physical and social environment.[5] The environment can also be a stressor, with a major impact on physical and mental health of entire generations. In war-ravaged nations, and nations where racial and economic disparities are rampant, chronic emotional stress can activate biologic mediators of inflammation with long-term effects on health and longevity. This framework also moves us from individual therapeutic/curative approaches to community-wide preventive and epide-miologic orientation and brings in much needed input from other disciplines like soci-ology, anthropology, economics, and political science. Finally, this framework helps in understanding which public health programs and regulatory approaches can yield the most impact on individuals and populations. Cumulative innovation has doubled life span, cut child mortality by three quarters, and improved quality of life for many chronic diseases. Yet, with the greatest gains in personalized medicine and disease management in a century at our hands, health challenges like prematurity and obesity continue unabated. This apparent paradox is but a huge opportunity to integrate these many approaches into a seamless offering for reproductive health promotion with a balanced portfolio of physical fitness, emotional health, and social cohesion. This would require combining behavioral changes with environmental modifications, with implementation at the individual, organizational, and community level. This would also require operational models to be socially relevant and adaptive. Success of such approaches can be quickly taken across the spectrum of health promotion, and across communities and nations to achieve global health.

I am delighted that Drs Fleishman and Iams have put together a comprehensive review of preterm birth in this edition of the *Clinics in Perinatology*. In addition to the authors, I would like to thank Kerry Holland and Elsevier for their support of this impor-tant topic.

Lucky Jain, MD, MBA
Department of Pediatrics
Emory University School of Medicine
2015 Uppergate Drive
Atlanta, GA 30322, USA

E-mail address:
ljain@emory.edu

REFERENCES

1. Ridley M. Humans: why they triumphed. Wall Street J 2010.
2. Mokdad AH, Marks JS, Stroup DF, et al. Actual causes of death in the United States, 2000. JAMA 2004;291:1238–45.
3. Fleishman AR, Oinuma M, Clark SL. Rethinking the definition of term pregnancy. Obstet Gynecol 2010;116:136–9.
4. Spong CY, Iams J, Goldenberg R, et al. Disparities in perinatal medicine: preterm birth, stillbirth, and infant mortality. Obstet Gynecol 2011;117:948–55.
5. Glamntz K, Bishop DB. The role of behavioral science theory in development and implementation of public health interventions. Annu Rev Public Health 2010;31: 399–418.

Preface
Understanding and Preventing Preterm Birth: the Power of Collaboration

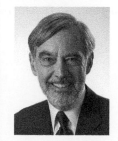 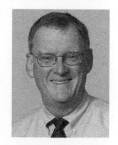

Alan R. Fleischman, MD   Jay D. Iams, MD
Guest Editors

This is an exciting time in perinatal medicine. While preterm birth remains a major public health problem and the leading cause of perinatal and infant mortality, progress in several areas has resulted in a decrease in the rate of prematurity and the amelioration of its impact on infants and families. Clinical research trials have shown improved outcomes for babies as the result of interventions applied during pregnancy to reduce the risk of preterm birth, and during labor and in the nursery to reduce neonatal morbidity. Perinatal quality improvement techniques are being applied to increase the use of prophylaxis with antenatal corticosteroids to decrease neonatal respiratory morbidity, to reduce nonmedically indicated inductions and cesarean deliveries associated with significant neonatal illness, unnecessary NICU admissions, and adverse long-term outcomes, and to decrease neonatal infections and enhance the care in NICUs. Finally, the collaborations represented by the authors of articles in this issue mirror the increased collaboration by pediatricians and obstetricians that is occurring throughout the country and will be necessary at every level of care to significantly decrease preterm birth and ultimately enhance the health of children in America.

Alan R. Fleischman, MD
March of Dimes
Albert Einstein College of Medicine
1275 Mamaroneck Avenue
White Plains, NY 10605, USA

Clin Perinatol 38 (2011) xvii–xviii
doi:10.1016/j.clp.2011.06.015
0095-5108/11/$ – see front matter © 2011 Elsevier Inc. All rights reserved.

perinatology.theclinics.com

Jay D. Iams, MD
Division of Maternal Fetal Medicine
Department of Obstetrics & Gynecology
The Ohio State University Medical Center
395 West 12th Avenue, Room 554
Columbus, OH 43210-1267, USA

E-mail addresses:
AFleischman@marchofdimes.com (A.R. Fleischman)
jay.iams@osumc.edu (J.D. Iams)

Epidemiology: The Changing Face of Preterm Birth

Mark A. Klebanoff, MD, MPH*, Sarah A. Keim, PhD, MA, MS

KEYWORDS

- Infant • Newborn • Preterm birth • Epidemiology
- Pregnancy complications

Preterm birth, defined by the World Health Organization as the delivery of an infant before 37 completed weeks (259 days) of gestational duration,[1] occurred in 12.3% of births in the United States in 2008.[2] It is the most common cause of perinatal[3] and infant[4] mortality in the United States, and this pressing problem has resisted most of medical science's best efforts to prevent it. In this article, the authors review the importance and time trends of preterm birth and the distinction between early and late preterm infants. The authors present some intriguing new epidemiologic findings about the familial recurrence of preterm birth and discuss the various approaches to classifying subtypes of preterm birth.

PRETERM BIRTH: DEFINITIONS, IMPORTANCE, AND COMPLEXITIES

Approximately one-third of infant mortality in the United States is attributable directly to preterm birth or as a result of complications occurring almost exclusively to the preterm infant.[4] Because of the recognition that previous rules for coding cause of death underestimated the contribution of preterm birth,[4] we now recognize that preterm birth and its attendant complications are the leading causes of infant mortality in the United States. Compared with infants born at term, surviving preterm infants are at an increased risk of long-term cognitive, motor, sensory, and behavioral deficits,[5] as well as of poor growth and long-term lung and gastrointestinal disease.[6] The Institute of Medicine has estimated the cost to society of preterm birth in the United States to be at least $26.2 billion in 2005; this estimate does not include the entire cost of medical care beyond early childhood, nor does it include the total cost of special educational services and lost productivity. It does not include any caregiver costs.[7]

Preterm birth is officially defined without a specific lower gestational age limit. Within the United States the lowest gestational duration at which a certificate of live birth or

The authors have nothing to disclose.

Department of Pediatrics, The Ohio State University College of Medicine and Research Institute at Nationwide Children's Hospital, 700 Children's Drive, Columbus, OH 43205, USA

* Corresponding author.

E-mail address: Mark.Klebanoff@nationwidechildrens.org

perinatology.theclinics.com

fetal death is required varies by state, although most states require reporting of all births and fetal deaths occurring at or more than 20 completed weeks' gestation.[8,9] The 20-week limit is arbitrary, and rather than being based on etiology, it was historically based on the timing of maternal perception of fetal movement and on the presumed theoretical lower limit of viability. However, the etiology of births at 16 to 20 weeks' gestation is similar to that of births at 20 to 25 weeks'. Women who experience a pregnancy loss at 16 to 20 weeks are at a comparable risk of a subsequent preterm birth as women who had a 20- to 25-week birth, and at a substantially greater risk of a subsequent preterm birth than are women who experienced a first-trimester pregnancy loss.[10–12] Thus, for both etiologic research and clinical management, consideration should be given to including pregnancies ending at 16 to 20 weeks' gestation as both a predictive factor and an etiologic clue.

Just as the lower limit of preterm birth is arbitrary, the upper limit of 36 weeks 6 days is perhaps even more arbitrary; not all infants born at or after 37 weeks' gestation are at a comparable risk. In the United States, from 1995 to 2001, gestational age-specific infant mortality was higher for infants born at 37 weeks' (2.3/1000 live-born infants) and 38 weeks' (1.7/1000) gestation than for infants born at 39 weeks' (1.4/1000) and 40 weeks' (1.4/1000) gestation.[13] As documented by Tita and colleagues,[14] the lowest incidence of a variety of neonatal complications in pregnancies with elective repeat cesarean delivery occurred at 39 or 40 weeks' gestation; infants delivered at 37 or 38 weeks were at an increased risk of neonatal morbidity compared with those born at 39 or 40 weeks. Because these deliveries were electively timed, the increased morbidity cannot be ascribed to an underlying condition that might cause a 37- or 38-week versus a 39- or 40-week birth; immaturity is the only possible explanation. In a study conducted in Belarus, the highest IQ at 6.5 years of age was observed among children born at 39 to 41 weeks' gestation; children born at 37 and 38 weeks gestation had IQ values that were 1.7 and 0.4 points lower, respectively; both differences were statistically significant.[15] Thus, as discussed in the articles by Iams and Donovan; Clark and Fleischman elsewhere in this issue, a cogent case can be made for redefining preterm birth to include babies born at 37 and 38 weeks' gestation. Of note, the American College of Obstetricians and Gynecologists recommends that inductions of labor conducted for logistical reasons not be done unless a well-documented gestational duration of at least 39 completed weeks has been reached.[16]

TIME TRENDS AND SUBCATEGORIES

Over the period from 1981 to 2006, preterm birth increased from 9.4% to 12.8% of all births, a 36% relative increase.[17] Part of the increase was attributable to an increase in the occurrence of multiple (twin and higher order) births[17]; approximately 57% of twin[18] and essentially all higher order births[19] are born before 37 weeks' gestation. However, even among singletons, preterm birth increased from 9.7% in 1990 to 11.1% in 2006.[17] Virtually all of the increase in singleton preterm birth over this era was seen among late (34–36 week) preterm births; the occurrence of birth at less than 34 weeks remained stable at 2.93% in 1990 and 2.96% in 2006.[17]

By convention, preterm birth has been dichotomized according to its clinical presentation: spontaneous (in which contractions, cervical softening and thinning, or spontaneous membrane rupture is the presenting event) versus indicated (in which, because of a complication of pregnancy that may impact maternal or fetal well-being, labor is induced or cesarean delivery is effected in the absence of labor or membrane rupture in a pregnancy that would not have otherwise ended in the immediate future). This dichotomy is not always easy to apply in practice.[20] It has not substantially improved our understanding of the causes of preterm birth,[21] and this taxonomy probably should be abandoned in favor of a more nuanced approach. However, it does serve to highlight the role of obstetric management in preterm birth. Although the data source is imperfect to answer this question, the review of birth certificates for the United States has indicated that virtually all of the increase in singleton preterm births since 1989, when the birth certificate was changed to allow the assessment of clinical presentation, was caused by an increase in indicated preterm birth (**Fig. 1**).[22] This finding suggests that either the indications to effect delivery before term (primarily hypertensive disorders and evidence of fetal compromise) have become more common or more commonly recognized or that the threshold for intervening once such conditions are discovered has lowered over time. Unfortunately, United States vital records do not contain sufficiently detailed data to study these possibilities further.

INFANTS OF 34 TO 36 WEEKS' GESTATION: NEAR TERM VERSUS LATE PRETERM

Not all preterm infants have equal risks of mortality and morbidity. The most important determinant of these outcomes is how remote from term the infant is born. In leading academic centers, survival of live-born preterm infants increases from less than 10% for babies born at the limit of viability (approximately 22 weeks' gestation) to greater than 90% for babies born at 28 weeks' gestation.[23] Survival of infants born alive at 34 weeks' gestation is currently greater than 98%[24]; even in the era before neonatal intensive care, infants born at 34 or more weeks' gestation usually survived and often did not have severe lung disease.[25,26] As a result, during the entire 40-year era of perinatal and neonatal intensive care, the focus has been primarily on pregnancies and infants of less than 34 weeks' gestation.[27] Beyond 34 weeks obstetric management changes; most efforts are no longer directed at prolonging gestation, and when there are complications, the threshold to effect delivery declines substantially.[28]

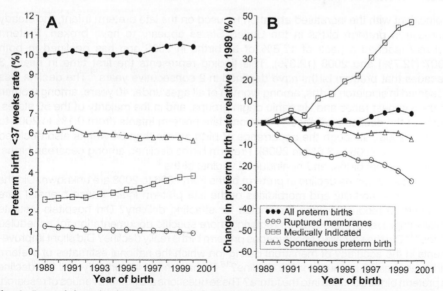

Fig. 1. Rates (*A*) and relative temporal changes since 1989 (*B*) of preterm birth less than 37 weeks (all races) as well as those resulting from ruptured membranes, medically indicated, and spontaneous preterm birth: United States (1989–2000). (*From* Ananth CV, Joseph KS, Oyelese Y, et al. Trends in preterm birth and perinatal mortality among singletons: United States, 1989 through 2000. Obstet Gynecol 2005;105:1086; with permission.)

Improvements in maternal, fetal, and neonatal care may have led to a cavalier attitude toward these more mature preterm infants; individual clinicians rarely see an infant of 34 or more weeks die. They are often admitted to the regular newborn nursery rather than the neonatal intensive care unit; and even their common designation as near-term infants may have resulted in the underestimation of their risks, with attendant less diligent evaluation, monitoring, and follow-up.[29] However, although individual infants may generally do well, over the past decade, clinicians and researchers have come to recognize that, in aggregate, infants of 34 to 36 weeks' gestation are not the same as term infants. They are nearly 3 times as likely as term infants to die in the first year of life, and congenital anomalies do not account for this elevated risk.[30] They are at an increased risk of numerous neonatal complications, including temperature instability, hypoglycemia, feeding difficulties, hyperbilirubinemia, neonatal respiratory distress syndrome, transient tachypnea of the newborn, and prolonged hospital stay.[31] Beyond the neonatal period, compared with term infants, those born at 34 to 36 weeks are at an increased risk of being readmitted to the hospital[32] and of developing neurodevelopmental disabilities.[33] Because approximately 70% of all preterm infants are born at 34 to 36 weeks' gestation,[17] the public health burden contributed by these infants is substantial.

With recognition of the increasing number of infants born at 34 to 36 weeks' gestation, and understanding that infants born at these late preterm gestational ages are not the same as infants born at term, came increases in both clinical and research attention. The most telling change is that these infants are no longer called near term. To convey the proper sense of vulnerability, a National Institutes of Health workshop recommended that infants born at 34 to 36 weeks' gestation be classified as late preterm to emphasize that "there is no such thing as a normal preterm infant."[29,31]

RECENT TRENDS IN PRETERM BIRTH

Coincident with the increased attention focused on the late preterm infant, the steady increase in preterm births in the United States appears to have broken. Preterm delivery reached a peak of 12.8% of all births in 2006 and has declined in both 2007 (12.7%) and 2008 (12.3%). This finding represents the first time in nearly 3 decades that preterm births have declined in 2 consecutive years.[2] The decline was observed in singleton births, among women of all ages under 40 years, among women of the 3 largest races and Hispanic origin groups, and in the majority of the 50 states. Much of the decline was observed among late preterm infants (from 9.1% in 2006 to 8.8% in 2008), although the occurrence of birth at less than 34 weeks also declined (from 3.7% in 2006 to 3.6% in 2008). Preterm births declined among cesarean births, induced vaginal births, and noninduced vaginal births.[2]

The reasons for the decline in preterm births from 2006 to 2008 are unknown. Did the focus on the mortality and morbidities of the late preterm infant cause prenatal care providers to reconsider their thresholds for effecting delivery? Did hospitals institute quality improvement procedures requiring more specific documentation for scheduled births?[34] Did the so-called spontaneous preterm births really decline? Did slight improvements in the accuracy of menstrual dating (on which the national estimates of preterm births are based) account for the decline?[35] Perhaps most importantly, will the decline in preterm births continue into the future? These questions are fruitful avenues of research.

WAS THE INCREASE IN PRETERM BIRTH GOOD OR BAD?

There is no question that, evaluated in cross section, an additional week of gestational duration improves the prognosis of a preterm infant. However, it does not necessarily follow that any given preterm fetus will benefit by being kept in utero an additional week, even if that could be accomplished. As noted previously, preterm birth is the leading cause of infant mortality in the United States. As documented in **Fig. 2,**[36] late preterm births steadily increased from 1981 to 2006, yet during this time the infant mortality rate declined from 11.9 to 6.7 per 1000 live births.[37] Undoubtedly, improvements in obstetric management, maternal and infant transport, and medical care of the preterm infant outweighed the increased occurrence of preterm births in that interval. When evaluating the impact of the specific increase of indicated preterm births, the considerations are more difficult. In considering whether to effect delivery in a complicated pregnancy that has not reached term, the prenatal caregiver must balance the known risks of delivery now against both the unknown benefits of allowing the fetus to continue to mature in utero and the unknown risks of allowing a compromised fetus to remain undelivered and possibly undergo physiologic deterioration. Is the prognosis for a mildly compromised infant born at, say, 35 weeks better than for

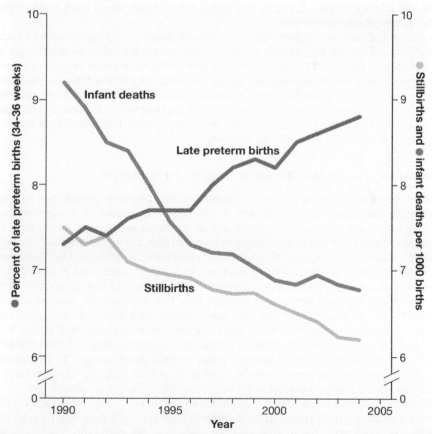

Fig. 2. Trends in late preterm birth, stillbirth, and infant mortality: United States (1990–2004). The left axis shows trends in stillbirth and infant mortality rates; the right axis shows trends in late preterm births (34–36 weeks). Late preterm birth rates are shown per 100 live births, stillbirth rates are per 1000 total births, and infant death rates are per 1000 live births. (*From* Ananth C, Gyamfi C, Jain L. Characterizing risk profiles of infants who are delivered at late preterm gestations: does it matter? Am J Obstet Gynecol 2005;199:330. Linked birth and infant death data, National Center for Health Statistics; with permission.)

a severely compromised one born at 37 weeks? At the most extreme, it seems obvious that a mildly compromised infant born at 35 weeks is preferable to a fetus that dies in utero at 37 weeks.

Thus, to evaluate more fully the impact of indicated preterm birth, we must consider both fetal and neonatal or infant death. In the United States, the fetal death rate declined from 7.83 per 1000 pregnancies of at least 20 weeks' gestation in 1985 to 6.22 per 1000 in 2005. The perinatal mortality rate (fetal deaths plus infant deaths up to 28 postnatal days per 1000 pregnancies of at least 20 weeks' gestation) fell from 14.57 in 1985 to 10.73 in 2005. Similar declines were observed when only pregnancies of at least 28 weeks were considered.[8] It is plausible, although far from proven, that the increase in indicated preterm births contributed to the net decrease in the combination of fetal and neonatal mortality observed over the past several decades, albeit at the cost of more infant and childhood morbidity. Joseph and colleagues[38] presented circumstantial evidence that this might be the case. Even so, given the change in frequency of indicated preterm births and the change in perinatal and infant mortality, it seems that many pregnancies would have been ended early for every death prevented.

A recent publication suggests that, on average, pregnancies complicated by so-called soft indications for preterm delivery might benefit by being allowed to go to term.[39] In one study,[40] 17% of all late preterm births were either elective or from a pregnancy regarded as high-risk but stable, and, thus, might have been preventable. Research to determine whether more aggressive obstetric management has contributed to the reduction in perinatal mortality and, if so, then which fetuses benefit from early delivery and which ones benefit from remaining in utero in the setting of specific pregnancy complications is urgently needed.

FAMILIAL PATTERN OF PRETERM BIRTH: INSIGHTS TO ETIOLOGY?

Several recent publications have shed interesting and, perhaps, unexpected light on the familial occurrence of preterm birth. It has been recognized for some time that women who were themselves preterm are at an increased risk of giving birth to a preterm infant, and that the more preterm a woman was, the higher the risk.[41] Recent research, based on multigenerational data from Denmark, Sweden, and Scotland, has extended this work to include other relatives. In a study conducted in Denmark,[42] women who were preterm at birth were at a 40% increased risk of preterm birth compared with women born at term (relative risk, 1.4). Interestingly, women born at term but who had a full sibling who was born preterm were also at an increased risk (relative risk 1.4) of preterm birth, as were women whose maternal half sibling was born preterm (relative risk 1.4). Women whose paternal half sibling was born preterm were not at an increased risk of having a preterm infant (relative risk 1.1). The female partners of men who were born preterm, or who came from a sibship where at least 1 child was born preterm, were not at an increased risk of having a preterm birth.

Studies conducted in Sweden[43] and Aberdeen, Scotland[44] reached essentially the same conclusion: the tendency to have preterm birth is transmitted only through the female line, even when the mother was not preterm at her own birth. These results are incompatible with any classic mendelian or polygenic model. Imprinting, in which only genes inherited from the grandmother to the mother or the mother to the fetus are active, could account for the observed familial transmission. Mitochondrial DNA, which is inherited by all children only from their mother, is the only other genetic explanation for these results.[42] These 2 possibilities could be distinguished only when data on the next generation of births become available. The observed results are compatible with the intriguing nongenetic explanation that a woman acquires risk factors from her mother at the time of birth or during her childhood living at home. Examples of such characteristics might be dietary preferences or personal hygienic behaviors, such as douching.[45]

Additional support for the possibility that early life events can predispose a woman to preterm birth comes from the work of Collins and colleagues,[46] who reported that the social class of the neighborhood in which a pregnant woman grew up is as strongly associated with her probability of having a preterm infant as the social class of the neighborhood where she lives during the pregnancy. Miller and colleagues[47] reported that individuals who grew up in low social class circumstances demonstrated decreased glucocorticoid and increased proinflammatory signaling as adults many decades later. Taken together, this body of work suggests that rather than being simply a condition of pregnancy, the roots of preterm birth may go back to the time the pregnant woman was born and perhaps earlier. Perhaps we should regard preterm birth as a life-course condition.[48]

CLASSIFICATION OF PRETERM BIRTH: PRESENTATION VERSUS MECHANISM VERSUS ETIOLOGY?

Understanding the pathophysiology leading to preterm birth is important both to clinicians who might use this information to tailor treatments to individual circumstances and to researchers who can make more rapid progress when studying homogeneous entities.[49] Given that there are possible benefits to subclassifying preterm birth, the first approaches were based on the primary clinical presentation: spontaneous onset of labor, spontaneous membrane rupture in the absence of labor, and indicated preterm birth as defined earlier in this article.[50] At the time of publication of this approach, each presentation was thought to have specific clinical management issues: How can contractions be stopped and pregnancy, thereby, prolonged? Do the benefits of prolonging pregnancy in the setting of ruptured membranes outweigh the risks (infectious and other), assuming pregnancy can be prolonged in that setting? Which maternal or fetal complications warrant delivery when it is unlikely that delivery would occur spontaneously in the immediate future?

Because intrauterine infection is a common cause of both spontaneous labor and spontaneous membrane rupture, many investigators combined these 2 presentations under the rubric of spontaneous preterm birth.[51,52] Is the dichotomy of spontaneous versus indicated preterm birth etiologically useful? As previously noted, risk factors for spontaneous and indicated preterm birth have not been consistently different.[53] Historically, both research and clinical management have focused on contractions, but over the past 2 decades we have come to recognize that contractions are merely a late event in the common pathway that began weeks earlier with chorio-decidual membrane activation and cervical dilation or effacement.[54] In other words, labor is the end result of the process of parturition. Thus, cervical shortening,[55] the presence of fetal fibronectin (a marker of membrane disruption) in cervical/vaginal secretions,[56] and evidence of infection or inflammation[57,58] are associated with the subsequent occurrence of preterm birth in women who have intact membranes and are not experiencing contractions. The lengthy time of the parturition process leading to spontaneous labor is the likely reason why tocolytic drugs delay labor for, at most, several days but do not reduce either preterm birth or neonatal mortality and morbidity.[59]

Separating preterm birth into spontaneous or indicated focuses on clinical presentation, and separating it into membrane activation, cervical change, placental abruption, preeclampsia, fetal compromise, and so forth focuses on the presumed mechanism. Recent research has attempted to integrate clinical and historical data with results of placental examinations to focus on more fundamental etiologies that might cause the mechanisms and clinical presentation. The goal is to derive etiologically homogeneous subtypes of preterm birth that are not necessarily based on clinical presentation. One group[60] used factor analysis to assess clustering of clinical, demographic, and placental pathologic characteristics of infants born at less than 28 weeks' gestation. One cluster was characterized by histologic chorioamnionitis and recovery of microbes from the placenta; the clinical correlates were preterm labor, preterm premature rupture of membranes, placental abruption, and cervical insufficiency.[60] The second cluster, characterized by lack of inflammation but evidence of placental dysfunction (thrombosis, infarcts, syncytial knots, and decidual hemorrhage/fibrin), was associated with preeclampsia and preterm birth for a fetal indication.[60] These results provide some support for a dichotomy between spontaneous and indicated preterm birth, although because abruption is a common indication for a preterm delivery,[61] they also suggest some overlap in etiology.

Another research group explored a variety of laboratory and placental pathologic characteristics and related them to clinical presentation. Elevated midpregnancy urinary catecholamine values (presumed by the investigators to represent psychosocial stress) were reported to be associated with spontaneous preterm birth; the association was strengthened after pregnancies with histologic chorioamnionitis were excluded.[62] This finding suggests that sympathetic activation might be a cause of spontaneous preterm birth that is distinct from infection. This same group reported that evidence of placental hemorrhage (disk-impacting blood clot or microscopic hemorrhage with or without a clinical diagnosis of placental abruption) was associated with increased risks of both spontaneous and indicated preterm births.[63] Placental vascular pathology was subdivided into constructs of maternal hemorrhage, maternal thrombosis, lack of physiologic conversion of the spiral arteries, fetal hemorrhage, and fetal thrombosis.[64] Interestingly, maternal or fetal hemorrhage and the lack of conversion of the spiral arteries were all associated with both spontaneous and indicated preterm birth; the other 2 constructs were associated only with indicated preterm birth.[64] More than 20 years ago, Naeye[65] noted a strong association between pathologic evidence of low placental blood flow (infarcts, small villi, and syncytial knots) and spontaneous preterm birth, even in the absence of preeclampsia, among women in the Collaborative Perinatal Project. Finally, women with a history of spontaneous preterm birth are at an increased risk of indicated preterm birth in a subsequent pregnancy.[52] Taken together, these reports suggest that although spontaneous and indicated preterm birth may have somewhat different underlying etiologies, they also share many common ones.

SUMMARY

Preterm birth and its associated complications are the leading cause of infant mortality in the United States. After steadily increasing from 1981 until 2006, mainly caused by increases in the occurrence of multiple births and of induction of labor or cesarean delivery of pregnancies at 34 to 36 weeks' gestation, preterm births reached a peak of 12.8% of all births and declined slightly in each of the past 2 years. At the same time that preterm induction and cesarean births were increasing, perinatal mortality, particularly at late preterm gestational ages, declined, suggesting that the increase in the so-called indicated preterm births may have contributed to a net benefit in mortality, albeit very inefficiently and at the expense of increased neonatal morbidity. Further research is urgently needed to explore whether this is the case, and, if so, to refine which pregnancies may benefit from being delivered early. Such research will probably need to be based on large databases with more detail than contained in vital records or to employ new and imaginative study designs.

New familial studies of preterm birth suggest either that imprinted maternal or mitochondrial genes are of etiologic importance or that environmental or familial factors experienced by a girl during her childhood are potential determinants of preterm birth. From a research perspective, perhaps we should be looking before the time that a woman is pregnant to view preterm birth from a life-course perspective.

Although the separation of spontaneous and indicated preterm births may reflect different clinical management concerns, it is becoming clear that not only does this dichotomy fail to capture the underlying mechanisms leading to preterm birth but it also may be defining groups with substantial etiologic overlap. Establishing a homogeneous phenotype will probably be necessary for real progress to be made in understanding the etiology of preterm birth. New research employing statistical techniques to analyze the clustering of factors has the exciting potential to combine data from clinical, biochemical, and placental pathologic observations in a form of discovery science that may enable the identification of homogeneous groups of pregnant women sharing common processes, all of which end in preterm birth. Such discoveries may form the basis for a leap of knowledge that could lead to new treatments to prevent preterm birth, which to date has resisted almost all of our best efforts to prevent it.

REFERENCES

1. World Health Organization. The prevention of perinatal mortality and morbidity. Geneva (Switzerland): WHO Technical Report Series; 1970. Report 457.
2. Martin JA, Osterman MJ, Sutto PD. Are preterm births on the decline in the United States? Recent data from the National Vital Statistics System. NCHS data brief, no 39. Hyattsville (MD): National Center for Health Statistics; 2010.
3. McCormick MC. The contribution of low birth weight to infant mortality and childhood morbidity. N Engl J Med 1985;312:82–90.
4. Callaghan WM, MacDorman MF, Rasmussen SA, et al. The contribution of preterm birth to infant mortality in the United States. Pediatrics 2006;118:1566–73.
5. Saigal S, Doyle LW. An overview of mortality and sequelae of preterm birth from infancy to adulthood. Lancet 2008;371:261–9.
6. Wood NS, Costeloe K, Gibson AT, et al. The EPICure study: growth and associated problems in children born at 25 weeks of gestational age or less. Arch Dis Child Fetal Neonatal Ed 2003;88:F492–500.
7. Institute of Medicine. Societal Costs of Preterm Birth. In: Behrman RE, Stith Butler A, editors. Preterm Birth: Causes, Consequences, and Prevention. Washington, DC: The National Academies Press; 2007. p. 398–429.
8. MacDorman MF, Kirmeyer S. Fetal and perinatal mortality, United States, 2005. National vital statistics reports, vol. 57, no 8. Hyattsville (MD): National Center for Health Statistics; 2009.
9. Wingate MS, Barfield WD. Racial and ethnic variations in temporal changes in fetal deaths and first day infant deaths. Matern Child Health J 2010. [Epub ahead of print].
10. Edlow AG, Srinivas SK, Elovitz MA. Second trimester loss and subsequent pregnancy outcomes: what is the real risk. Am J Obstet Gynecol 2007;197:581, e1–6.
11. Srinivas SK, Ernst LM, Edlow AG, et al. Can placental pathology explain second trimester pregnancy loss and subsequent pregnancy outcomes. Am J Obstet Gynecol 2008;199:402, e1–5.

12. Goldenberg RL, Mayberry SK, Copper RL, et al. Pregnancy outcome following a second-trimester loss. Obstet Gynecol 1993;81:444–6.
13. Zhang X, Kramer MS. Variations in mortality and morbidity by gestational age among infants born at term. J Pediatr 2009;154:358–62.
14. Tita AT, Landon MB, Spong CY, et al. Timing of elective repeat cesarean delivery at term and neonatal outcomes. N Engl J Med 2009;360:111–20.
15. Yang S, Platt RW, Kramer MS. Variation in child cognitive ability by week of gestation among healthy term births. Am J Epidemiol 2010;171:399–406.
16. ACOG Committee on Practice Bulletins – Obstetrics. Induction of labor. ACOG practice bulletin No. 107. Obstet Gynecol 2009;114:386–97.
17. Martin JA, Hamilton BE, Sutton PD, et al. Births: final data for 2006. National vital statistics reports, vol. 57, no 7. Hyattsville (MD): National Center for Health Statistics; 2009.
18. Burton A, Ananth CV. Contributions of ischaemic placental disease to preterm birth in twin gestations. J Matern Fetal Neonatal Med 2010;23:1183–6.
19. Elliott JP. High-order multiple gestations. Semin Perinatol 2005;29:305–11.
20. Iams JD, Berghella V. Care for women with prior preterm birth. Am J Obstet Gynecol 2010;203:89–100.
21. Savitz DA. Invited commentary: disaggregating preterm birth to determine etiology. Am J Epidemiol 2008;168:990–2.
22. Ananth CV, Joseph KS, Oyelese Y, et al. Trends in preterm birth and perinatal mortality among singletons, 1989 through 2000. Obstet Gynecol 2005;105:1084–91.
23. Stoll BJ, Hansen NI, Bell EF, et al. Neonatal outcomes of extremely preterm infants from the NICHD Neonatal Research Network. Pediatrics 2010;126:443–56.
24. Donovan EF, Besl J, Paulson J, et al. Infant death among Ohio resident infants born at 32 to 41 weeks of gestation. Am J Obstet Gynecol 2010;203:58.e1–5.
25. Usher RH, Allen AC, McLean FH. Risk of respiratory distress syndrome related to gestational age, route of delivery and maternal diabetes. Am J Obstet Gynecol 1971;111:826–32.
26. Hardy JB, Drage JS, Jackson EC. The first year of life. Baltimore (MD): The Johns Hopkins Press; 1979. p. 54–66.
27. Cunningham FG, Leveno KJ, Bloom S, et al, editors. Williams' obstetrics. 23rd edition. New York (NY): McGraw-Hill; 2010. p. 803.
28. Fuchs K, Gyamfi C. The influence of obstetric practices on late prematurity. Clin Perinatol 2008;35:343–60.
29. Raju TNK, Higgins RD, Stark AR, et al. Optimizing care and outcome for late-preterm (near-term) infants: a summary of the workshop sponsored by the National Institute of Child Health and Human Development. Pediatrics 2006; 118:1207–14.
30. Kramer MS, Demissie K, Yang H, et al. The contribution of mild and moderate preterm birth to infant mortality. JAMA 2000;284:843–9.
31. Raju TN. The problem of late-preterm (near-term) births: a workshop summary. Pediatr Res 2006;60:775–6.
32. Shapiro-Mendoza CK, Tomashek KM, Kotelchuck M, et al. Effects of late-preterm birth and maternal medical conditions on newborn morbidity risk. Pediatrics 2008;121:e223–32.
33. Petrini JR, Dias T, McCormick MC, et al. Increased risk of adverse neurological development for late preterm infants. J Pediatr 2009;154:169–76.
34. The Ohio Perinatal Quality Collaborative Writing Committee. A statewide initiative to reduce inappropriate scheduled births at $36^{0/7}$ – $38^{6/7}$ weeks' gestation. Am J Obstet Gynecol 2010;202:243, e1–8.

35. Kramer MS, McLean FH, Boyd ME, et al. The validity of gestational age estimate by menstrual dating in term, preterm, and postterm gestations. JAMA 1988;260:3306–8.
36. Ananth CV, Gyamfi C, Jain L. Characterizing risk profiles of infants who are delivered at late preterm gestations: does it matter? Am J Obstet Gynecol 2008;199: 329–31.
37. Heron MP, Hoyert DL, Murphy SL, et al. Deaths: final data for 2006. National vital statistics reports, vol. 57, no 14. Hyattsville (MD): National Center for Health Statistics; 2009.
38. Joseph KS, Demissie K, Kramer MS. Obstetric intervention, stillbirth, and preterm birth. Semin Perinatol 2002;26:250–9.
39. Laughon SK, Reddy U, Sun L, et al. Precursors for late preterm birth in singleton gestations. Obstet Gynecol 2010;116:1047–55.
40. Holland MG, Refurezo JS, Ramin SM, et al. Late preterm birth: how often is it avoidable? Am J Obstet Gynecol 2009;201:404.e1–4.
41. Porter TF, Fraser AM, Hunter CY, et al. The risk of preterm birth across generations. Obstet Gynecol 1997;90:63–70.
42. Boyd HA, Poulsen G, Wohlfahrt J, et al. Maternal contributions to preterm delivery. Am J Epidemiol 2009;170:1358–64.
43. Svensson AC, Sandin S, Cnattingius S, et al. Maternal effects for preterm birth: a genetic epidemiologic study of 630,000 families. Am J Epidemiol 2009;170:1365–72.
44. Bhattacharya S, Raja EA, Mirazo ER, et al. Inherited predisposition to spontaneous preterm delivery. Obstet Gynecol 2010;115:1125–33.
45. Fiscella K, Franks P, Kendrick JS, et al. Risk of preterm birth that is associated with vaginal douching. Am J Obstet Gynecol 2002;186:1345–50.
46. Collins JW Jr, David RJ, Rankin KM, et al. Transgenerational effect of neighborhood poverty on low birthweight among African Americans in Cook County, Illinois. Am J Epidemiol 2009;169:712–7.
47. Miller GE, Chen E, Fok AK, et al. Low early-life social class leaves a biological residue manifested by decreased glucocorticoid and increased proinflammatory signaling. Proc Natl Acad Sci U S A 2009;106:14716–21.
48. Kuh D, Ben-Shlomo Y, editors. A life-course approach to chronic diseases epidemiology. Oxford (UK): Oxford University Press; 1997.
49. Klebanoff MA, Shiono P. Top down, bottom up, and inside out: reflections on preterm birth. Paediatr Perinat Epidemiol 1995;9:125–9.
50. Savitz DA, Blackmore CA, Thorp JM. Epidemiologic characteristics of preterm delivery: etiologic heterogeneity. Am J Obstet Gynecol 1991;162:467–71.
51. Meis PJ, Michielutte R, Peters TJ, et al. Factors associated with preterm birth in Cardiff, Wales. II: indicated and spontaneous preterm birth. Am J Obstet Gynecol 1995;173:597–602.
52. Meis PJ, Goldenberg RL, Mercer BM, et al. The preterm prediction study: risk factors for indicated preterm birth. Am J Obstet Gynecol 1998;178:562–7.
53. Savitz DA, Dole N, Herring AH. Should spontaneous and medically indicated preterm births be separated for studying aetiology? Paediatr Perinat Epidemiol 2005;19:97–105.
54. Romero R, Mazor M, Munoz H, et al. The preterm labor syndrome. Ann N Y Acad Sci 1994;734:414–29.
55. Iams JD, Goldenberg RL, Meis PJ, et al. The length of the cervix and the risk of spontaneous premature delivery. N Engl J Med 1996;334:567–72.
56. Goldenberg RL, Mercer BM, Meis PJ, et al. The preterm prediction study: fetal fibronectin testing and spontaneous preterm birth. Obstet Gynecol 1996;87(5 Pt 1): 643–8.

57. Sorokin Y, Romero R, Mele L, et al. Maternal serum interleukin-6, C-reactive protein, and matrix metalloproteinase-9 concentrations as risk factors for preterm birth <32 weeks and adverse neonatal outcomes. Am J Perinatol 2010;27: 631–40.
58. Horowitz S, Mazor M, Romero R, et al. Infection of the amniotic cavity with Ureaplasma urealyticum in the mid trimester of pregnancy. J Reprod Med 1995;40: 375–9.
59. Haas DM, Imperiale TF, Kirkpatrick PR, et al. Tocolytic therapy: a meta-analysis and decision analysis. Obstet Gynecol 2009;113:585–94.
60. McElrath TF, Hecht JL, Dammann O, et al. Pregnancy disorders that lead to delivery before the 28th week of gestation: an epidemiologic approach to classification. Am J Epidemiol 2008;168:980–9.
61. Ananth CV, Vintzileos AM. Maternal-fetal conditions necessitating a medical intervention resulting in preterm birth. Am J Obstet Gynecol 2006;195:1557–63.
62. Holzman C, Senagore P, Tian Y, et al. Maternal catecholamine levels in midpregnancy and risk of preterm delivery. Am J Epidemiol 2009;170:1014–24.
63. Gargano JW, Holzman CB, Senagore PK, et al. Evidence of placental haemorrhage and preterm delivery. BJOG 2010;117:445–55.
64. Kelly R, Holzman C, Senagore P, et al. Placental vascular pathology findings and pathways to preterm delivery. Am J Epidemiol 2009;170:148–58.
65. Naeye RL. Pregnancy hypertension, placental evidences of low uteroplacental blood flow, and spontaneous premature delivery. Hum Pathol 1989;20:441–4.

The Contribution of Maternal Stress to Preterm Birth: Issues and Considerations

Pathik D. Wadhwa, MD, PhD[a,c,]*, Sonja Entringer, PhD[b,c],
Claudia Buss, PhD[b,c], Michael C. Lu, MD, MPH[d]

KEYWORDS

- Stress • Preterm birth • Psychosocial
- Maternal-placental-fetal endocrine
- Immune • Vascular • Genetic

Preterm birth represents the most significant problem in maternal–child health in the United States. It is the leading cause of infant mortality and morbidity; its prevalence is unacceptably high and has not decreased over the past 40 years; and its etiology is unknown in a substantial proportion of cases.[1] The ongoing search to better elucidate its underlying causes and pathophysiologic mechanisms has identified maternal stress as a variable of interest. The question of the role of stress in preterm birth is, however, complex and challenging for many reasons. First, the basic physiologic and pathophysiologic mechanisms that underlie the timing of onset of human parturition and preterm birth, respectively, are not yet well understood. Second, the study of stress processes in pregnancy is complicated by the effects that pregnancy-related alterations in maternal physiology produce on central and peripheral systems implicated in the experience of and psychobiological responses to stress. This article

---

The preparation of this manuscript was supported in part by US PHS (NIH) grants RO1 HD-060628 and PO1 HD-047609 to PDW, RO1 HD-065825 to SE, and RO1 MH-091351 to CB. The authors have nothing to disclose.

[a] Departments of Psychiatry & Human Behavior, Obstetrics & Gynecology, and Epidemiology, University of California, Irvine, School of Medicine, 3177 Gillespie Neuroscience Research Facility, Irvine, CA 92697, USA

[b] Department of Pediatrics, University of California, Irvine, School of Medicine, 333 The City Drive (West), Suite 1200, Orange, CA 92868, USA

[c] University of California, Irvine, Development, Health and Disease Research Program (DHDR), 333 The City Drive (West), Suite 1200, Orange, CA 92868, USA

[d] Department of Obstetrics & Gynecology, David Geffen School of Medicine, University of California Los Angeles, Box 951772, 36-070B CHS, Los Angeles, CA 90095-1772, USA

* Corresponding author. Departments of Psychiatry & Human Behavior, Obstetrics & Gynecology, and Epidemiology, University of California, Irvine, School of Medicine, 3177 Gillespie Neuroscience Research Facility, Irvine, CA 92697.

E-mail address: pwadhwa@uci.edu

Clin Perinatol 38 (2011) 351–384
doi:10.1016/j.clp.2011.06.007
0095-5108/11/$ – see front matter © 2011 Elsevier Inc. All rights reserved.

does not purport to serve as a comprehensive review of all of the available findings on maternal stress and preterm birth; several reviews on this topic are available elsewhere.[2–9] Instead, select key issues and questions are addressed that warrant further consideration and discussion.

RATIONALE FOR CONSIDERING A ROLE FOR MATERNAL STRESS IN PRETERM BIRTH

The rationale for considering a role for stress in preterm birth derives partly from concepts in evolutionary biology and developmental plasticity. The mother and her developing fetus both play an obligatory, active role in the process of human parturition. The length of gestation and timing of onset of mammalian parturition represent a phenotype that emerges as a consequence of the culmination of intrauterine development. Development is a plastic process, wherein a range of different phenotypes can be expressed from a given genotype (contained within the fertilized zygote). The unfolding of all developmental processes across the multicontoured landscape from genotype to phenotype is context-dependent, wherein the developing embryo/fetus responds to, or is acted on by, conditions in the internal or external environment. Key environmental conditions that have shaped evolutionary selection and developmental plasticity include not only variation in energy substrate availability (ie, nutrition) but also challenges that have the potential to impact the structural or functional integrity and survival of the organism (ie, stress). Based on this consideration, it is likely and plausible that prenatal stress represents an important aspect of the intrauterine environment that would be expected to influence many, if not all, developmental outcomes.[10] Some evidence shows that preterm birth may be a maternal adaptation to limit the energetic costs of a pregnancy in the face of adverse conditions, or a fetal adaptation to an unfavorable intrauterine environment when other facultative measures have been unsuccessful.[11] Moreover, the application of a prenatal stress and stress biology framework offers an excellent model system for the study of intrauterine development and associated developmental, birth, and subsequent health-related phenotypes, because it is increasingly apparent that the developing fetus acquires and incorporates information about the nature of its environment partly via the same biologic systems that, in an already-developed individual, mediate adaptation and central and peripheral responses to endogenous and exogenous stress (eg, the maternal-placental-fetal [MPF] neuroendocrine and immune systems[12]).

From the perspective of the maternal compartment, another compelling rationale for considering a role for maternal stress as a contributor to preterm birth derives from the effort to elucidate and better understand the underlying reasons for the well-documented, persistent, and large socioeconomic and racial/ethnic disparities in the population distribution of preterm birth. Many of the factors that disproportionally affect socially disadvantaged individuals, such as prenatal care, diet/nutrition, and health-related behaviors, have been shown to play a limited role in accounting for these disparities.[13–16] The search for alternate explanations has led to the hypothesis that high levels of maternal stress may partly, independently, or in combination with other factors, explain these disparities, because the experience of social disadvantage and minority racial/ethnic status is characterized by higher levels of psychosocial stress and lack of resources, and because stress and stress-related biologic processes have been implicated in a wide array of adverse reproductive and other health outcomes.[13,17]

PSYCHOSOCIAL STRESS AND PRETERM BIRTH: A BRIEF OVERVIEW

The belief that a mother's emotional or psychological state during pregnancy may influence the development of her fetus has existed since ancient times across all cultures. Empirical studies examining the effects of prenatal psychosocial stress first appeared in the literature in the mid-1950s. Much of the earlier work in this area, however, was limited by major conceptual and methodological problems. Over the past 2 decades, larger, better-designed studies have presented more consistent findings. A rapidly growing body of empirical evidence, based on these prospective, population-based studies in pregnant women of different sociodemographic, racial/ethnic, and national backgrounds, now provides support for the premise that women experiencing high levels of psychosocial stress during pregnancy are at significantly increased risk for shortened gestation and preterm delivery, even after accounting for the effects of other established sociodemographic, biophysical, biomedical, and behavioral risk factors.[2,4,6,9,18–20] Although the tremendous heterogeneity in study designs, study populations, methodology, and measures makes comparisons of effect size difficult to interpret across studies, pregnant women reporting high levels of psychosocial stress seem to have, on average, a 25% to 60% increased risk for preterm birth compared with women reporting low levels of stress.

Based on these findings, several researchers and public health experts are now increasingly highlighting the need for a new, integrative research and clinical practice agenda, with an emphasis on biopsychosocial processes, including the impact of maternal stress, to address the problem of preterm birth.[21] In fact, recent guidelines for obstetric practice issued by the American College of Obstetricians and Gynecologists recommend performing psychosocial screening at least once during each trimester of pregnancy.[21] However, before specific clinical guidelines and interventions can be developed for primary, secondary, and tertiary prevention, the authors suggest that some critical issues warrant further consideration.

ISSUES AND QUESTIONS

At the population level, maternal stress seems to represent a significant risk factor for shortened gestation and increased risk of preterm birth, and the magnitude of the effect size may be similar to that of many other established sociodemographic, obstetric, and behavioral risk factors. However, in any individual pregnancy, the specificity and sensitivity of maternal stress as a predictor of adverse birth outcomes is clearly modest, at best. Some, but certainly not all, women who experience high levels of stress during pregnancy deliver preterm, and the challenge of identifying which particular women (or subgroups of women) and in what circumstances (context) and at which stages of gestation these women are particularly susceptible to the potentially detrimental effects of prenatal stress has yet to be satisfactorily addressed. The authors suggest that these issues must be addressed before the present research findings can be translated into a public health and clinical framework. Many of these issues have been previously discussed; this article highlights and expands on some specific aspects related to study design and methodology, stressor specificity, outcome specificity, the nature of the relationship, potential interactions with other individual-level or contextual-level factors, and critical periods of susceptibility.

Study Design and Methodology

The same study design and methodology issues applicable for rigorous epidemiologic, genetic, and clinical studies of putative risk factors for preterm birth remain applicable for studies of maternal psychosocial stress. The importance of a prospective design (to minimize ascertainment bias), appropriate study population (to ensure adequate variability in the distribution of the exposures and outcomes of interest), well-defined and characterized measures of the birth phenotype (accurate dating of pregnancy and ascertainment of whether the birth was preceded by spontaneous labor or membranes rupture, or whether it was induced or followed elective cesarean section), comprehensive assessment of psychosocial stress and related constructs, and measurement of covariates and potential confounding variables, is emphasized.

Accurate dating of pregnancy using last menstrual period in combination with early ultrasound and standardization across studies remains a critical issue.[22] Another related issue pertains to the use of the conventional definition of preterm birth as occurring at less than 37 completed weeks gestation. Recognizing this cutoff is somewhat arbitrary, some recent studies have reported that the effects of length of gestation on infant morbidity and mortality risk extend continuously across the normal range of pregnancy duration, instead of merely being a function of preterm birth.[23,24] Thus, to assess potential effects across the entire distribution instead of at only one tail of the distribution, the value of including measures of gestational length along a continuum (quantitative trait) in addition to the conventional, clinical, categorical classification is emphasized.

Most human studies of the effects of prenatal stress necessarily use a correlational design. The caveat that correlation cannot establish causality is well recognized. Obviously, randomly assigning humans to high stress exposure is not ethically possible, and studies of interventions to lower stress may not provide the same information as those that would induce additional stress. Although the use of experimental manipulations in animal models confers many benefits, one of their major limitations, particularly in the area of preterm birth research, is the considerable interspecies variation in physiologic processes underlying parturition and in the developmental time line (discussed later). Thus, the use of well-designed prospective studies in representative populations with serial, longitudinal assessments to determine the nature and strength of the association of naturally occurring variation in stress with subsequent birth outcomes after measuring and statistically adjusting for effects of other established sociodemographic, behavioral, and environmental risk factors can go a long way to provide the best possible evidence that either supports or refutes an underlying causal model (Bradford Hill, in his seminal 1965 paper,[25] first articulated considerations regarding association and causation, and others subsequently elaborated on these[26–28]).

Finally, the importance of good clinical phenotyping of preterm births is emphasized. Preterm birth is a heterogeneous entity in terms of the extent to which the birth is preterm (mild, moderate, or severe), and in terms of the precipitating events (induced or elective preterm birth, or spontaneous preterm birth after either preterm labor or preterm rupture of membranes). Therefore, it is important to recognize and examine the possibility that the contribution of maternal stress may vary between these different categories of preterm birth. For example, maternal stress would be hypothesized to have its largest marginal (main) effects on near-term spontaneous births, followed by near-term indicated births. In contrast, an important conditional (moderator) effect of maternal stress (eg, interaction with intrauterine infection) would be hypothesized for earlier (moderate to severe) preterm births.

Characterization and Assessment of Maternal Stress

A question that frequently arises regarding the putative effects of maternal stress on preterm birth risk concerns the elucidation of the aspects or domains of maternal stress that may be particularly salient. Although no universally accepted definition of psychosocial stress exists, stress is clearly not a unidimensional construct but rather "a person-environment interaction," in which there is a perceived discrepancy between environmental demands and the individual's psychological, social, or biologic resources.[29] This transactional view of the stress construct calls for the identification of stressful stimuli, subjects' appraisal of these stimuli, and their emotional responses. As described in a recent review,[4] most human studies of prenatal stress have used measures of major life event stress (eg, death of a family member), catastrophic community-wide disasters (eg, earthquakes, acts of terrorism), chronic stress, daily hassles, perceived stress, symptoms of depression or general anxiety, and pregnancy-specific anxiety. Although firm conclusions are difficult to draw, this and other reviews indicate that stressors such as major negative life events and catastrophes confer greater risk for preterm birth than less-severe chronic stressful exposures and depressive symptoms.[30-32] Moreover, measures of stress that focus on pregnancy-related concerns (pregnancy-specific anxiety) seem to be stronger predictors of preterm birth risk than measures of general anxiety.[33-37] The authors' review of pregnancy-specific psychosocial measures[35,36,38-48] suggests that the major constructs that encompass pregnancy-specific stress relate to (1) feelings about being pregnant (positive and negative), (2) pregnancy-specific concerns or anxiety about the health of the unborn baby, labor, and delivery, and about body size/image, (3) pregnancy-specific support (emotional, enacted), (4) pregnancy-related symptoms, and (5) attitudes toward the current pregnancy (intendedness, wantedness).

The distinction between various components or dimensions of psychological stress as discrete entities may be somewhat arbitrary. Different components of psychological stress are not randomly distributed; they tend to co-occur. An acute circumstance, such as a stressful life event (eg, death of a family member), produces chronic psychological distress that could vary considerably across individuals in the nature, intensity, and duration of its psychological and physiologic consequences. Moreover, in some instances, acute psychological stressors may represent the culmination of a preceding period of increased and chronic psychological distress (eg, if the death of the family member followed a period of long hospitalization). Chronic stress may partly reflect external events, and may partly reflect more persistent psychological attributes of the individual that are minimally related to external events.[49]

A substantial body of previous research has identified certain key dimensions of psychological stress that may be particularly salient in terms of their potential for producing unfavorable psychological and physiologic consequences, especially the dimensions of predictability and controllability (these are addressed in the classical studies by Weiss[50,51] and are reviewed by Sapolsky[52] and Koolhaas and colleagues[53]). In addition to these dimensions, yet another dimension of stressful experience may warrant further consideration: that of lability, or variability, or changeability, over time. In considering the cumulative effects of psychological stress, the authors of this article hypothesize that the number and magnitude of psychological "ups" and "downs" experienced by the individual over the given period of interest will produce an impact on the likelihood of stress-related health outcomes that is either independent of, or interacts with, the overall mean level of stress over that particular period. This concept is akin to that of the negative consequences of poor glycemic control, wherein among a group of individuals with the same average level of hyperglycemia, those whose blood sugar levels fluctuate a great deal around the mean (number and magnitude of highs and lows) are at greater risk for hyperglycemia-related complications than those who maintain a more consistent or stable level of hyperglycemia. The authors note that the common approach to assessment of psychological stress using self-reported retrospective recall measures does not lend itself well to the assessment of the dimensions of predictability or lability of stress over time.

Other psychological factors that may influence the relationship between maternal stress and preterm birth include maternal psychopathology (eg, development of posttraumatic stress disorder after a severe stressor),[54] personality traits, social support, and coping processes. Moreover, stress may not entirely be an individual-level phenomenon but may also be linked to the individual's social-structural context (eg, experience of racism,[55,56] neighborhood characteristics[57–59]). Thus, the construct of prenatal psychosocial stress and the social-structural context within which stress is experienced by the individual are areas that clearly need further refinement in the effort to better understand the role of prenatal stress in preterm birth.

Another issue that sometimes arises from broad and overgeneralized assertions that "stress is bad for you and your baby" is the concern that this may inadvertently be contributing to yet another reason for increasing anxiety and worry among pregnant women: the worry about being worried. The authors believe that this is a reasonable and justifiable concern, and caution against overinterpretation or over-generalization of findings in this area of research. They do note that although some studies have reported a protective or beneficial effect of mild of moderate stress during pregnancy on certain child neurodevelopmental outcomes[49,60] (which, paren-thetically, is consistent with the expectation of a fetal adaptation to accelerate devel-opment in the context of unfavorable circumstances), no studies have found a protective or beneficial effect of maternal stress on the risk of adverse birth outcomes such as preterm birth.

The authors submit that two key limitations to current approaches to characterizing and assessing maternal stress in pregnancy relate to (1) the problem of retrospective recall measures and (2) the lack of attention to the issue of psychobiological stress reactivity.

The problem of retrospective recall measures

With the exception of studies on exposure to natural disasters, wars, or acts of terrorism, human studies in the stress and pregnancy outcomes area (including studies that use a prospective design) have relied almost exclusively on self-reported retrospective recall measures of stress. Respondents are typically asked to rate, on average, how stressed or depressed or anxious they have felt over the past week or month or since the beginning of their pregnancy. These traditional, self-report recall measures are prone to numerous systematic biases that undermine their validity. These measures rely on autobiographical memory (ie, in time and place) as opposed to semantic memory (ie, independent of time and place), and on the respondents' ability to first integrate and then summarize states and events across the reporting period. Autobiographical memory requires the use of certain heuristic strategies for recall or reconstruction that introduce not only random error but also systematic biases.[61,62] A key example of a biasing cognitive heuristic is the "avail-ability heuristic," wherein more salient events that are easily available in memory are given greater weight. Furthermore, emotional states and arousal at the time of encod-ing and recall can bias past memories. Also, the recency effect bias refers to better recall of more recent experience. In addition, most psychosocial and behavioral measures involve global assessment of events or states over time. Self-reports of global assessments, as opposed to reports of specific-event recall, are known to be particularly susceptible to all these biases, because they involve not only recall but also integration and summarization of these states and events across the reporting period. Thus, because of all these biases associated with the use of retrospective recall measures of psychosocial stress and related constructs in the context of this area of research, whether the modest effect sizes observed in the literature are a func-tion of "true" weak or small effects of prenatal stress on birth outcomes or of defi-ciency in measurement procedures is difficult to establish.

Psychobiological stress responsivity

The likelihood of occurrence of a stress-related adverse health outcome is a well-established function of not only the amount of actual or perceived stress exposure over time but also that individual's biologic propensity to respond to stress. The concept of biologic stress reactivity refers to characteristics of the biologic response (eg, magnitude, duration) to a unit of stress exposure. Evoked physiologic responses to behavioral challenge provide reliable and valid measures of an individual's propensity for biologic perturbation during stress, and these measures have proven useful in other health domains in predicting risk of stress-related outcomes.[63,64] Most studies of prenatal stress and birth outcomes have considered only the prenatal stress exposure or experience side of the equation, but have neglected the issue of individual differences in biologic stress reactivity in pregnancy. The principle of measuring response to a controlled stimulus certainly is not new; it is, in fact, widely used in an array of settings, including the diagnostic laboratory (glucose tolerance test, dexamethasone suppression test), the behavioral medicine laboratory (cold pressor test, social evaluation threat [eg, Trier Social Stress Test[65]]), and even in clinical obstetric practice (eg, pharmacologic [glucose], physical [nipple stimulation, sound], or endocrine [oxytocin] challenges). However, only few studies have used this approach in evaluating stress and stress processes in human pregnancy.[66–68] The authors' use of this approach has shown that a progressive attenuation occurs of not only maternal biologic but also psychological responses to stress over the course of gestation,[66] and that after accounting for the effects of other established risk factors, individual differences in the degree (trajectory) of this attenuation is a significant predictor of shortened length of gestation and risk of earlier delivery.[69] Thus, the authors submit that the use of standardized behavioral or psychological probes, using appropriate and ecologically valid stimuli, to assess individual differences in the responsivity of stress-related maternal or fetal biologic systems at various time points over the course of gestation may prove useful in identifying individuals who may be particularly susceptible to the deleterious effects of stress.

Critical Periods of Susceptibility

Fetal development is a logarithmic process, with rapid mitosis at early stages and cellular hypertrophy and accumulation of fat, glycogen, and connective tissue later in gestation. It is well established that several sensitive or critical periods occur in development, and critical periods during pregnancy of altered vulnerability to the effects of prenatal stress may also occur. These periods may be related to the times in gestation corresponding to specific developmental events, or to time-specific changes in maternal or fetal physiologic responses to stress over the course of gestation.[70,71] Although this premise of susceptible periods is well supported in the animal literature, a relatively small number of human studies of prenatal stress have incorporated multiple assessments of stress across gestation and tested hypotheses about time-specific effects.

The state of pregnancy is associated with major alterations in maternal biology, including changes in stress-sensitive endocrine, immune, and vascular processes and control mechanisms (feedback loops). Furthermore, evidence suggests that the state of pregnancy is associated with alterations in maternal biologic responsivity to a stimulus or stressor. Evoked physiologic responses to pharmacologic and physical challenges have been studied in pregnant women, and results generally suggest maternal responses are dampened in pregnancy, particularly in the later stages of gestation. For example, administration of exogenous corticotrophin-releasing hormone (CRH) in late but not mid-pregnancy failed to evoke a significant pituitary or adrenal response,[72,73] and administration of dexamethasone produced less suppression of cortisol production.[74] Similarly, autonomic responses (heart rate, blood pressure) to a variety of challenges, including exercise, orthostatic challenge, and the cold pressure test, are attenuated in pregnancy.[75–77] Moreover, maternal appraisals of psychological stress seem to progressively decrease as pregnancy advances.[78–80]

The authors recently conducted a longitudinal study of psychological and biologic responses to a standardized laboratory stressor at three time points in a population of pregnant and nonpregnant women. Findings suggest that timing of stressor exposure in pregnancy had a significant impact on the magnitude of the autonomic stress response, with greater biologic stress responses in earlier compared with later gestation. Furthermore, as pregnancy advanced, the cortisol response to awakening progressively decreased,[66] and a larger cortisol-awakening response in late pregnancy and a reduced attenuation of this response from early to late gestation were significantly associated with shorter gestational length.[69]

Bidirectional relationship between the maternal and fetal compartments: implications for causality of effects

What drives these changes in maternal responses to stress over gestation and hence potentially alters the developing fetus and birth outcomes? An implicit assumption regarding the direction of causality is that it is unidirectional in nature, in that potentially unfavorable circumstances in a pregnant women's life that are perceived or appraised by the maternal brain as stressful may then influence maternal physiology, which, in turn, may impact the developing fetus via direct or indirect biologic mechanisms. However, the pregnancy-related alterations in maternal physiology are known to originate from the fetal and not maternal compartment (the placenta is an organ of fetal origin). Because these observed variations in maternal physiology (that have consequences for maternal stress responses and fetal susceptibility to maternal stress exposure) originate from, and are sustained by, the developing fetoplacental unit over gestation, this suggests the intriguing possibility of reciprocal, bidirectional causality. In this scenario, variations in processes that underlie fetal growth, maturation, and development result in variations in maternal physiology, which, in turn, influence or moderate the effects of maternal stress exposure on the developing fetus, including perhaps, subsequent changes in maternal physiology and fetal susceptibility to maternal stress (**Fig. 1**). The object (fetus) of the influence (maternal stress) is the cause of the process that produces the influence (changes in maternal stress responsivity); this process is dynamic, recursive, and bidirectional between the fetal and maternal compartment over the course of gestation.[10]

The Role of Context: Potential Interaction Effects of Maternal Stress

Preterm birth is a multifactorial outcome. At the individual level, the major risk categories include sociodemographic, historical, biophysical, obstetric, behavioral, psychosocial, genetic, and other environmental factors. Studies of the effects of maternal stress and related psychosocial processes on preterm birth generally treat these other risk factors as potential confounding variables and attempt to account (adjust) for their putative effects through either study design (subject selection criteria) or statistical adjustment. However, emerging concepts of causation for complex common disorders, including preterm birth, suggest that it is not only possible but in fact probable that causation does not reside in any single factor or in the additive effects of numerous factors, but rather lies at the interface between multiple risk factors (interaction, or multiplicative effect).[81,82] The authors consider, by way of example and illustration of this critically important concept, two conditions that are

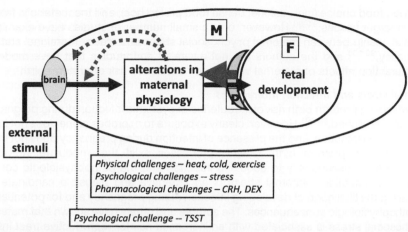

Fig. 1. Maternal physiology and fetal development: a case of reciprocal determinism. External conditions during pregnancy that are appraised by the maternal brain as stressful may result in stress-related alterations in maternal physiology that, in turn, may influence fetal development and birth outcomes. However, the state of pregnancy itself produces progressive changes in maternal physiology that have been shown to alter maternal peripheral (physiologic) responses to a variety of physical, psychological, and pharmacologic challenges, and also maternal central (psychological) responses to a social stressor. These pregnancy-related changes in maternal physiology (that alter maternal psychological and physiologic responses to exogenous stressors) originate from the fetal–placental compartment. Hence, the fetus, the object of maternal stress-related physiologic perturbations, is also the initiator of alterations in maternal physiology that progressively dampen maternal responses to exogenous (and likely endogenous) challenges, a case of reciprocal determinism. F, fetal; M, maternal; P, placental compartment.

important in their own right from the standpoint of preterm birth, and for which a high plausibility exists of interaction effects with maternal stress, namely nutrition and infection.

Prenatal stress and nutrition interactions
The two fundamental processes that are believed to shape evolutionary selection and developmental plasticity are variation in energy substrate availability (nutrition) and challenges that have the potential to impact the structural or functional integrity and survival of the organism (stress). Preterm birth may represent a maternal adaptation to limit the energetic costs of a pregnancy in the face of adverse conditions, or a fetal adaptation to an unfavorable intrauterine environment when other facultative measures have been unsuccessful.[11] Maternal nutrition, assessed with indicators of body size such as body mass index (BMI), nutritional intake, or serum measures of nutritional biomarkers, is a well-established risk factor for preterm birth.[83,84] Growing evidence supports the concept of a bidirectional interaction between nutrition and stress, such that the effects of nutrition on health may vary as a function of stress, or that the effects of stress on health may vary as a function of nutritional status. For example, several experimental studies in animals have shown that nutritional manipulations, particularly in the preconception or early pregnancy period, may produce their effects on maternal and fetal outcomes, including preterm birth, via alterations in stress biology (cortisol, inflammatory cytokines).[85–93] Conversely, studies in animals and humans of stress induction (through exposure to laboratory-based social stressors or endocrine stress analogs) have shown effects on feeding

behavior, food choice (high-calorie, dense food preference), and the metabolic fate of food in target tissues.[94–98] However, only a small number of studies have examined the relationship between maternal psychosocial stress and diet or nutritional state in pregnancy,[99,100] and the authors are not aware of any studies that have modeled the interaction effects of maternal stress and nutrition on risk of preterm birth.

Prenatal stress and infection interactions

The effects on preterm birth risk of intrauterine or systemic infection during pregnancy are well established.[83,101] However, clearly exposure to microbes alone does not inevitably result in infection, and the presence of infection during pregnancy does not inevitably result in preterm birth. Clearly, processes exist that modulate individual differences in susceptibility to acquiring infection and the pathophysiologic consequences of infection. Maternal stress is an attractive and plausible candidate for increasing the likelihood of developing infection during pregnancy and for potentiating its pathophysiologic consequences. The authors and others have shown that maternal psychosocial stress is associated with an increased risk for reproductive tract infection during pregnancy.[102,103] Moreover, biologic stress mediators such as CRH may potentiate inflammation in the context of antigen stimulation (infection).[104] However, the synergistic effects of high psychosocial stress and reproductive tract or intrauterine infection on preterm birth risk have not yet been examined.

STRESS PATHWAYS TO PRETERM BIRTH

The influence of psychosocial factors on health outcomes is mediated either directly via physiologic pathways, indirectly via behavioral pathways, or both.[19,105–107] The influence of psychosocial stress on increasing the propensity for engaging in a wide array of unhealthy behaviors, including key behavioral risk factors for preterm birth such as poor diet/nutrition and smoking, is well established in studies of the general population and pregnant women.[36,108] One important issue that has yet to be addressed is the possibility of an interaction between maternal stress and nutrition, wherein the effect of stress on preterm birth risk varies as a function of the nutritional status of the mother, or that the effect of nutritional status on preterm birth risk varies as a function of maternal stress and stress biology during pregnancy.

BIOLOGIC PATHWAYS TO PARTURITION

Human parturition involves the time- and context-dependent interplay of several systems and signaling molecules within the maternal, placental, and fetal tissues. Events leading to parturition start early in pregnancy, occur sequentially, and involve feedback systems. Clinical and experimental evidence broadly supports the concept that preterm birth is determined by multiple genetic and environmental factors that reflect the interactions among one or more of several pathophysiologic processes, which may ultimately share common biologic pathways leading to uterine contractions, cervical changes, and rupture of membranes. These pathways include (1) early or excessive activation of the MPF neuroendocrine axis; (2) decidual/chorioamniotic/fetal inflammation caused by ascending genitourinary tract or systemic infection; (3) uteroplacental vascular lesions caused by coagulopathy, hypertension, or abruption/decidual hemorrhage; and (4) pathologic distention of the uterus, caused by multiple gestation.[1,33,109–112] The authors recognize the possibility that these pathways may not represent all potential routes to preterm birth, and also note that these pathways are unlikely to be mutually exclusive and distinct but rather have substantial overlap and interaction between them.

The MPF Endocrine, Immune, and Vascular Systems in Mammalian Pregnancy

Pregnancy produces major alterations in neuroendocrine, immune, and vascular function, including changes in hormone and cytokine levels and control mechanisms (feedback loops) that are crucial in providing a favorable environment within the uterus and fetal compartment for growth, differentiation, and maturation, and in conveying signals when the fetus is ready for extrauterine life. Starting very early in gestation, the placenta, which is the first fetal organ to develop and function, produces hormones, neuropeptides, growth factors, and cytokines, and appears to function in a manner resembling that of compressed hypothalamic-pituitary-target systems.[113] Glucocorticoid physiology (cortisol in humans) has received extensive and well-placed consideration as a critical endocrine mediator of fetal development and birth outcomes, with an emphasis on not only hormone production but also hormone action mediated by tissue-specific glucocorticoid receptor expression, sensitivity, and affinity, and by maternal–fetal transfer mediated by the activity of the placental 11β-hydroxysteroid dehydrogenase enzyme system.[114] Less well recognized is the potential and perhaps equally important role of the peptide CRH. In primates, but not other mammals, the placenta synthesizes and releases CRH in large amounts into the fetal and maternal circulations. In contrast to the inhibitory influence on hypothalamic CRH production, cortisol stimulates placental CRH production,[115] and this positive feedback loop results in a progressive amplification of CRH and cortisol production over the course of gestation.[116]

With respect to the immune axis, one of the major endeavors of pregnancy-related alterations in immune function is to achieve and maintain the optimal balance between tolerating the fetal semiallograft while not suppressing maternal immune responses to an extent that increases maternal or fetal susceptibility to infection. Thus, a generalized reduction of maternal immune responsiveness occurs during pregnancy, mediated by hormonal changes (eg, increased levels of progesterone), trophoblast expression of key immunomodulatory molecules, and a progressive switch from a T-helper cell type 1 (TH_1)/T-helper cell type 2 (TH_2) balance to a predominantly T-helper 2–type pattern of cytokines.[117] A recent study of the longitudinal modulation of the cytokine profile across human pregnancy reported an overall decrease in proinflammatory cytokine trajectories in the innate and adaptive arms of the immune system and an increase in counter-regulatory cytokines as pregnancy progresses.[118]

Cardiovascular adaptations in pregnancy include anatomic changes and changes in blood volume, cardiac output, and systemic vascular resistance, all of which result in conditions that are normal in pregnancy but would constitute signs of cardiovascular dysfunction in the nonpregnant state.[119] The study of cardiovascular changes associated with pregnancy has relevance, because related disorders (eg, hypertension, preeclampsia) are one of the major indicators for elective preterm delivery.[1,83]

Interactions Among MPF Neuroendocrine, Immune/Inflammatory, and Vascular Pathways in Pregnancy

Although distinct neuroendocrine, immune/inflammatory, and vascular pathways have been described, growing evidence suggests that these and other physiologic systems involved in pregnancy are highly interrelated, and that they extensively regulate and counterregulate one another. The potential complexity of the interrelationships among these physiologic systems is seen when considering the role of infection in the cause of adverse fetal developmental and birth outcomes. For example, inflammatory cytokines that are produced in response to infection, such as tumor necrosis factor α (TNF-α), interleukin (IL)-1β, and IL-6, can activate components of the

MPF–neuroendocrine system that also increase the risk of premature birth.[120–123] Conversely, it is also known that hypothalamic-pituitary-adrenal (HPA) axis hormones such as CRH and cortisol influence the production of cytokines and modulate the inflammatory response to infection.[124–126] Central CRH, acting via glucocorticoids and catecholamines, inhibits inflammation, whereas CRH directly secreted by peripheral nerves and mast cells stimulates local inflammation.[127] Moreover, researchers have postulated that acute and chronic infections may be risk factors for uteroplacental vasculopathies that may be associated with premature birth.[110] Impaired nutrient and oxygen exchange associated with uteroplacental vasculopathy may stress the fetus and result in increased production of placental–fetal hormones such as CRH, whereas placental CRH, in turn, may influence fetal–placental circulation.[128] Thus, the relationship of a well-defined risk factor, such as prenatal infection, to adverse birth outcomes is likely to involve complex interactions among the endocrine, immune, and vascular systems.

Stress Biology in Human Pregnancy

Stress biology refers to the set of biologic adaptations in response to challenges or demands that threaten or are perceived to be a potential threat to the stability of the internal milieu of the organism. The nervous, endocrine, immune, and vascular systems play a major role in adaptations to stress. There are no direct neural, vascular, or other connections between the mother and her developing fetus; all communication between the maternal and fetal compartments is mediated via the placenta, an organ of fetal origin.

Based on the physiology of stress and parturition and the evidence linking maternal stress to earlier delivery, the authors have proposed a biobehavioral framework of stress and adverse birth outcomes.[12] Substantial evidence in nonpregnant humans and animals shows that stress activates the neuroendocrine system and produces exaggerated inflammatory responses and alterations in vascular hemodynamics[129,130]; however, these associations cannot be assumed to also be present in the pregnant state, because the changes in endocrine, immune, and vascular physiology have consequences for attenuating the responsivity of these systems to stress. The authors' model proposes a major role for placental CRH in mediating the effects of maternal stress, because not only is this system known to play an important role in human parturition but it also provides a biologically plausible link between known environmental risk factors and preterm birth, including in the context of racial/ethnic disparities. For instance, (1) placental production of CRH, which is a key activator of the HPA axis, has been proposed to be an early event that regulates the subsequent cascade of fetal, placental, and maternal physiologic processes involved in human parturition[111,131]; (2) variations in markers of MPF neuroendocrine activity, such as placental CRH and estriol concentrations in early to mid-gestation, significantly predict subsequent differences in the timing of onset of parturition and risk of preterm birth[132]; (3) large racial/ethnic differences have been observed in both the production of MPF hormones and the magnitude of their effect on risk of preterm birth[133,134]; (4) significant racial/ethnic differences have been reported in relative allele frequencies in various regions of the CRH gene[135]; (5) MPF neuroendocrine activity is altered by obstetric risk conditions and also by exposure to environments that reflect adverse social and behavioral conditions[136,137]; and (6) the effects of the infection/inflammation and uteroplacental vasculopathy may be modulated partly by the activity of placental CRH and other elements of the MPF neuroendocrine pathway.[17,131,138]

Prenatal psychosocial stress and MPF endocrine function
Placental CRH, the key mediator of stress-related MPF endocrine function in primates, is stress-sensitive. A series of in vitro studies by Petraglia and colleagues[139–141] have shown that CRH is released from cultured human placental cells in a dose–response manner in response to all of the major biologic effectors of stress, including cortisol, inflammatory cytokines, and hypoxia. Other in vivo studies have found significant correlations among maternal pituitary-adrenal stress hormones (eg, adrenocortico-tropic hormone [ACTH], cortisol) and placental CRH levels.[142–144] Moreover, maternal psychosocial stress is significantly correlated with maternal pituitary-adrenal hormone levels (eg, ACTH, cortisol[145–148]) that are known to stimulate placental CRH secretion. Some,[136,137,149] but not all studies,[150,151] also have reported direct associations between maternal psychosocial stress and placental CRH function. One recent study found an association between placental CRH and preterm birth only in women with high chronic stress.[152] A recent report suggests that a maternal stress signal—elevated cortisol early in pregnancy—is associated with a significant and precocious rise in placental CRH later in pregnancy, and that this effect is associated with risk for preterm delivery.[153] Thus, substantial in vitro and in vivo evidence indicates that the placenta detects and responds to a variety of maternal physiologic and psychological stress signals in a manner consistent with promoting earlier parturition.

One of the challenges in human pregnancy research is the identification of biomarkers that reflect long-term or cumulative stress exposure. In this context, measures of cortisol in hair samples seem to be a promising candidate biomarker. Two recent studies have reported significant associations between measures of maternal psychosocial stress in pregnancy and hair cortisol levels.[33,154]

Prenatal psychosocial stress and immune function
Studies have reported that elevated psychosocial stress in pregnant women is asso-ciated with higher circulating levels of inflammatory markers, such as C-reactive protein (CRP) and the proinflammatory cytokines IL-1b, IL-6, and TNF-α, and lower circulating levels of the antiinflammatory cytokine IL-10 and ex vivo endotoxin (lipo-polysaccharide)-stimulated levels of IL-1b and IL-6.[155–158] Another recent study of proinflammatory responses to an in vivo antigen challenge (influenza virus vaccination) in pregnant women reported an association between depressive symptoms and sensitization of the inflammatory cytokine responses.[156] Some studies also have reported associations between maternal psychosocial stress and reproductive tract infection (bacterial vaginosis), which is a risk factor for preterm birth.[102,103]

Prenatal psychosocial stress and vascular function
Vascular disorders in pregnancy, such as pregnancy-induced hypertension and preeclampsia, are the major indications for elective preterm delivery. Findings suggest that maternal psychosocial stress is significantly associated with increased risk of hypertensive disorders in pregnancy.[159–164] In one study, blood pressure responses to a laboratory-based psychosocial stressor in pregnant women predicted the length of gestation and infant birth weight[165]; however, this effect was not apparent when blood pressure responses were assessed in the nonpregnant state and related to birth outcomes in subsequent pregnancies.[151] Reduced aortic blood flow velocity and elevated uteroplacental Doppler flow velocity waveform indices have been associated with adverse birth outcomes and impaired neonatal status.[67] A few studies have reported that among pregnant women, high anxiety is associated with reduced uterine,[166] fetal, and umbilical blood flow and pulsatility patterns indicative of fetal hypoxia and compensatory redistribution of blood flow to the fetal brain.[167,168]

Placental CRH seems to play an important role in the context of cardiovascular physiology in pregnancy. Several studies have reported an association between CRH and hypertensive disorders.[169–171] Furthermore, elevated levels of CRH have been shown to correlate significantly with abnormal uteroplacental flow waveforms.[172,173] Although not conclusive, the reported data support the notion of stress-related vascular pathophysiology contributing to preterm birth.

Multivariable pathway models linking maternal psychosocial stress, biologic function, and preterm birth

Although the evidence discussed provides biologic plausibility for the concept that psychosocial stress may contribute to preterm birth risk via its effects on several stress-sensitive biologic processes implicated in parturition, tests of pathway (meditational) models to show these linkages have generally been unsuccessful. Many reasons are possible for this difficulty in generating findings to support these hypothesized linkages, including weaknesses in the conceptualization and operationalization of psychosocial stress, of the biologic processes of interest (eg, single time-point biomarkers, biomarkers in systemic circulation as a proxy for local [tissue-specific] biology, biomarkers assessed at basal state as a proxy for biologic responses to challenge), or of the study design (use of cross-sectional assessments to depict biologic processes that are characterized by progressive alterations over time/course of gestation). These issues notwithstanding, the authors submit that another major limitation may relate to the oversimplistic manner in which these processes are believed to operate. Consider, for example, a conceptual model frequently evoked in the stress and preterm birth literature, in which variation in maternal psychosocial stress in pregnancy is hypothesized to correlate with variation in maternal cortisol in pregnancy, which in turn is hypothesized to correlate with variation in gestational age at birth. No known instance exists in biology at which a simple, one-to-one correspondence is present between a specific psychological and a specific biologic state. In the example considered here, cortisol production in vivo is influenced not only by the psychological state of the individual but also concurrently by a host of other conditions, such as variations in the nutritional milieu, physical activity, infection/inflammation, hypoxia, sleep, chronobiological state, and, in the case of pregnancy, by the stage of gestation. Moreover, the effects of psychological stress on cortisol production likely vary as a consequence of these other conditions (ie, an interactional, conditional, or effect–modification model). Second, no instance in biology is known when perturbation within a particular biologic system remains constrained within that system. Regardless of the nature of the initiating stressor (eg, psychological, nutritional, infectious), once a perturbation is produced within the endocrine system, it will inevitably produce secondary perturbations in the brain and immune, vascular, and other endocrine-related systems. The nature and magnitude of these secondary perturbations will then, through negative or positive feedback loops, alter the nature, magnitude, and time-course of the initial stress-initiated perturbation (in this case, of the endocrine system). Thus, the effect of stress-related endocrine function on the outcome of interest (preterm birth) will vary as a function of the state of the immune and vascular systems and their feedback effects on the endocrine system (again, an interactional, conditional, or effect–modification model). Therefore, conceptualizations of simple one-to-one correspondence between variation in psychological and biologic systems and health outcomes that do not measure and account for the effects of and interactions with other important states or contexts on a particular biologic system, or of the impact of secondary perturbations in other closely linked biologic systems on the primary biologic system of interest, would be hard-pressed to show evidence to support a pathway or mediational model. Adoption and implementation of a systems biology approach will be required to uncover the complex web of interrelationships and pathways inherent in in vivo human models of complex multifactorial disorders such as preterm birth (**Fig. 2**).

Applicability of animal models for research on prenatal stress and preterm birth
Although the use of experimental manipulations using animal models confers many benefits, one of their limitations, particularly in the area of preterm birth research, is the considerable interspecies variation that exists in physiologic processes underlying parturition and in the developmental time line. Consider, for example, the comparative endocrinology of mammalian pregnancy. One of the major challenges in elucidating the endocrinology of human parturition arises from the existence of large interspecies differences in the endocrinology of pregnancy, even among closely related mammals. In most mammals, the shift over the course of gestation in the balance from a progesterone-dominant to an estrogen-dominant milieu to promote labor is effected by the direct conversion of progesterone to estrogen in the placenta via a mechanism regulated by the fetal HPA axis. Maturation of the fetal HPA axis results in rising concentrations of fetal cortisol, which in turn induces placental expression of the enzyme 17α-hydroxylase (P450 cytochrome system) required for the conversion of progesterone to estrogen. However, unlike most other mammals, primates cannot convert

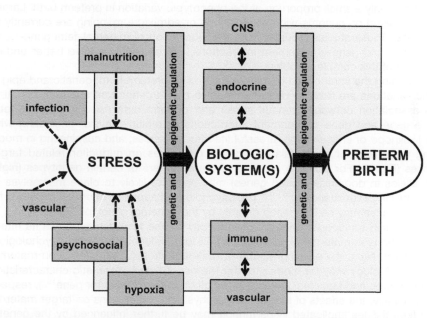

Fig. 2. Contribution of maternal stress and stress biology to preterm birth: a matter of context. No one-to-one correspondence exists between psychosocial stress and a stress-sensitive biology; the nature, magnitude, and duration of the effects of maternal psychosocial stress during pregnancy on any given stress-sensitive biologic system are likely altered by the context of other conditions/stressors, such as those related to nutrition, infection, and hypoxia. Similarly, the nature, magnitude, and duration of the effects of a given stress-sensitive biologic system in pregnancy on maternal and fetal target systems involved in parturition are likely altered by the secondary perturbations in other closely related biologic systems and their feedback effects on the primary biologic system under consideration.

progesterone to estrogen because they lack the placental enzyme 17α-hydroxylase required for this purpose. Instead, the primate placenta uses another precursor hormone, dehydroepiandrosterone sulfate, produced by the fetal adrenal zone, to synthesize estrogen (estriol[174–176]). A second major difference in the endocrinology of pregnancy is that primates are the only mammals that produce the neuropeptide CRH in the placenta.[177,178] However, even among primates, large differences exist in the pattern of production, activity, and regulation of placental CRH between New and Old World monkeys and humans. In particular, the baboon exhibits a mid-gestational peak in secretion.[179] Studies in other primates also indicate differences in production of the CRH-binding protein.[178] Great apes (chimpanzees and gorillas) are the only primates in which patterns of placental CRH production in pregnancy are similar to those seen in humans, with a clear exponential increase over the entire course of gestation.[176]

GENETIC AND EPIGENETIC CONSIDERATIONS

The ascertainment of genetic contributors to preterm birth is an area of active and intense investigation. Studies in humans of familial aggregation suggest a heritable component for preterm birth. The major component of this heritability is clearly polygenic (as opposed to of classical Mendelian origin).[1] Studies using a candidate gene approach have yielded limited success; they have been difficult to replicate and have explained only a small proportion of the phenotypic variation in preterm birth. Larger studies based on genome-wide associations or admixture mapping are currently in progress. These studies, coupled with the elucidation of maternal–fetal gene–gene (epistasis) and gene–environment interactions, will be required for a better understanding of this complex problem.[1,180–186]

Regarding the contribution of maternal stress to preterm birth, genetic and epigenetic variations are likely to be determined to play an important role in moderating the association between prenatal stress and preterm birth risk via maternal–fetal gene–gene and gene–environment interactions at multiple levels, originating with the likelihood of encountering stressful life circumstances, and culminating in modifying the effects of stress-related biologic processes on parturition-related target tissues (**Fig. 3**). For example, women who are carriers of certain genotypes (high-risk alleles in dopamine-related genes) may be more likely to place themselves in stressful life circumstances.[187–189] The psychological appraisal of potentially stressful circumstances may be influenced directly by the maternal genotypic variation (eg, in the serotonin transporter gene[190]) or indirectly by the fetal genotype (via its effect on alterations in maternal physiology that, in turn, influence maternal psychological appraisals). Next, the ensuing effects of maternal stressful experience on maternal and fetal biology may be moderated by the genetic and epigenetic characteristics of the mother and fetus (eg, variants in the glucocorticoid receptor gene[191]), respectively. Finally, the effects of stress-related physiologic alterations on target maternal and fetal tissues implicated in parturition may be further influenced by the genetic and epigenetic makeup of the mother and fetus, respectively.

To date, only a few studies have systematically addressed the issue of a genetic predisposition for susceptibility to psychosocial stress and related psychobiological states. For example, the authors and others have described that certain polymorphisms in the promoter region of the gene encoding the glucocorticoid receptor are associated with changes in the regulation of the HPA axis at different levels, including the basal level; in feedback regulation; and in response to a psychosocial stressor.[191] Because several genes that code for proteins are involved in the regulation of the stress

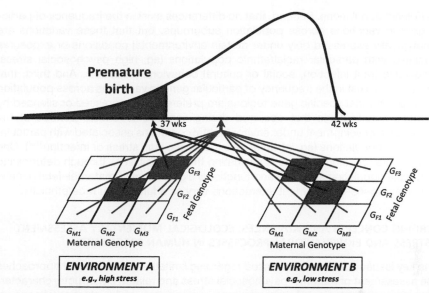

Fig. 3. Maternal–fetal gene–environment interactions in human parturition. Combinations of genes (epistasis), rather than single genes or single gene variants, likely produce effects on complex health and disease risk outcomes. For birth outcomes such as preterm birth, combinations of genes of the mother and the fetus must be considered (maternal–fetal genetic interactions). The effects of certain maternal–fetal genetic combinations may vary as a function of environmental context (eg, maternal stress level, gene–environment interactions).

response are also involved in the physiology of pregnancy and parturition (eg, CRH, cortisol, IL-6), individual differences in genetic variation may be another factor underlying susceptibility in terms of the potentially adverse effects of maternal stress on pregnancy outcomes. The participation of placental CRH as a central molecule in regulating various aspects of pregnancy, fetal development, and birth outcomes was discussed earlier. Thus, DNA sequence variations in the CRH gene, the CRH receptor genes, the glucocorticoid receptor gene, and other genes encoding key enzymes and binding proteins in their biosynthetic pathways may have important implications in this context.

Genetic and epigenetic mechanisms have been proposed to explain the observed racial/ethnic disparities in preterm birth, particularly with respect to the hypothesized contribution of prenatal stress. The observed racial/ethnic disparity in preterm birth is commonly assumed to reflect the burden of adverse societal conditions associated with minority racial/ethnic status in the United States. Prenatal stress is a plausible mediator of the effects of race/ethnicity on preterm birth via one or both of two possibilities: greater cumulative exposure to stress and greater vulnerability to the effects of stress (arising from differences in psychobiological responses to stress).

The characterization of racial/ethnic differences in DNA sequence or epigenetic variation in genes associated with the stress response will prove particularly informative in this regard. For instance, the authors and others have previously reported significant racial/ethnic differences in stress-related hormonal states in human pregnancy.[17,134] These racial/ethnic differences in neuroendocrine function in pregnancy may, in turn, reflect one or more of three possibilities. First, that particular genetic variations associated with pathophysiology are more frequent in specific racial/ethnic populations. Second, that no differences exist in the frequency of particular genetic variations across population subgroups, but that these variations are phenotypically expressed only under certain environmental conditions or exposures associated with particular racial/ethnic populations (eg, high psychosocial stress, reproductive tract infection, social or cultural behavioral practices). And third, that no differences exist in the frequency of particular genetic variations across population subgroups, but that specific gene regions are preferentially expressed or silenced by epigenetic modifications that occurred during sensitive or critical periods of the mother's own development under environmental conditions associated with particular racial/ethnic populations (eg, intrauterine exposure to high stress or infection[192]). One of the authors' ongoing projects is evaluating these possibilities through determining whether the population structure and functional significance of maternal–fetal genetic variation and gene–environment interactions vary as a function of race/ethnicity.

EMERGING CONCEPTS AND ADVANCES: ECOLOGICAL MOMENTARY ASSESSMENT OF STRESS AND BIOBEHAVIORAL PROCESSES IN HUMAN PREGNANCY

Some key issues have been discussed regarding limitations of traditional approaches in the assessment of maternal psychosocial stress and related constructs, characterization of psychobiological stress responses in pregnancy, and evaluation of context-specific effects in the link between prenatal stress, stress-related biologic processes, and preterm birth. The authors propose that recent technological and methodological advances now afford the opportunity to address many of these issues and limitations through the application of the ecological momentary assessment (EMA) approach to the study of maternal stress and stress biology in human pregnancy. EMA methods emphasize the longitudinal, repeated collection of information about respondents' momentary or current state, affect, experience, behavior, and biology in real time.[193] These methods serve to minimize biases inherent in retrospective recall approaches, because immediate reports of a respondent's current state or activity do not require retrieval from memory and other processing, and are accordingly far less subject to distortions and biases. In addition to obtaining more-accurate summary estimates over time, this methodology allows for the computation of indices of other potentially important dimensions, such as variability (lability), context-specificity, and dynamic measures of temporal linkages between psychosocial states and biological processes. EMA methods provide greater ecological validity than laboratory-based measures because they are collected in naturalistic settings as respondents go about their normal, day-to-day activities. Although individual differences in reactivity to a controlled stimulus in a laboratory setting seem to be relatively stable across tasks and time, associations between reactivity in the laboratory and in naturalistic settings have generally been only moderate,[194,195] because laboratory measures are not obtained at comparable conditions of behavior state and activity in natural, everyday settings.[196] Because aggregation and assessment at multiple time points increase the range of stimuli sampled and reduce measurement error, EMA results are more reliable, and variations in values across settings and situations can be assessed.[62,197–200] EMA techniques also require that assessments be timed to ensure they span a wide range of times and locations, therefore tapping into the respondent's full repertoire of states and behaviors. Last, repeated observations of states and responses not only allow the assessment of within-subject variation (to reliably compute measures of variability or lability of psychological and physiologic states over time) but also measure how a target variable covaries with situational antecedents.[63] The authors suggest that EMA approaches can be used to compute measures of biologic stress reactivity that reflect the degree of biologic perturbation produced by a unit change in psychological stress (using a within-subject specific criterion), after accounting for the effects of other important influences on biology, including time of day, diet, physical activity, and sleep. For example, some of the authors' recent findings suggest that EMA-derived measures of maternal psychosocial stress are better predictors of cortisol levels in pregnancy than traditional measures, and that EMA-derived measures of cortisol during pregnancy are better predictors of birth outcomes (length of gestation) than cortisol assessed in the clinical setting.[69,201] Therefore, the authors suggest that EMA-based measures of real-time, ambulatory, repeated sampling of psychological, behavioral, and biologic states during pregnancy are promising for addressing critical questions and gaining new, more-precise information about the magnitude and context-specificity of the effects of maternal psychosocial stress and biologic stress reactivity on pregnancy and birth outcomes.

A LIFE COURSE PERSPECTIVE

The authors submit it may be important to adopt a life course perspective in considering the issue of the contribution of maternal stress to preterm birth. The life course perspective conceptualizes reproductive and birth outcomes as the product of not only the 9 months of pregnancy, but of the entire life course of the mother from her own conception onward (or even before her own conception), and leading up to the index pregnancy.[202,203] The suggestion that maternal health before pregnancy may have important bearing on pregnancy outcomes is not new,[204] but a growing body of evidence is beginning to shed light on the mechanisms through which life course factors, including stress, might influence birth outcomes, such as preterm birth. Two broad mechanisms have been postulated: early programming and cumulative pathways.

The early programming model suggests that a stimulus or insult (eg, stress), operating at a critical or sensitive period, can result in a permanent or long-term change in the structure or function of the organism that becomes manifest in health and disease risk in later life.[205-207] For example, animal and human studies have shown that exposure to maternal stress during pregnancy and in early childhood can program the stress reactivity of her offspring, and that this effect persists well into adulthood.[208-210] This process may be mediated by epigenetic alterations in the glucocorticoid receptor gene in the developing brain.[211,212] Exposure to stress hormones during sensitive periods of immune maturation in early life may also influence immune programming, leading to altered immune responses in later life.[213] In a series of recent reports on a population of young adults exposed specifically during intrauterine life to high maternal psychosocial stress, the authors found that prenatal stress exposure was associated with significant dysregulation of metabolic, immune, endocrine, and cognitive function consistent with increased risk for obesity, insulin resistance and diabetes, allergy and atopic disorders, and dementia.[214-217]

Animal studies support the plausibility that these alterations may be transmitted across generations by nongenomic mechanisms.[218] Thus, hypothetically, preterm birth may result from not only maternal stress but also stress of the grandmother during her pregnancy, which may program the mother's endocrine and immune stress responses in utero; programmed stress hyperreactivity could put the mother at greater risk for preterm delivery when she herself becomes pregnant.[202]

The cumulative pathways model suggests that throughout the life course, exposures and insults gradually accumulate through episodes of illness or injury, adverse environmental conditions, and risky behaviors, leading to declines in health and function over time.[219] This risk accumulation creates wear and tear, or "allostatic load," on the body's regulatory processes that are central to the maintenance of allostasis.[220] Allostatic load refers to the cumulative physiologic toll resulting from chronic overactivity or underactivity of allostatic systems. This effect may result from overexposure to stress hormones, as often occurs in chronic and repeated stress. Overexposure to glucocorticoids can adversely impact an individual's central nervous system, immune system, and metabolism. For example, studies have found that animals and humans subjected to chronic and repeated stress exhibit elevated basal cortisol levels and dysregulated HPA response to natural or experimental stressors.[221,222] This HPA dysregulation may reflect the loss of feedback inhibition via downregulation of glucocorticoid receptors in the brain.[221] Similarly, chronically elevated levels of cortisol may also lead to not only relative immune suppression but also immune-inflammatory dysregulation from the loss of counterregulation by the HPA axis.[223] Thus, HPA and immune/inflammatory dysregulation are two of several possible pathways through which cumulative stress over the life course may lead to increased vulnerability to preterm birth as a consequence of stress or infection in pregnancy.

The life course perspective suggests that vulnerability to preterm birth may be traced not only to stress exposure during pregnancy but also to host stress responses (eg, psychobiological, autonomic, endocrine, and immune/inflammatory stress reactivity) that have been patterned by early programming and cumulative pathways mechanisms over the life course. Some evidence supports these concepts of the developmental origins of preterm birth, or of the link between allostatic load and preterm birth. Among pregnant women, a history of exposure to early life trauma or abuse has been associated with not only an increased risk of preterm birth[224] but also a higher likelihood of depression,[225] reproductive tract infection,[226] altered cortisol activity,[227] and engaging in preterm birth–related risky behaviors.[228] A recent report provides evidence among African American women of an association between preterm birth risk and a three-way interaction of lifetime experience of racism, depressive symptoms, and stress in pregnancy.[229] Another study showed that nonpregnant women with a previous history of infection-related preterm birth exhibited higher antigen-stimulated proinflammatory cytokine (TNF) levels; however, this study was unable to determine whether the proinflammatory trait preceded or followed the occurrence of a preterm birth.[230] Thus, the life course perspective suggests a need to expand the time horizon for preterm birth research, to assess precursors (including stress) at points more distant temporally than has been examined in most previous research, and to understand not only disease pathways but also predisease pathways, defined as the "early and long-term biologic, behavioral, psychological and social precursors to disease."[231] The life course perspective also suggests the need for a new prevention paradigm in preterm birth, one that emphasizes not only risk reduction during pregnancy but also health promotion and optimization of women's health before conception and over the life course. Accordingly, studies are currently underway to test the effects of preconceptional health interventions on pregnancy and birth outcomes.[232–234]

The life course perspective also offers another way to look at the issue of racial/ethnic disparities in preterm birth. The cause of these persisting racial disparities remains largely unexplained. Most extant studies have focused on differential exposures to risk and protective factors during pregnancy, such as genetic or socioeconomic differences, maternal behaviors, prenatal care use, psychosocial stress, and perinatal infections. These factors during pregnancy, however, may not adequately account for the racial gap in preterm birth. Disparities in birth outcomes (including preterm birth) may represent the consequences of not only differential exposures during pregnancy but also more important differential accumulation of protective and risk factors over the life course.[202] The life course perspective offers an explanatory model for how chronic stressors, such as lifelong experience of racism, "get under the skin" to affect the physiology of the pregnant mother and the developmental biology of the child from conception onward.[235] It provides the biologic basis for the "weathering hypothesis"—that the effects of social inequality on the health of populations may compound with age, leading to growing gaps in health status through young and middle adulthood that can eventually affect fetal health.[236]

SUMMARY

The question of the contribution of maternal stress to preterm birth is a challenging issue. Concepts in evolutionary biology and developmental plasticity support a rationale for considering a role for maternal stress in preterm birth. Evidence from population-based epidemiologic and clinical studies suggests that after accounting for the effects of other established sociodemographic, obstetric, and behavioral risk factors, women reporting higher levels of psychological stress during pregnancy are at significantly increased risk of preterm birth. However, at the individual level, the specificity and sensitivity of maternal stress as predictors of preterm birth risk are, at best, modest. To translate population-level findings to public health and clinical practice applications, it is critical to identify which subgroups of women may be particularly susceptible to the potentially detrimental effects of high prenatal stress, and under what circumstances and at which stages of gestation. Determining this will require progress on three major fronts. First, the limitations in current approaches to characterizing and assessing maternal stress must be addressed, including the problems inherent in retrospective recall measures of stress and the failure to consider the role of individual differences in maternal psychobiological stress responsivity. Second, the possibility must be considered that the effects of maternal stress may be mostly conditional or context-dependent. The authors suggest that maternal nutrition and infection are candidate processes of considerable interest in this context. Third, the biologic pathways through which maternal stress may impact human parturition must be understood better. The authors suggest that MPF neuroendocrine, immune/inflammatory, and vascular processes are attractive candidate pathways because they are responsive to stress and participate in the physiology of parturition. Multivariable conditional models will be required to elucidate the context-dependent effects of maternal stress during pregnancy on these candidate biologic systems and on their interactive effects on parturition. Studies of stress-related genetic and epigenetic processes that incorporate the maternal and fetal genomes and consider gene–gene (epistasis) and gene–environment interactions are emphasized.

The authors contend that recent technological and methodological advances now afford the opportunity to address many of these limitations through the adoption of the EMA approach to the study of maternal stress and stress biology in human pregnancy. EMA methods emphasize the longitudinal, repeated collection of information about momentary or current states, affects, experiences, behaviors, and biology in real time and in naturalistic settings. Finally, the authors espouse a life course perspective that conceptualizes reproductive and birth outcomes as the product of circumstances and events not only during gestation but also over the entire life course of the mother, beginning at the time of her own conception (or before) and leading up to the index pregnancy.

The authors note that large, national, multicenter studies are currently underway evaluating the association of genetic and environmental determinants in early development to maternal and child health outcomes, including preterm birth (eg, the U.S. National Children's Study[237] and the National Institute of Child Health and Human Development Study of Preterm Birth in Nulliparous Women), and they expect that findings from these studies will provide a better understanding of how maternal stress contributes to preterm birth.

REFERENCES

1. Muglia LJ, Katz M. The enigma of spontaneous preterm birth. N Engl J Med 2010;362(6):529–35.
2. Beydoun H, Saftlas AF. Physical and mental health outcomes of prenatal maternal stress in human and animal studies: a review of recent evidence. Paediatr Perinat Epidemiol 2008;22(5):438–66.
3. Chambliss LR. Intimate partner violence and its implication for pregnancy. Clin Obstet Gynecol 2008;51(2):385–97.
4. Dunkel Schetter C. Psychological science on pregnancy: stress processes, biopsychosocial models, and emerging research issues. Annu Rev Psychol 2011; 62:531–58.
5. Hodnett ED, Fredericks S, Weston J. Support during pregnancy for women at increased risk of low birthweight babies. Cochrane Database Syst Rev 2010; 6:CD000198.
6. Paarlberg KM, Vingerhoets AJ, Passchier J, et al. Psychosocial factors and pregnancy outcome: a review with emphasis on methodological issues. J Psychosom Res 1995;39(5):563–95.
7. Shah PS, Zao J, Ali S. Maternal marital status and birth outcomes: a systematic review and meta-analyses. Matern Child Health J 2010. [Epub ahead of print].
8. Hobel CJ, Goldstein A, Barrett ES. Psychosocial stress and pregnancy outcome. Clin Obstet Gynecol 2008;51(2):333–48.
9. Alder J, Fink N, Bitzer J, et al. Depression and anxiety during pregnancy: a risk factor for obstetric, fetal and neonatal outcome? A critical review of the literature. J Matern Fetal Neonatal Med 2007;20(3):189–209.
10. Entringer S, Buss C, Wadhwa PD. Prenatal stress and developmental programming of human health and disease risk: concepts and integration of empirical findings. Curr Opin Endocrinol Diabetes Obes 2010;17(6):507–16.
11. Pike IL. Maternal stress and fetal responses: evolutionary perspectives on preterm delivery. Am J Human Biol 2005;17(1):55–65.
12. Wadhwa PD. Psychoneuroendocrine processes in human pregnancy influence fetal development and health. Psychoneuroendocrinology 2005;30(8):724–43.
13. Giscombe CL, Lobel M. Explaining disproportionately high rates of adverse birth outcomes among African Americans: the impact of stress, racism, and related factors in pregnancy. Psychol Bull 2005;131(5):662–83.
14. McGrady GA, Sung JF, Rowley DL, et al. Preterm delivery and low birth weight among first-born infants of black and white college graduates. Am J Epidemiol 1992;136(3):266–76.
15. Schoendorf KC, Hogue CJ, Kleinman JC, et al. Mortality among infants of black as compared with white college-educated parents. N Engl J Med 1992;326(23): 1522–6.
16. Ventura SJ, Martin JA, Curtin SC, et al. Births: final data for 1998. Natl Vital Stat Rep 2000;48(3):1–100.
17. Wadhwa PD, Culhane JF, Rauh V, et al. Stress, infection and preterm birth: a biobehavioural perspective. Paediatr Perinat Epidemiol 2001;15(Suppl 2):17–29.

18. Institute of Medicine. Committee on understanding premature birth and assuring healthy outcomes, board on health sciences policy. Preterm birth: causes, consequences, and prevention. Washington, DC: The National Academies Press; 2007.
19. Adler NE, Rehkopf DH. U.S. disparities in health: descriptions, causes, and mechanisms. Annu Rev Public Health 2008;29:235–52.
20. Shah PS, Shah J. Maternal exposure to domestic violence and pregnancy and birth outcomes: a systematic review and meta-analyses. J Womens Health (Larchmt) 2010;19(11):2017–31.
21. ACOG. ACOG committee opinion no. 343: psychosocial risk factors: perinatal screening and intervention. Obstet Gynecol 2006;108(2):469–77.
22. Lynch CD, Zhang J. The research implications of the selection of a gestational age estimation method. Paediatr Perinat Epidemiol 2007;21(Suppl 2):86–96.
23. Tita AT, Landon MB, Spong CY, et al. Timing of elective repeat cesarean delivery at term and neonatal outcomes. N Engl J Med 2009;360(2):111–20.
24. Zhang X, Kramer MS. Variations in mortality and morbidity by gestational age among infants born at term. J Pediatr 2008;154(3):358–62.
25. Hill AB. The environment and disease: association or causation? Proc R Soc Med 1965;58:295–300.
26. Hoefler M. The Bradford Hill considerations on causality: a counterfactual perspective. Emer Themes Epidemiol 2005;2:11.
27. Phillips CV, Goodman KJ. The missed lessons of Sir Austin Bradford Hill. Epidemiol Perspect Innov 2004;1(1):3.
28. Ward AC. The role of causal criteria in causal inferences: Bradford Hill's "aspects of association". Epidemiol Perspect Innov 2009;6:2.
29. Lazarus RS, Folkman S. Stress, appraisal, and coping. New York: Springer; 1984.
30. Zhu P, Tao F, Hao J, et al. Prenatal life events stress: implications for preterm birth and infant birthweight. Am J Obstet Gynecol 2010;203(1):34.e1–8.
31. Khashan AS, McNamee R, Abel KM, et al. Rates of preterm birth following antenatal maternal exposure to severe life events: a population-based cohort study. Hum Reprod 2009;24(2):429–37.
32. Xiong X, Harville EW, Mattison DR, et al. Exposure to Hurricane Katrina, posttraumatic stress disorder and birth outcomes. Am J Med Sci 2008;336(2):111–5.
33. Kramer MS, Lydon J, Seguin L, et al. Stress pathways to spontaneous preterm birth: the role of stressors, psychological distress, and stress hormones. Am J Epidemiol 2009;169(11):1319–26.
34. Roesch SC, Dunkel-Schetter C, Woo G, et al. Modeling the types and timing of stress in pregnancy. Anxiety Stress Coping 2004;17:87–102.
35. Wadhwa PD, Sandman CA, Porto M, et al. The association between prenatal stress and infant birth weight and gestational age at birth: a prospective investigation. Am J Obstet Gynecol 1993;169(4):858–65.
36. Lobel M, Cannella DL, Graham JE, et al. Pregnancy-specific stress, prenatal health behaviors, and birth outcomes. Health Psychol 2008;27(5):604–15.
37. Dole N, Savitz DA, Hertz-Picciotto I, et al. Maternal stress and preterm birth. Am J Epidemiol 2003;157(1):14–24.
38. Collins NL, Dunkel-Schetter C, Lobel M, et al. Social support in pregnancy: psychosocial correlates of birth outcomes and postpartum depression. J Pers Soc Psychol 1993;65(6):1243–58.
39. Curry MA, Burton D, Fields J. The prenatal psychosocial profile: a research and clinical tool. Res Nurs Health 1998;21(3):211–9.

40. DiPietro JA, Christensen AL, Costigan KA. The pregnancy experience scale-brief version. J Psychosom Obstet Gynaecol 2008;29(4):262–7.
41. DiPietro JA, Ghera MM, Costigan K, et al. Measuring the ups and downs of pregnancy stress. J Psychosom Obstet Gynaecol 2004;25(3/4):189–201.
42. Huizink AC, Mulder EJ, Robles de Medina PG, et al. Is pregnancy anxiety a distinctive syndrome? Early Hum Dev 2004;79(2):81–91.
43. Rini CK, Dunkel-Schetter C, Wadhwa PD, et al. Psychological adaptation and birth outcomes: the role of personal resources, stress, and sociocultural context in pregnancy. Health Psychol 1999;18(4):333–45.
44. Sable MR, Wilkinson DS. Impact of perceived stress, major life events and pregnancy attitudes on low birth weight. Fam Plann Perspect 2000;32(6):288–94.
45. Speizer IS, Santelli JS, Afable-Munsuz A, et al. Measuring factors underlying intendedness of women's first and later pregnancies. Perspect Sex Reprod Health 2004;36(5):198–205.
46. Yali AM, Lobel M. Coping and distress in pregnancy: an investigation of medically high risk women. J Psychosom Obstet Gynaecol 1999;20(1):39–52.
47. Zambrana RE, Dunkel-Schetter C, Collins NL, et al. Mediators of ethnic-associated differences in infant birth weight. J Urban Health 1999;76(1):102–16.
48. Alderdice F, Lynn F. Factor structure of the Prenatal distress questionnaire. Midwifery 2010. [Epub ahead of print].
49. Dipietro JA, Novak MF, Costigan KA, et al. Maternal psychological distress during pregnancy in relation to child development at age two. Child Dev 2006;77(3):573–87.
50. Weiss JM. Somatic effects of predictable and unpredictable shock. Psychosom Med 1970;32(4):397–408.
51. Weiss JM. Effects of coping behavior in different warning signal conditions on stress pathology in rats. J Comp Physiol Psychol 1971;77(1):1–13.
52. Sapolsky R. Why zebras don't get ulcers: a guide to stress, stress-related diseases, and coping. New York: W.H. Freeman & Co; 1994. p. 1–19, 283–5.
53. Koolhaas JM, de Boer SF, Buwalda B, et al. Individual variation in coping with stress: a multidimensional approach of ultimate and proximate mechanisms. Brain Behav Evol 2007;70(4):218–26.
54. Lipkind HS, Curry AE, Huynh M, et al. Birth outcomes among offspring of women exposed to the September 11, 2001, terrorist attacks. Obstet Gynecol 2010; 116(4):917–25.
55. Kramer MR, Hogue CR. What causes racial disparities in very preterm birth? A biosocial perspective. Epidemiol Rev 2009;31:84–98.
56. Dominguez TP. Race, racism, and racial disparities in adverse birth outcomes. Clin Obstet Gynecol 2008;51(2):360–70.
57. Collins JW Jr, David RJ. Urban violence and African-American pregnancy outcome: an ecologic study. Ethn Dis 1997;7(3):184–90.
58. O'Campo P, Burke JG, Culhane J, et al. Neighborhood deprivation and preterm birth among non-Hispanic Black and White women in eight geographic areas in the United States. Am J Epidemiol 2008;167(2):155–63.
59. Culhane JF, Elo IT. Neighborhood context and reproductive health. Am J Obstet Gynecol 2005;192(5 Suppl):S22–9.
60. Davis EP, Sandman CA. The timing of prenatal exposure to maternal cortisol and psychosocial stress is associated with human infant cognitive development. Child Dev 2010;81(1):131–48.
61. Gorin AA, Stone AA. Recall biases and cognitive errors in retrospective self-reports: a call for momentary assessments. In: Baum A, Revenson T, Singer J,

editors. Handbook of health psychology. Mahwah (NJ): Lawrence Erlbaum; 2001. p. 405–13.

62. Shiffman S, Stone AA, Hufford MR. Ecological momentary assessment. Annu Rev Clin Psychol 2008;4:1–32.

63. Barnett PA, Spence JD, Manuck SB, et al. Psychological stress and the progression of carotid artery disease. J Hypertens 1997;15(1):49–55.

64. al'Absi M, Bongard S. Neuroendocrine and behavioral mechanisms mediating the relationship between anger expression and cardiovascular risk: assessment considerations and improvements. J Behav Med 2006;29(6):573–91.

65. Kirschbaum C, Pirke KM, Hellhammer DH. The 'Trier Social Stress Test'—a tool for investigating psychobiological stress responses in a laboratory setting. Neuropsychobiology 1993;28(1–2):76–81.

66. Entringer S, Buss C, Shirtcliff EA, et al. Attenuation of maternal psychophysiological stress responses and the maternal cortisol awakening response over the course of human pregnancy. Stress 2010;13(3):258–68.

67. McCubbin JA, Lawson EJ, Cox S, et al. Prenatal maternal blood pressure response to stress predicts birth weight and gestational age: a preliminary study. Am J Obstet Gynecol 1996;175(3 Pt 1):706–12.

68. de Weerth C, Buitelaar JK. Physiological stress reactivity in human pregnancy–a review. Neurosci Biobehav Rev 2005;29(2):295–312.

69. Buss C, Entringer S, Reyes JF, et al. The maternal cortisol awakening response in human pregnancy is associated with the length of gestation. Am J Obstet Gynecol 2009;201(4):398, e1–8.

70. Brunton PJ. Resetting the dynamic range of hypothalamic-pituitary-adrenal axis stress responses through pregnancy. J Neuroendocrinol 2010;22(11):1198–213.

71. Douglas AJ. Baby on board: do responses to stress in the maternal brain mediate adverse pregnancy outcome? Front Neuroendocrinol 2010;31(3):359–76.

72. Schulte HM, Weisner D, Allolio B. The corticotrophin releasing hormone test in late pregnancy: lack of adrenocorticotrophin and cortisol response. Clin Endocrinol (Oxf) 1990;33(1):99–106.

73. Sasaki A, Shinkawa O, Yoshinaga K. Placental corticotropin-releasing hormone may be a stimulator of maternal pituitary adrenocorticotropic hormone secretion in humans. J Clin Invest 1989;84(6):1997–2001.

74. Odagiri E, Ishiwatari N, Abe Y, et al. Hypercortisolism and the resistance to dexamethasone suppression during gestation. Endocrinol Jpn 1988;35(5):685–90.

75. Ekholm EM, Erkkola RU. Autonomic cardiovascular control in pregnancy. Eur J Obstet Gynecol Reprod Biol 1996;64(1):29–36.

76. de Weerth C, Buitelaar JK. Cortisol awakening response in pregnant women. Psychoneuroendocrinology 2005;30(9):902–7.

77. Wolfe LA, Weissgerber TL. Clinical physiology of exercise in pregnancy: a literature review. J Obstet Gynaecol Can 2003;25(6):473–83.

78. Glynn LM, Wadhwa PD, Dunkel-Schetter C, et al. When stress happens matters: effects of earthquake timing on stress responsivity in pregnancy. Am J Obstet Gynecol 2001;184(4):637–42.

79. Glynn LM, Schetter CD, Wadhwa PD, et al. Pregnancy affects appraisal of negative life events. J Psychosom Res 2004;56(1):47–52.

80. Glynn LM, Schetter CD, Hobel CJ, et al. Pattern of perceived stress and anxiety in pregnancy predicts preterm birth. Health Psychol 2008;27(1):43–51.

81. Clayton DG. Prediction and interaction in complex disease genetics: experience in type 1 diabetes. PLoS Genet 2009;5(7):e1000540.

82. Hunter DJ. Gene-environment interactions in human diseases. Nat Rev Genet 2005;6(4):287–98.
83. Goldenberg RL, Culhane JF, Iams JD, et al. Epidemiology and causes of preterm birth. Lancet 2008;371(9606):75–84.
84. Torloni MR, Betran AP, Daher S, et al. Maternal BMI and preterm birth: a systematic review of the literature with meta-analysis. J Matern Fetal Neonatal Med 2009;22(11):957–70.
85. Bloomfield FH, Oliver MH, Hawkins P, et al. Periconceptional undernutrition in sheep accelerates maturation of the fetal hypothalamic-pituitary-adrenal axis in late gestation. Endocrinology 2004;145(9):4278–85.
86. Chadio SE, Kotsampasi B, Papadomichelakis G, et al. Impact of maternal undernutrition on the hypothalamic-pituitary-adrenal axis responsiveness in sheep at different ages postnatal. J Endocrinol 2007;192(3):495–503.
87. Bispham J, Gopalakrishnan GS, Dandrea J, et al. Maternal endocrine adaptation throughout pregnancy to nutritional manipulation: consequences for maternal plasma leptin and cortisol and the programming of fetal adipose tissue development. Endocrinology 2003;144(8):3575–85.
88. Ford SP, Zhang L, Zhu M, et al. Maternal obesity accelerates fetal pancreatic beta-cell but not alpha-cell development in sheep: prenatal consequences. Am J Physiol Regul Integr Comp Physiol 2009;297(3):R835–43.
89. Lingas R, Dean F, Matthews SG. Maternal nutrient restriction (48 h) modifies brain corticosteroid receptor expression and endocrine function in the fetal guinea pig. Brain Res 1999;846(2):236–42.
90. Dwyer CM, Stickland NC. The effects of maternal undernutrition on maternal and fetal serum insulin-like growth factors, thyroid hormones and cortisol in the guinea pig. J Dev Physiol 1992;18(6):303–13.
91. Shen Q, Li ZQ, Sun Y, et al. The role of pro-inflammatory factors in mediating the effects on the fetus of prenatal undernutrition: implications for schizophrenia. Schizophr Res 2008;99(1–3):48–55.
92. Tamashiro KL, Terrillion CE, Hyun J, et al. Prenatal stress or high-fat diet increases susceptibility to diet-induced obesity in rat offspring. Diabetes 2009;58(5):1116–25.
93. Gonzalez-Bono E, Rohleder N, Hellhammer DH, et al. Glucose but not protein or fat load amplifies the cortisol response to psychosocial stress. Horm Behav 2002;41(3):328–33.
94. Epel E, Lapidus R, McEwen B, et al. Stress may add bite to appetite in women: a laboratory study of stress-induced cortisol and eating behavior. Psychoneuroendocrinology 2001;26(1):37–49.
95. Hitze B, Hubold C, van Dyken R, et al. How the selfish brain organizes its supply and demand. Front Neuroenergetics 2010;2:7.
96. George SA, Khan S, Briggs H, et al. CRH-stimulated cortisol release and food intake in healthy, non-obese adults. Psychoneuroendocrinology 2010;35(4):607–12.
97. Tataranni PA, Larson DE, Snitker S, et al. Effects of glucocorticoids on energy metabolism and food intake in humans. Am J Physiol 1996;271(2 Pt 1):E317–25.
98. la Fleur SE, Akana SF, Manalo SL. Interaction between corticosterone and insulin in obesity: regulation of lard intake and fat stores. Endocrinology 2004;145(5):2174–85.
99. Hurley KM, Caulfield LE, Sacco LM, et al. Psychosocial influences in dietary patterns during pregnancy. J Am Diet Assoc 2005;105(6):963–6.

100. Han YS, Ha EH, Park HS, et al. Relationships between pregnancy outcomes, biochemical markers and pre-pregnancy body mass index. Int J Obes (Lond) 2011;35(4):570–7.

101. Romero R, Gotsch F, Pineles B, et al. Inflammation in pregnancy: its roles in reproductive physiology, obstetrical complications, and fetal injury. Nutr Rev 2007;65(12 Pt 2):S194–202.

102. Culhane JF, Rauh V, McCollum KF, et al. Exposure to chronic stress and ethnic differences in rates of bacterial vaginosis among pregnant women. Am J Obstet Gynecol 2002;187(5):1272–6.

103. Culhane JF, Rauh V, McCollum KF, et al. Maternal stress is associated with bacterial vaginosis in human pregnancy. Matern Child Health J 2001;5(2):127–34.

104. Agelaki S, Tsatsanis C, Gravanis A, et al. Corticotropin-releasing hormone augments proinflammatory cytokine production from macrophages in vitro and in lipopolysaccharide-induced endotoxin shock in mice. Infect Immun 2002;70(11):6068–74.

105. Kristenson M, Eriksen HR, Sluiter JK, et al. Psychobiological mechanisms of socioeconomic differences in health. Soc Sci Med 2004;58(8):1511–22.

106. McEwen BS. Central effects of stress hormones in health and disease: understanding the protective and damaging effects of stress and stress mediators. Eur J Pharmacol 2008;583(2/3):174–85.

107. Schneiderman N, Ironson G, Siegel SD. Stress and health: psychological, behavioral, and biological determinants. Annu Rev Clin Psychol 2005;1:607–28.

108. Weisman CS, Hillemeier MM, Chase GA, et al. Preconceptional health: risks of adverse pregnancy outcomes by reproductive life stage in the Central Pennsylvania Women's Health Study (CePAWHS). Womens Health Issues 2006;16(4): 216–24.

109. Petraglia F, Imperatore A, Challis JR. Neuroendocrine mechanisms in pregnancy and parturition. Endocr Rev 2010;31(6):783–816.

110. Romero R, Espinoza J, Kusanovic JP, et al. The preterm parturition syndrome. BJOG 2006;113(Suppl 3):17–42.

111. Smith R. Parturition. N Engl J Med 2007;356(3):271–83.

112. Kalantaridou SN, Zoumakis E, Makrigiannakis A, et al. Corticotropin-releasing hormone, stress and human reproduction: an update. J Reprod Immunol 2010;85(1):33–9.

113. Liu JH, Rebar RW. Endocrinology of pregnancy. In: Creasy RK, Resnick HS, editors. Maternal-Fetal Medicine: principles and practice. Philadelphia: W. B. Saunders Company; 1999. p. 379–91.

114. Harris A, Seckl J. Glucocorticoids, prenatal stress and the programming of disease. Horm Behav 2011;59(3):279–89.

115. Cheng YH, Nicholson RC, King B, et al. Corticotropin-releasing hormone gene expression in primary placental cells is modulated by cyclic adenosine 3',5'-monophosphate. J Clin Endocrinol Metab 2000;85(3):1239–44.

116. Lowry PJ. Corticotropin-releasing factor and its binding protein in human plasma. Ciba Found Symp 1993;172:108–15 [discussion: 115–28].

117. Weetman AP. Immunity, thyroid function and pregnancy: molecular mechanisms. Nat Rev Endocrinol 2010;6(6):311–8.

118. Denney JM, Nelson EL, Wadhwa PD, et al. Longitudinal modulation of immune system cytokine profile during pregnancy. Cytokine 2011;53(2):170–7.

119. Abbas AE, Brodie B, Dixon S, et al. Incidence and prognostic impact of gastrointestinal bleeding after percutaneous coronary intervention for acute myocardial infarction. Am J Cardiol 2005;96(2):173–6.

120. Romero R, Gomez R, Ghezzi F, et al. A fetal systemic inflammatory response is followed by the spontaneous onset of preterm parturition. Am J Obstet Gynecol 1998;179(1):186–93.

121. Athayde N, Edwin SS, Romero R, et al. A role for matrix metalloproteinase-9 in spontaneous rupture of the fetal membranes. Am J Obstet Gynecol 1998; 179(5):1248–53.

122. Yoon BH, Romero R, Jun JK, et al. An increase in fetal plasma cortisol but not dehydroepiandrosterone sulfate is followed by the onset of preterm labor in patients with preterm premature rupture of the membranes. Am J Obstet Gynecol 1998;179(5):1107–14.

123. Yoon BH, Romero R, Park JS, et al. Microbial invasion of the amniotic cavity with Ureaplasma urealyticum is associated with a robust host response in fetal, amniotic, and maternal compartments. Am J Obstet Gynecol 1998;179(5):1254–60.

124. Chrousos GP. Stressors, stress, and neuroendocrine integration of the adaptive response. The 1997 Hans Selye Memorial Lecture. Ann N Y Acad Sci 1998;851: 311–35.

125. Haddad JJ, Saade NE, Safieh-Garabedian B. Cytokines and neuro-immune-endocrine interactions: a role for the hypothalamic-pituitary-adrenal revolving axis. J Neuroimmunol 2002;133(1/2):1–19.

126. McEwen BS, Biron CA, Brunson KW, et al. The role of adrenocorticoids as modulators of immune function in health and disease: neural, endocrine and immune interactions. Brain Res Brain Res Rev 1997;23(1/2):79–133.

127. Tsigos C, Chrousos GP. Hypothalamic-pituitary-adrenal axis, neuroendocrine factors and stress. J Psychosom Res 2002;53(4):865–71.

128. Clifton VL, Wallace EM, Smith R. Short-term effects of glucocorticoids in the human fetal-placental circulation in vitro. J Clin Endocrinol Metab 2002;87(6): 2838–42.

129. Chrousos GP, Gold PW. The concepts of stress and stress system disorders. Overview of physical and behavioral homeostasis. JAMA 1992;267(9):1244–52.

130. Elenkov IJ, Chrousos GP. Stress hormones, Th1/Th2 patterns, pro/anti-inflammatory cytokines and susceptibility to disease. Trends Endocrinol Metab 1999;10(9):359–68.

131. Smith R, Mesiano S, McGrath S. Hormone trajectories leading to human birth. Regul Pept 2002;108(2/3):159–64.

132. McLean M, Bisits A, Davies J, et al. A placental clock controlling the length of human pregnancy. Nat Med 1995;1(5):460–3.

133. Holzman C, Jetton J, Siler-Khodr T, et al. Second trimester corticotropin-releasing hormone levels in relation to preterm delivery and ethnicity. Obstet Gynecol 2001;97(5 Pt 1):657–63.

134. Glynn LM, Schetter CD, Chicz-DeMet A, et al. Ethnic differences in adrenocorticotropic hormone, cortisol and corticotropin-releasing hormone during pregnancy. Peptides 2007;28(6):1155–61.

135. Shimmin LC, Natarajan S, Ibarguen H, et al. Corticotropin releasing hormone (CRH) gene variation: comprehensive resequencing for variant and molecular haplotype discovery in monosomic hybrid cell lines. DNA Seq 2007;18(6):434–44.

136. Hobel CJ, Dunkel-Schetter C, Roesch SC, et al. Maternal plasma corticotropin-releasing hormone associated with stress at 20 weeks' gestation in pregnancies ending in preterm delivery. Am J Obstet Gynecol 1999;180(1 Pt 3):S257–63.

137. Erickson K, Thorsen P, Chrousos G, et al. Preterm birth: associated neuroendocrine, medical, and behavioral risk factors. J Clin Endocrinol Metab 2001;86(6): 2544–52.

138. Wadhwa PD, Glynn L, Hobel CJ, et al. Behavioral perinatology: biobehavioral processes in human fetal development. Regul Pept 2002;108(2/3):149–57.
139. Petraglia F, Calza L, Garuti GC, et al. New aspects of placental endocrinology. J Endocrinol Invest 1990;13(4):353–71.
140. Petraglia F, Sawchenko PE, Rivier J, et al. Evidence for local stimulation of ACTH secretion by corticotropin-releasing factor in human placenta. Nature 1987; 328(6132):717–9.
141. Petraglia F, Sutton S, Vale W. Neurotransmitters and peptides modulate the release of immunoreactive corticotropin-releasing factor from cultured human placental cells. Am J Obstet Gynecol 1989;160(1):247–51.
142. Chan EC, Smith R, Lewin T, et al. Plasma corticotropin-releasing hormone, beta-endorphin and cortisol inter-relationships during human pregnancy. Acta Endocrinol (Copenh) 1993;128(4):339–44.
143. Goland RS, Conwell IM, Warren WB, et al. Placental corticotropin-releasing hormone and pituitary-adrenal function during pregnancy. Neuroendocrinology 1992;56(5):742–9.
144. Wadhwa PD, Sandman CA, Chicz-DeMet A, et al. Placental CRH modulates maternal pituitary adrenal function in human pregnancy. Ann N Y Acad Sci 1997;814:276–81.
145. Wadhwa PD, Dunkel-Schetter C, Chicz-DeMet A, et al. Prenatal psychosocial factors and the neuroendocrine axis in human pregnancy. Psychosom Med 1996;58(5):432–46.
146. Valladares E, Pena R, Ellsberg M, et al. Neuroendocrine response to violence during pregnancy—impact on duration of pregnancy and fetal growth. Acta Obstet Gynecol Scand 2009;88(7):818–23.
147. Kivlighan KT, DiPietro JA, Costigan KA, et al. Diurnal rhythm of cortisol during late pregnancy: associations with maternal psychological well-being and fetal growth. Psychoneuroendocrinology 2008;33(9):1225–35.
148. Evans LM, Myers MM, Monk C. Pregnant women's cortisol is elevated with anxiety and depression - but only when comorbid. Arch Womens Ment Health 2008;11(3):239–48.
149. Latendresse G, Ruiz RJ. Maternal coping style and perceived adequacy of income predict CRH levels at 14–20 weeks of gestation. Biol Res Nurs 2010; 12(2):125–36.
150. Petraglia F, Hatch MC, Lapinski R, et al. Lack of effect of psychosocial stress on maternal corticotropin-releasing factor and catecholamine levels at 28 weeks' gestation. J Soc Gynecol Investig 2001;8(2):83–8.
151. Harville EW, Savitz DA, Dole N, et al. Stress questionnaires and stress biomarkers during pregnancy. J Womens Health (Larchmt) 2009;18(9):1425–33.
152. Guendelman S, Kosa JL, Pearl M, et al. Exploring the relationship of second-trimester corticotropin releasing hormone, chronic stress and preterm delivery. J Matern Fetal Neonatal Med 2008;21(11):788–95.
153. Sandman CA, Glynn L, Schetter CD, et al. Elevated maternal cortisol early in pregnancy predicts third trimester levels of placental corticotropin releasing hormone (CRH): priming the placental clock. Peptides 2006; 27(6):1457–63.
154. Kalra S, Einarson A, Karaskov T, et al. The relationship between stress and hair cortisol in healthy pregnant women. Clin Invest Med 2007;30(2):E103–7.
155. Coussons-Read ME, Okun ML, Schmitt MP, et al. Prenatal stress alters cytokine levels in a manner that may endanger human pregnancy. Psychosom Med 2005;67(4):625–31.

156. Christian LM, Franco A, Glaser R, et al. Depressive symptoms are associated with elevated serum proinflammatory cytokines among pregnant women. Brain Behav Immun 2009;23(6):750–4.
157. Paul K, Boutain D, Agnew K, et al. The relationship between racial identity, income, stress and C-reactive protein among parous women: implications for preterm birth disparity research. J Natl Med Assoc 2008;100(5):540–6.
158. Coussons-Read ME, Okun ML, Nettles CD. Psychosocial stress increases inflammatory markers and alters cytokine production across pregnancy. Brain Behav Immun 2007;21(3):343–50.
159. Klonoff-Cohen HS, Cross JL, Pieper CF. Job stress and preeclampsia. Epidemiology 1996;7(3):245–9.
160. Marcoux S, Berube S, Brisson C, et al. Job strain and pregnancy-induced hypertension. Epidemiology 1999;10(4):376–82.
161. Landsbergis PA, Hatch MC. Psychosocial work stress and pregnancy-induced hypertension. Epidemiology 1996;7(4):346–51.
162. Wergeland E, Strand K. Working conditions and prevalence of pre-eclampsia, Norway 1989. Int J Gynaecol Obstet 1997;58(2):189–96.
163. Qiu C, Williams MA, Calderon-Margalit R, et al. Preeclampsia risk in relation to maternal mood and anxiety disorders diagnosed before or during early pregnancy. Am J Hypertens 2009;22(4):397–402.
164. Leeners B, Neumaier-Wagner P, Kuse S, et al. Emotional stress and the risk to develop hypertensive diseases in pregnancy. Hypertens Pregnancy 2007; 26(2):211–26.
165. Chang Q, Natelson BH, Ottenweller JE, et al. Stress triggers different pathophysiological mechanisms in younger and older cardiomyopathic hamsters. Cardiovasc Res 1995;30(6):985–91.
166. Vythilingum B, Geerts L, Fincham D, et al. Association between antenatal distress and uterine artery pulsatility index. Arch Womens Ment Health 2010; 13(4):359–64.
167. Huneke B, Ude C. Uteroplacental and fetal arterial Ultrasound Doppler Flow Velocity measurements in unselected pregnancies as a screening test at 32 to 34 gestational weeks. Z Geburtshilfe Neonatol 2002;206(2):57–64 [in German].
168. Sjostrom K, Valentin L, Thelin T, et al. Maternal anxiety in late pregnancy: effect on fetal movements and fetal heart rate. Early Hum Dev 2002;67(1–2): 87–100.
169. Teixeira JM, Fisk NM, Glover V. Association between maternal anxiety in pregnancy and increased uterine artery resistance index: cohort based study. BMJ 1999;318(7177):153–7.
170. Jeske W, Soszynski P, Lukaszewicz E, et al. Enhancement of plasma corticotropin-releasing hormone in pregnancy-induced hypertension. Acta Endocrinol (Copenh) 1990;122(6):711–4.
171. Perkins AV, Linton EA, Eben F, et al. Corticotrophin-releasing hormone and corticotrophin-releasing hormone binding protein in normal and pre-eclamptic human pregnancies. Br J Obstet Gynaecol 1995;102(2):118–22.
172. Warren WB, Gurewitsch ED, Goland RS. Corticotropin-releasing hormone and pituitary-adrenal hormones in pregnancies complicated by chronic hypertension. Am J Obstet Gynecol 1995;172(2 Pt 1):661–6.
173. Harville EW, Savitz DA, Dole N, et al. Stress and placental resistance measured by Doppler ultrasound in early and mid-pregnancy. Ultrasound Obstet Gynecol 2008;32(1):23–30.

174. Jaffe RB. Role of human fetal adrenal gland in the initiation of parturition. In: Smith R, editor. The endocrinology of parturition. Newcastle (Australia): Karger; 2001. p. 75–85.

175. Mesiano S. Roles of estrogen and progesterone in human parturition. In: Smith R, editor. The endocrinology of parturition. Newcastle (Australia): Karger; 2001. p. 86–104.

176. Smith R. The timing of birth. Sci Am 1999;280(3):68–75.

177. Robinson BG, Emanuel RL, Frim DM, et al. Glucocorticoid stimulates expression of corticotropin-releasing hormone gene in human placenta. Proc Natl Acad Sci U S A 1988;85(14):5244–8.

178. Bowman ME, Lopata A, Jaffe RB, et al. Corticotropin-releasing hormone-binding protein in primates. Am J Primatol 2001;53(3):123–30.

179. Smith R, Chan EC, Bowman ME, et al. Corticotropin-releasing hormone in baboon pregnancy. J Clin Endocrinol Metab 1993;76(4):1063–8.

180. Chaudhari BP, Plunkett J, Ratajczak CK, et al. The genetics of birth timing: insights into a fundamental component of human development. Clin Genet 2008;74(6):493–501.

181. Himes KP, Simhan HN. Genetic susceptibility to infection-mediated preterm birth. Infect Dis Clin North Am 2008;22(4):741–53, vii.

182. Anum EA, Springel EH, Shriver MD, et al. Genetic contributions to disparities in preterm birth. Pediatr Res 2009;65(1):1–9.

183. Plunkett J, Muglia LJ. Genetic contributions to preterm birth: implications from epidemiological and genetic association studies. Ann Med 2008;40(3):167–95.

184. Pennell CE, Jacobsson B, Williams SM, et al. Genetic epidemiologic studies of preterm birth: guidelines for research. Am J Obstet Gynecol 2007;196(2):107–18.

185. Crider KS, Whitehead N, Buus RM. Genetic variation associated with preterm birth: a HuGE review. Genet Med 2005;7(9):593–604.

186. Menon R, Fortunato SJ, Thorsen P, et al. Genetic associations in preterm birth: a primer of marker selection, study design, and data analysis. J Soc Gynecol Investig 2006;13(8):531–41.

187. Derringer J, Krueger RF, Dick DM, et al. Predicting sensation seeking from dopamine genes. A candidate-system approach. Psychol Sci 2010;21(9): 1282–90.

188. Hamidovic A, Dlugos A, Skol A, et al. Evaluation of genetic variability in the dopamine receptor D2 in relation to behavioral inhibition and impulsivity/sensation seeking: an exploratory study with d-amphetamine in healthy participants. Exp Clin Psychopharmacol 2009;17(6):374–83.

189. Adriani W, Boyer F, Gioiosa L, et al. Increased impulsive behavior and risk proneness following lentivirus-mediated dopamine transporter over-expression in rats' nucleus accumbens. Neuroscience 2009;159(1):47–58.

190. Szily E, Bowen J, Unoka Z, et al. Emotion appraisal is modulated by the genetic polymorphism of the serotonin transporter. J Neural Transm 2008;115(6): 819–22.

191. Derijk RH, de Kloet ER. Corticosteroid receptor polymorphisms: determinants of vulnerability and resilience. Eur J Pharmacol 2008;583(2/3):303–11.

192. Burris HH, Collins JW Jr. Race and preterm birth–the case for epigenetic inquiry. Ethn Dis 2010;20(3):296–9.

193. Stone AA, Shiffman S. Ecological momentary assessment (EMA) in behavioral medicine. Ann Behav Med 1994;16:199–202.

194. Walker SP, Permezel M, Brennecke SP, et al. Blood pressure in late pregnancy and work outside the home. Obstet Gynecol 2001;97(3):361–5.

195. Kamarck TW, Muldoon MF, Shiffman S, et al. Experiences of demand and control in daily life as correlates of subclinical carotid atherosclerosis in a healthy older sample. Health Psychol 2004;23(1):24–32.

196. van Doornen LJ, van Blokland RW. The relationship between cardiovascular and catecholamine reactions to laboratory and real-life stress. Psychophysiology 1992;29(2):173–81.

197. Kamarck TW, Debski TT, Manuck SB. Enhancing the laboratory-to-life generalizability of cardiovascular reactivity using multiple occasions of measurement. Psychophysiology 2000;37(4):533–42.

198. Kamarck TW, Muldoon MF, Shiffman SS, et al. Experiences of demand and control during daily life are predictors of carotid atherosclerotic progression among healthy men. Health Psychol 2007;26(3):324–32.

199. Schwartz JE, Warren K, Pickering TG. Mood, location and physical position as predictors of ambulatory blood pressure and heart rate: application of a multi-level random effects model. Society of Behavioral Medicine. Ann Behav Med 1994;16:210–20.

200. Shiffman S. Real-time self-report of momentary states in the natural environment: computerized ecological momentary assessment. In: Stone AA, Turkkan JJ, Bachrach CA, et al, editors. The science of self-report: implications for research and practice. Mahwah (NJ): Lawrence Erlbaum Associates; 2000. p. 277–96.

201. Entringer S, Buss C, Andersen J, et al. Ecological momentary assessment (EMA) of maternal cortisol profiles over a multiple-day period predict the length of human gestation. Psychosom Med 2011. [Epub ahead of print].

202. Lu MC, Halfon N. Racial and ethnic disparities in birth outcomes: a life-course perspective. Matern Child Health J 2003;7(1):13–30.

203. Misra DP, Guyer B, Allston A. Integrated perinatal health framework. A multiple determinants model with a life span approach. Am J Prev Med 2003;25(1):65–75.

204. Kermack WO, McKendrick AG, McKinlay PL. Death-rates in Great Britain and Sweden: expression of specific mortality rates as products of two factors, and some consequences thereof. J Hyg (Lond) 1934;34(4):433–57.

205. Gluckman PD, Hanson MA, Cooper C, et al. Effect of in utero and early-life conditions on adult health and disease. N Engl J Med 2008;359(1):61–73.

206. Swanson JM, Entringer S, Buss C, et al. Developmental origins of health and disease: environmental exposures. Semin Reprod Med 2009;27(5):391–402.

207. Wadhwa PD, Buss C, Entringer S, et al. Developmental origins of health and disease: brief history of the approach and current focus on epigenetic mechanisms. Semin Reprod Med 2009;27(5):358–68.

208. Seckl JR. Physiologic programming of the fetus. Clin Perinatol 1998;25(4):939–62, vii.

209. Hertzman C. The biological embedding of early experience and its effects on health in adulthood. Ann N Y Acad Sci 1999;896:85–95.

210. Suomi SJ. Early determinants of behaviour: evidence from primate studies. Br Med Bull 1997;53(1):170–84.

211. Meaney MJ, Szyf M. Environmental programming of stress responses through DNA methylation: life at the interface between a dynamic environment and a fixed genome. Dialogues Clin Neurosci 2005;7(2):103–23.

212. Weaver IC, Champagne FA, Brown SE, et al. Reversal of maternal programming of stress responses in adult offspring through methyl supplementation: altering epigenetic marking later in life. J Neurosci 2005;25(47):11045–54.

213. Coe LC. Psychosocial factors and psychoneuroimmunology within a lifespan perspective. In: Keating DP, Hertzman C, editors. Developmental health and the wealth of nations: social, biological and educational dynamics. New York: Guilford Stress; 1999. p. 201–19.

214. Entringer S, Buss C, Kumsta R, et al. Prenatal psychosocial stress exposure is associated with subsequent working memory performance in young women. Behav Neurosci 2009;123(4):886–93.

215. Entringer S, Kumsta R, Hellhammer DH, et al. Prenatal exposure to maternal psychosocial stress and HPA axis regulation in young adults. Horm Behav 2009;55(2):292–8.

216. Entringer S, Kumsta R, Nelson EL, et al. Influence of prenatal psychosocial stress on cytokine production in adult women. Dev Psychobiol 2008;50(6):579–87.

217. Entringer S, Wust S, Kumsta R, et al. Prenatal psychosocial stress exposure is associated with insulin resistance in young adults. Am J Obstet Gynecol 2008;199(5):498,e1–7.

218. Champagne F, Meaney MJ. Like mother, like daughter: evidence for non-genomic transmission of parental behavior and stress responsivity. Prog Brain Res 2001;133:287–302.

219. Power C, Matthews S. Origins of health inequalities in a national population sample. Lancet 1997;350(9091):1584–9.

220. McEwen BS. Protective and damaging effects of stress mediators. N Engl J Med 1998;338(3):171–9.

221. Sapolsky RM. Social subordinance as a marker of hypercortisolism. Some unexpected subtleties. Ann N Y Acad Sci 1995;771:626–39.

222. Kristenson M, Kucinskiene Z, Bergdahl B, et al. Increased psychosocial strain in Lithuanian versus Swedish men: the LiVicordia study. Psychosom Med 1998;60(3):277–82.

223. Chrousos GP. The stress response and immune function: clinical implications. The 1999 Novera H. Spector Lecture. Ann N Y Acad Sci 2000;917:38–67.

224. Noll JG, Schulkin J, Trickett PK, et al. Differential pathways to preterm delivery for sexually abused and comparison women. J Pediatr Psychol 2007;32(10):1238–48.

225. Chung EK, Mathew L, Elo IT, et al. Depressive symptoms in disadvantaged women receiving prenatal care: the influence of adverse and positive childhood experiences. Ambul Pediatr 2008;8(2):109–16.

226. Cammack AL, Buss C, Entringer S, et al. The association between early life adversity and bacterial vaginosis during pregnancy. Am J Obstet Gynecol 2011. [Epub ahead of print].

227. Shea AK, Streiner DL, Fleming A, et al. The effect of depression, anxiety and early life trauma on the cortisol awakening response during pregnancy: preliminary results. Psychoneuroendocrinology 2007;32(8–10):1013–20.

228. Chung EK, Nurmohamed L, Mathew L, et al. Risky health behaviors among mothers-to-be: the impact of adverse childhood experiences. Acad Pediatr 2010;10(4):245–51.

229. Misra D, Strobino D, Trabert B. Effects of social and psychosocial factors on risk of preterm birth in black women. Paediatr Perinat Epidemiol 2010;24(6):546–54.

230. Amory JH, Hitti J, Lawler R, et al. Increased tumor necrosis factor-alpha production after lipopolysaccharide stimulation of whole blood in patients with previous preterm delivery complicated by intra-amniotic infection or inflammation. Am J Obstet Gynecol 2001;185(5):1064–7.

231. National Research Council (U.S.). Committee on future directions for behavioral and social sciences research at the national institute of health. New horizons in health: an integrative approach. Washington, DC: National Academy Press; 2001.
232. Downs DS, Feinberg M, Hillemeier MM, et al. Design of the Central Pennsylvania Women's Health Study (CePAWHS) strong healthy women intervention: improving preconceptional health. Matern Child Health J 2009;13(1):18–28.
233. Weisman CS, Hillemeier MM, Downs DS, et al. Preconception predictors of weight gain during pregnancy: prospective findings from the Central Pennsylvania Women's Health Study. Womens Health Issues 2010;20(2):126–32.
234. Webb DA, Coyne JC, Goldenberg RL, et al. Recruitment and retention of women in a large randomized control trial to reduce repeat preterm births: the Philadelphia Collaborative Preterm Prevention Project. BMC Med Res Methodol 2010; 10:88.
235. Collins JW Jr, David RJ, Handler A, et al. Very low birthweight in African American infants: the role of maternal exposure to interpersonal racial discrimination. Am J Public Health 2004;94(12):2132–8.
236. Geronimus AT. Black/white differences in the relationship of maternal age to birthweight: a population-based test of the weathering hypothesis. Soc Sci Med 1996;42(4):589–97.
237. Landrigan PJ, Trasande L, Thorpe LE, et al. The National Children's Study: a 21-year prospective study of 100,000 American children. Pediatrics 2006;118(5): 2173–86.

The Role of Inflammation and Infection in Preterm Birth

Jamie A. Bastek, MD[a,b,c,1], Luis M. Gómez, MD[a,b,c,1], Michal A. Elovitz, MD[a,b,*]

KEYWORDS

- Preterm birth • Inflammation • Infection • Animal model
- Biomarkers

Preterm birth is defined as delivery before 37 weeks' gestation. In 2010, the incidence of preterm birth in the United States was 12.3%[1] and ranged from 8% to 12% in developed countries.[2] Despite decades of prematurity research, the incidence of preterm birth has remained essentially constant—if not increased—in recent years. The clinical presentations associated with preterm birth are diverse and include preterm labor (PTL), membrane rupture, and cervical dilatation as well as cramping or spotting. As such, preterm birth actually represents a syndrome. Consequently, it is theorized that there are several molecular pathways associated with triggering preterm parturition. Although research has demonstrated potential roles for disruptions in endocrine, immune, and other biochemical pathways in precipitating preterm birth, the precise pathogenesis remains unknown. As a result, the preterm birth rate has remained relatively constant and effective therapeutic strategies remain elusive.

Although there is still much to unravel, there is a growing body of evidence that demonstrates that inflammation and/or infection may be a primary causal mechanism of preterm birth.[3–8] This article explores the epidemiologic, clinical, and animal data that exist to support this conceptual paradigm.

Financial support: none.
Financial disclosures and conflicts of interest: The authors have nothing to disclose.
[1] Drs Bastek and Gómez share first authorship.
[a] Maternal and Child Health Research Program, Philadelphia, PA, USA
[b] Department of Obstetrics and Gynecology, Center for Research on Reproduction and Women's Health, University of Pennsylvania, Philadelphia, PA, USA
[c] Department of Maternal-Fetal Medicine, 3400 Spruce Street, 2000 Courtyard Building, Philadelphia, PA 19104, USA
* Corresponding author. Department of Maternal-Fetal Medicine, Hospital of the University of Pennsylvania, 421 Curie Boulevard, 1353 BRB 2/3, Philadelphia, PA 19104.
E-mail address: melovitz@obgyn.upenn.edu

Clin Perinatol 38 (2011) 385–406
doi:10.1016/j.clp.2011.06.003
0095-5108/11/$ – see front matter

EPIDEMIOLOGIC AND CLINICAL DATA TO SUPPORT THE ROLE OF INFLAMMATION AND INFECTION IN THE PATHOGENESIS OF PRETERM BIRTH

In 1950, Knox and Hoerner[9] published their findings that "infection in the female reproductive tract can cause premature rupture of the membranes and induce premature labor." Despite this initial suggestion of a relationship between infection/inflammation and spontaneous preterm birth more than 60 years ago, the rate of prematurity continues to rise and highly sensitive, clinically useful diagnostic techniques as well as effective therapeutic interventions remain at a loss.

In the 1960s, investigators focused on the association between preterm birth and extrauterine maternal infections, such as malaria[10,11] and pyelonephritis.[12,13] Today, it continues to be recognize that these extrauterine infections as well as asymptomatic bacteriuria, pneumonia, and appendicitis probably dispose women to preterm birth.[14,15] Although periodontal disease has been perhaps the most controversial extrauterine source of intrauterine bacterial infection, the most recent data suggest that the association between periodontal disease and preterm birth is not causal.[16–20]

Over the past 20 years, a growing body of evidence has emerged to suggest that intrauterine infection and/or inflammation (as opposed to systemic infection) leads to activation of localized inflammatory pathways and plays a critical role in at least 25% to 40% of preterm births.[3,4,8,21,22] Some of the strongest evidence to support the role of intrauterine infection as a cause of preterm birth has been generated by pathologic placental assessment. Studies performed in 1980,[23] 1990,[24] and 2000[25] have all demonstrated an inversely proportional relationship between histologic chorioamnionitis, defined as neutrophil infiltration of the fetal membranes, and gestational age at delivery. Specifically, whereas only 10% of preterm births between 33 and 36 weeks have evidence of localized inflammation, this percentage increases with progressively earlier gestational age at delivery. Greater than 85% of pregnancies delivering before 28 weeks and 94% of deliveries between 21 and 24 weeks are complicated by histologic chorioamnionitis.[23–25]

There are several hypotheses regarding how intrauterine infection might occur. Although some theories describe the possibility of hematogenous dissemination of microorganisms through the placenta, accidental introduction of microorganisms at the time of invasive procedures and/or retrograde flow of microorganisms through the fallopian tubes, the most common pathway is believed to involve the ascent of microorganisms from the vagina and cervix into the uterine cavity.[8,21–25] This conceptualized pathway of ascending intrauterine infection is theorized to occur in several stages. During early stages, changes occur in the microbial flora of the vagina and/or cervix. Vaginal organisms then ascend into the choriodecidual space. Subsequently, some microorganisms migrate between the chorion and amnion and infect the intrauterine cavity. Ultimately the fetus becomes infected, marking the most advanced and serious stage of ascending intrauterine infection.[2,8,26] As rates of culture proved neonatal sepsis are low[27] in preterm neonates, it is plausible that the initial stages may be sufficient for preterm parturition to occur.

Once microorganisms have entered the cervix, uterus, and/or amnion, there are several possible signaling pathways that may be initiated, which can either individually or collectively promote preterm parturition. A likely pathway is the activation of the innate immune system. First, bacteria or even bacterial by-products, such as lipopolysaccharide (LPS), are detected by immune system pattern recognition receptors, specifically the toll-like receptors (TLRs).[28] TLRs, in particular TLR-2 and TLR-4, are expressed in the uterus,[29] cervix,[29] amniotic epithelium,[30] and the decidua.[31] When TLRs are ligated, they activate several immune pathways, which stimulate the release of proinflammatory cytokines and other inflammatory mediators.[30,31]

Although interleukin (IL)-1 was the first inflammatory cytokine to be associated with infection-mediated PTL, subsequent studies corroborate the role of other members of the interleukin family, including IL-1α and IL-1β,[5,32–35] IL-6,[36–41] and IL-8[6,42–46] as well as tumor necrosis factor α (TNF-α)[7,47–56] in preterm birth. These cytokines, which are produced by a variety of cells in the cervix, uterus, and amnion in response to bacterial infection, along with microbial endotoxin, stimulate the amnion, chorion, decidua, and myometrium to release prostaglandin (PG)[5,32–35,57,58] and the amnion and chorion to release matrix metalloproteinases (MMPs).[2,8,57–59] PG release then initiates uterine contractility, leading to cervical dilatation and the potential for membrane exposure and further intrauterine microbial migration. MMPs stimulate cervical ripening and contribute to rupture of fetal membranes. Despite the elegance of this proposed theory of prematurity, several factors complicate this potential causal mechanism between infection and prematurity.

First, on a clinical level, an intrauterine infection can be difficult to diagnose—at least with standard clinical testing. For example, although microbial invasion of the amniotic cavity is present in 12.8% of women with PTL and intact membranes,[21] 32% of preterm premature rupture of membranes (PPROM),[21] and 51% of cervical insufficiency,[60,61] most women with evidence of histologic chorioamnionitis do not demonstrate signs of systemic illness or inflammation.[25] One study showed that only 14% of women with histologic chorioamnionitis developed signs of an overt infection,[23] whereas another reported that only 5% to 10% of women with histologic chorioamnionitis were diagnosed with fever, uterine tenderness, and an elevated white blood cell count.[62] Maternal serum cultures in women with histologic chorioamnionitis are usually negative.[63,64] Furthermore, amniotic fluid polymerase chain reaction (PCR)—which is not a conventional detection technique—must often be used to detect the intrauterine presence of genital mycoplasmas found most frequently in spontaneous PTL and PPROM, including *Ureaplasma urealyticum* and *Mycoplasma hominis*.[2,65,66] Conventional culture techniques are also unable to detect the presence of intrauterine virus as a potential cause of infection. And, although historically the evidence that viruses predisposed women to preterm birth was considered sparse,[2] new data suggest that placental adenovirus is strongly associated with histologic chorioamnionitis and preterm birth.[67] It remains to be seen whether further studies will reveal that other viruses are also associated with preterm birth.

Another factor that complicates the relationship between infection, inflammation, and preterm birth is that intrauterine colonization is not necessarily associated with a clinically significant intrauterine infection that precipitates labor. It is possible that due to individual variations in the immunologic response to foreign microorganisms, the inflammatory cascade—and subsequent labor—may be triggered in some women (diagnosed with an infection) and not triggered in others (assumed to be simply colonized). For example, when intrauterine bacteria were detected using PCR in the setting of negative conventional culture, only 31% of patients delivered preterm.[68] The assumption was made that these women were merely colonized with *Escherichia coli* and that they thus had not mounted a clinically significant immune response that would be recognized as an overt infection. Similarly, another study demonstrated that bacteria were cultured from the chorioamnion of 15% of nonlaboring women with intact membranes[8] whereas a third used fluorescent in situ hybridization to detect bacterial DNA in the membranes of 70% of women undergoing elective cesarean delivery at term.[69]

Additional evidence of the dissociation between mere colonization and significant infection is seen with studies of vaginal microorganisms. Despite the associations reported between vaginal colonization with *Gardnerella vaginalis*, *Neisseria gonorrhoeae*,

Chlamydia trachomatis, group B streptococcus, and *Trichomonas vaginalis*, a causal relationship between these organisms and preterm has not been proved and is controversial.[57] As a result, although treatment is advisable from a public health standpoint, there are no data to support that treatment of vaginal colonization actually decreases the risk of preterm birth.[57,70,71] Furthermore, although organisms, such as *Neisseria gonorrhoeae* and *Chlamydia trachomatis*, have been isolated from the amniotic cavity of women who delivered preterm, most of the women in these studies presented with ruptured membranes.[72,73] This fact, combined with data that demonstrate that neither *Neisseria gonorrhoeae* nor *Chlamydia trachomatis* binds to fetal membranes,[74] suggest that intrauterine infection with such organisms may have been opportunistic and not causal.[3,57]

Even if one were to be able to distinguish a priori the difference between which women might experience a clinically significant intrauterine infection and those who might be merely colonized by foreign microorganisms, differences in the amount of time it takes for an individual to mount a potential immune response prevent a clear association between the time of microbial invasion and delivery. For example, many women theorized as having subclinical intrauterine infection before 20 weeks' gestation remain asymptomatic until after 20 weeks' gestation, when the membranes become more adherent to the decidua. After the membranes adhere, a subclinical infection can develop with subsequent preterm birth within the next 8 to 10 weeks.[8] Furthermore, women with intrauterine infection detected by PCR at the time of midtrimester amniocentesis often do not experience PTL or PPROM until weeks later.[75-77] Collectively, these data call into question how inflammation or infection of pregnancy is currently (clinically) diagnosed. Whether or not looking for improved methods to detect microbial invasion is the right research approach, and whether there is a need to investigate the presence of pathogenic organisms using more sophisticate techniques remain urgent research questions.

It seems natural to conclude that if acute infection were at the epicenter of spontaneous preterm birth, then treatment of infection with antibiotics should mitigate this outcome. The administration of antibiotics to those at risk for preterm birth with intact membranes has not been found to decrease the risk of preterm birth, delivery within 48 hours, or perinatal mortality, however.[78-80] Even when analyses were restricted to those antibiotics that are most effective against anaerobes, including metronidazole and clindamycin, there was still no significant reduction in the preterm birth rate.[57,78] In another study, when antibiotics were administered to women with positive fetal fibronectin (fFN) under the assumption that bacterial invasion of the chorion had precipitated the release of fFN into the cervicovaginal fluids, there was no improvement in the rate of preterm birth. Furthermore, when antibiotics were administered to women with both a positive fFN and a history of prior preterm birth, their risk of recurrent preterm birth actually increased.[81-84]

There are several possible explanations as to why antibiotics have been unsuccessful in preventing preterm birth to date. First, it is possible that the antibiotics studied have not been appropriate for the invading microorganisms or have not been administered for sufficient time to clear the infection. Second, the inciting infection may be transient and cleared by the innate immune response even before the initiation of antibiotics. In such a scenario, the inflammation created by the activated immune system to clear the infection—and not the presence of an invading microorganism itself—could be what actually triggers the onset of labor. Alternatively, if the invading microorganism is still present and has not yet been cleared by the innate immune response when antibiotic treatment is initiated, it is possible that the antibiotics could kill the microorganism and thus lead to a greater inflammatory response. Whether the truth lies with one of these or an alternative theory, current evidence does not support the use of antibiotics to prevent preterm birth.

Finally, the relationship between intrauterine infection, inflammation, and subsequent preterm birth seems to be complicated by individual genetic susceptibilities. Although recent genome-wide association studies have been negative,[85] predisposition to preterm birth seems to have some hereditary component, as evidenced by the fact that women whose sisters had a preterm birth are 80% more likely to deliver preterm themselves.[86] Recent studies suggest that bacterial exposure, such as bacterial vaginosis (BV), may only be a risk for preterm birth in genetically susceptible women. Specifically, women who carry a specific polymorphism in TNF-α and have BV are at significantly increased risk of preterm birth over women with only a single exposure.[87] Likewise, asymptomatic BV may act as an environmental exposure that modifies the risk of spontaneous preterm birth in women with susceptible single nucleotide polymorphisms (SNPs) in genes that regulate the maternal inflammatory response.[88] Furthermore, although neither white nor black women with a particular IL-6 SNP were at increased risk of preterm birth, black women with this specific SNP and BV infection had a twofold increase in the risk of prematurity.[89] These data demonstrate the existence of a significant gene-environment interaction and that identification of high-risk subgroups might be necessary for effective preventative or treatment strategies.

Despite these difficulties with which obstetricians must grapple in an effort to understand the potential causality between intrauterine infection and prematurity, infection and inflammation are of even greater concern for the fetus. As discussed previously, the later stages of the pathway of ascending intrauterine infection involving potential fetal infection are generally considered the most advanced and serious stages.[2,26] This is due to the adversity of outcomes with which preterm infants exposed to intrauterine infection are faced. Overall, the risk of fetal bacteremia is significantly greater in the setting of maternal PPROM with positive rather than negative amniotic fluid cultures.[90] Controlling for gestational age at delivery and neonatal birth weight, there is a significant association between clinically apparent in utero infection and neonatal respiratory distress syndrome, sepsis, and seizures.[56,91] The association between infection and neonatal adverse outcome persists regardless of whether or not there are overt signs of maternal disease: subclinical in utero infection was significantly associated with increased risk of neonatal respiratory distress syndrome, intraventricular hemorrhage, necrotizing enterocolitis, and multisystem organ failure.[56,92] Finally, preterm Infants exposed to clinical chorioamnionitis have a nearly 2-fold increase in the risk of long-term neurologic sequelae, such as cerebral palsy,[93,94] whereas elevated amniotic fluid levels of IL-6 and IL-8 have been associated with cerebral palsy at 3 years.[95] More recent studies suggest that very preterm infants have a wide spectrum of neurobehavioral disorders and that prematurity is associated with an increased risk for attention-deficit/hyperactivity disorder emotional disorders and autism spectrum disorders in childhood.[96–99] Whether an ex-preterm child is at risk solely from prematurity or from exposure to inflammation in addition to prematurity is not currently known. If inflammation, independent of prematurity, places preterm infants at risk for neurobehavioral disorders, such as autism, however, this could greatly affect potential intervention strategies.

The fetal immune-mediated response to this intrauterine inflammatory insult has been referred to as the fetal inflammatory response syndrome.[100] Defined as an elevated fetal plasma concentration of IL-6 (>11 pg/mL) and confirmed histopathologically by funisitis and chronic vasculitis,[101] fetal inflammatory response syndrome is associated with increased rates of severe neonatal morbidity and decreased latency to delivery regardless of the inflammatory state of the amniotic fluid.[100,102] Thus, it seems that activation of the fetal immune system can also contribute to the propagation of prematurity independent of other maternal events.

There are imperfections in the model associating intrauterine infection, the generation of an inflammatory response by the innate immune system, and subsequent preterm birth. This calls into question whether it is the presence of intrauterine infection—or simply an inflammatory response—that is the keystone to spontaneous preterm birth. If it is inflammation and not infection that is both necessary and sufficient for spontaneous preterm birth, then inflammatory biomarkers must exist that can help risk-stratify patients for preterm birth. Furthermore, if the primary mechanism is inflammation and not infection, then shifting the focus of therapy from anti-infectious agents to immunomodulating agents could aid in the successful treatment of the preterm birth syndrome.

Biomarkers of inflammation, such as certain members of the IL family, MMPs, and white blood cells, have been studied in both the amniotic fluid and maternal serum for an association with preterm birth.[5,36,42,103–107] Despite many small studies that suggest that several ILs and MMPs may hold promise in the risk stratification of preterm birth, a 2010 systematic review of 17 studies and more than 6000 patients designed to estimate the association between inflammatory cytokines and the risk of spontaneous preterm birth in asymptomatic women found that only IL-6 in cervicovaginal fluid and IL-6 and C-reactive protein in amniotic fluid were significantly associated with preterm birth.[108] Specifically, IL-6 detected in cervicovaginal fluid was associated with a 3-fold increase, whereas IL-6 detected in amniotic fluid was associated with a 4.5-fold increase, in the risk of preterm birth.[108] Amniotic fluid levels of C-reactive protein were associated with a nearly 8-fold increased risk of preterm birth.[108] There was no significant association between levels of plasma IL-6 or C-reactive protein and prematurity.[108] Although other biomarkers were studied, including IL-1, IL-2, IL-8, IL-10, and TNF-α, there was insufficient evidence to suggest an association between levels of these biomarkers and preterm birth in asymptomatic women.[108]

Although some investigators continue to study the association between levels of IL-6 and TNF-α obtained at midtrimester amniocentesis,[109] the search for a promising immune-mediated biomarker of prematurity continues. Since 2009, several novel biomarkers obtained at midtrimester amniocentesis have been demonstrated as associated with increased risk of prematurity, including IL-18,[110] soluble HLA-G,[111] and complement split products C3a, C4a, and C5a.[112] Recent serum studies have examined other potential biomarkers, such as high sensitivity C-reactive protein and placental growth factor,[113] and also found an association with preterm birth.

Despite the promise of these and other biomarkers, the routine use of most of these markers is clinically difficult. For example, although multiple studies might corroborate that an elevated level of a particular biomarker is associated with an increased risk of preterm birth, many of them fail to share a standardized cut-point. Furthermore, the presence of such biomarkers does not lend insight into when the anticipated preterm birth event might occur nor is there a specific successful intervention to prevent preterm birth if a patient is deemed at higher risk.

Perhaps the most clinically successful biomarker has been cervicovaginal fFN. A unique glycoprotein, fFN, has been described as "trophoblast glue" that promotes cellular adhesion at uterine-placental and decidual-fetal membrane interfaces.[114,115] Typically absent from cervicovaginal fluid between 24 and 37 weeks' gestation, the presence of fFN may signify infectious-mediated choriodecidual disruption and subsequent preterm birth with clinical and/or histologic chorioamnionitis within 7 weeks.[2,83] In clinical practice, however, fFN is used most for its strong negative predictive value because the positive predictive value is somewhat poor.[116] Despite its clinical utility and its demonstrated validity as a biomarker of prematurity, however, there is still one significant drawback to fFN: a continued lack of effective therapies to prevent impending preterm birth.

Immunomodulating agents have shown varying degrees of success in helping mitigate preterm birth. Perhaps the best large-scale clinical example of how immune modulation may potentially reduce the risk of preterm birth was seen in the 2003 Maternal-Fetal Medicine Units Network trial on 17α-hydroxyprogesterone caproate (17P).[3,117] Although 17P was initially used in the trial for its presumed tocolytic effect by promoting myometrial quiescence, recent studies suggest that 17P might have anti-inflammatory properties.[118,119] If 17P does, in fact, have immunomodulating properties (similar to other progestational agents, such as medroxyprogesterone acetate [MPA]), this study's suggestion of such targeted therapy may hold promise for preventing PTB. The immunomodulating properties of 17P need to be confirmed in human studies.

Other immune-modulators that have not gained the same widespread popularity for use as 17P include IL-10, which suppresses the production of proinflammatory cytokines by other cells and decreases the incidence of preterm birth and adverse neonatal outcomes,[120,121] and macrophage inhibiting factor, which may prevent preterm birth and adverse perinatal outcomes.[120] Although glucocorticoids have been administered to help mitigate the adversity of obstetric outcomes with antiphospholipid antibody syndrome[122] and in the treatment of other adverse pregnancy outcomes, such as preeclampsia, these potentially promising agents have not yet been trialed in the prevention of preterm birth.

Before these and other immunomodulating agents are administered in an attempt to prevent preterm birth, however, it must be remembered that spontaneous preterm birth is an end result of activation of the maternal immune system even if just at the local (uterus/cervix) level. Therefore, if the process of preterm birth has evolved to ensure maternal survival, then use of immune-modulators to impede preterm birth may cause greater harm than good for the mother. Furthermore, whether such immune-modulators could have an adverse impact on the developing fetus and/or quell the maternal immune response without down-regulating the fetal immune system must also be investigated before the widespread administration of these medications for this purpose.[3]

ANIMAL EXPERIMENTS DATA TO SUPPORT THE ROLE OF INFLAMMATION AND INFECTION IN THE PATHOGENESIS OF PRETERM BIRTH
The Search for a Valid Animal Model for the Study of Spontaneous Preterm Birth

Because the study of inflammation and infection in human pregnancies and fetuses is subject to ethical factors, the use of animal models is a valuable resource that allows for strict control of environmental, genetic, pharmacologic, maternal, and fetal variables otherwise difficult to regulate in human studies. Rodents, pigs, sheep, and simian models have facilitated the investigation of the role of inflammation and infection in spontaneous preterm birth.[4,123–126] Studies in animal models have shown that preterm parturition is preceded by an inflammatory response at the cervical and vaginal level.[127,128] The use of animal models, nonetheless, is not free of challenges; models that are applicable for a particular mechanism of preterm birth may not be suitable for another. For instance, sheep are better mechanical ventilation models than mice because the alveolar development in sheep occurs in the antenatal period whereas in mice it happens predominantly in the postnatal period.[129] Another area of difficulty in different animal species is the dissimilarities in placental function. Unlike human and sheep that maintain pregnancy by placental production of progesterone, the placenta in mice is not an important source of progesterone; therefore, mice may not arise as appropriate models for studying the effects of placental dysfunction on progesterone synthesis.[129] Dissimilarities in placentation among various animal models may translate into significant differences in the colonization of microbes in fetal membranes and amniotic fluid.[130]

Understanding these limitations, rodents constitute efficient models for infection and/or inflammation associated preterm birth. Advantages of this model include a short pregnancy length (19 to 22 days), well-characterized genomes, and well-defined immune systems, which are similar to that of humans. Mice have the advantage of different routes of easy access for the administration of inflammatory/infectious agents (described by Elovitz and colleagues elsewhere in this issue).[131] Furthermore, mice are amenable to genetic modification. Experiments in knockout models have demonstrated the relevance of multiple signaling in infection/inflammation–associated preterm birth. In addition, a wide array of antibodies and microarray platforms is available for rodent models. Similar concepts apply to rabbit models (average pregnancy length 30 days). Although nonhuman primates have the advantage of anatomy and pregnancy length similarity with humans, they are expensive, their housing is complicated, and their study requires consideration of ethical factors. Sheep are useful for investigating the effect of inflammation in pregnancy because the mother and fetus can be chronically instrumented.[132,133] Reports have demonstrated, however, that decidual or uterine infection may cause a mild increase in uterine contractility but do not seem to trigger prematurity in sheep.[133] Thus, they are useful models for studying fetal responses to amniotic fluid pathogens or inflammation but may not be suited to investigating mechanisms leading to preterm parturition. Although their pregnancy physiology is well characterized, their immunology and genetics are not as well understood as in rodents. Furthermore, there is a limited availability of antibodies and molecular resources for the use of sheep models in the investigation of preterm birth.

Induction of Preterm Birth in Animal Models

Research in animal models has rendered valuable information in the role of inflammation and infection in spontaneous preterm birth. Various animal models have demonstrated that bacteria or bacterial by-products can induce preterm birth. In 1991, Romero and colleagues[35] were able to induce preterm birth in mice within 24 hours of exposure to systemic recombinant human IL-1. Experiments on rabbit models demonstrated that intracervical and intrauterine administration of *Escherichia coli* at day 21 of pregnancy-induced inflammation, preterm delivery, and pregnancy loss.[134,135] The concept of a temporal evolving inflammatory/infection process after intrauterine infection (ie, infection in the uterus and fetal membranes preceding PTL and fetal infection) arose from experiments in rabbits[80,136] and has been replicated recently in rhesus monkey models.[137]

Research in these nonhuman primates has shown that chronic intraamniotic exposure to group B streptococcus results in uterine contractions and elevated levels of TNF-α, IL-1β, and IL-6 followed by increases in PGE2 and PGF2α.[138] Subsequent research has shown that although infectious microorganisms are able to elicit PTL, they are not necessary once inflammatory changes occur.[139] Furthermore, in the absence of bacteria, an inflammatory state can be sufficient to evolve into spontaneous preterm birth. For instance, intra-amniotic infusion of the inflammatory cytokine IL-1β correlates with increased expression of IL-6, IL-8, and TNF-α, leading to increased uterine activity and PTL.[140,141] Why does an inflammatory state occur in the absence of infectious microorganisms? It could be that the offending microbe initially provokes an inflammatory response and is later eradicated by the host immune system. Alternatively, the microorganism itself may be unable to cause infection but in the presence of the maternal immune and genetic environment is capable to elicit an inflammatory response.[4]

Systemic Versus Local Intrauterine Inflammation Models for Preterm Birth

The systemic injection of LPS in mice results in elevated maternal serum and amniotic fluid concentrations of inflammatory chemokines and cytokines (TNF-α, IL-1, and IL-6, among others).[35,142] The induction of PTL in mice after systemic LPS exposure varies, however, on strains.[127] This has prompted the use of standardized mice models of localized intrauterine to allow comparisons between strains.[143] Local intrauterine infection/inflammation models using microbes or bacterial by-products provide more consistent results. Using attenuated E coli, Hirsch and colleagues[144] demonstrated that injection bacteria into a ligated uterine horn in pregnant mice resulted in preterm birth of the opposite noninjected horn. A reproducible model of intrauterine inflammation has been proposed by Elovitz and colleagues,[4,128,130] which involves intrauterine (local) injection of bacterial by-products, such as LPS (rather than injection of live or killed bacteria)— again confirming that inflammation, not infection, is sufficient to induce preterm birth.[4,128,130]

As proposed previously, a maternal response is necessary for the development of preterm birth. Maternal TLR4, for instance, recognizes LPS and is required for LPS-induced preterm birth.[128,130,145] The specificity of TLR signaling in preterm birth was outlined by Elovitz and colleagues[128]; using a mouse model of localized intrauterine inflammation, the investigators demonstrated that infusion of purified LPS resulted in preterm birth in wild-type mice but not in mice expressing mutant TLR4 receptors. Mice that were TLR4 deficient but not TLR2 deficient failed to deliver prematurely after intraamniotic infection with Fusobacterium nucleatum.[146] Expression of TLR4 and TLR2 mRNA are differentially upregulated in the uterus and placenta after exposure to LPS.[130] Another important mediator in the maternal inflammatory response is the protein myeloid differentiation primary response gene 88 (MyD88). MyD88 is primarily responsible for the activation of nuclear factor κB (NF-κB).[147] Mice deficient in MyD88 exhibit an attenuated inflammatory response induced by LPS.[148] MyD88 knockout mice models are resistant to preterm delivery after LPS exposure compared with wild-type mice.[149] Finally, the importance of maternal IL-1 and TNF-α synergistic signaling in mice was outlined recently by Hirsch and colleagues[56]: by using mice lacking the type 1 receptors for IL-1 and TNF-α they found significant lower rates of preterm delivery in response to heat-killed E coli in IL-1/TNF knockout mice compared with wild-type pregnant mice controls. Collectively, these findings demonstrate that in addition to potential inflammatory signaling in the fetus, the maternal host environment plays an essential role in the immune response after bacterial exposure and is necessary for inflammation/infection-induced preterm birth.

What Animal Models Indicate About the Pathogenesis of Inflammation-Induced Preterm Birth

Clinical and animal studies suggest that premature cervical remodeling (leading to cervical shortening and/or cervical ripening) may be the primary event in the pathogenesis of preterm birth.[150,151] The cervix is composed mostly of extracellular matrix elements (collagen, elastin, proteoglycans, and hyaluronan) in addition to stroma, smooth muscle, and epithelial cells. Cervical ripening before dilation requires changes in the composition and structure of the extracellular matrixleading to an increase in the hyaluronan synthase, glycosaminoglycans, and hyaluronan before parturition.[152] The process of cervical remodeling has been considered traditionally an inflammatory event where leukocytes invade the stromal matrix and release proteases that digest collagen and other components of the extracellular matrix.[153–155] This concept has recently been challenged. Recent animal data demonstrate that inflammation is not needed for cervical remodeling. Using a noninfectious model of preterm birth, mice exposed to mifepristone failed to show an increase in the expression of cytokines or other immune mediators.[151] Similarly, no change or influx of immune cells was observed in term cervical remodeling in mice studies.[156]

Although inflammation may not be required for parturition, it does seem sufficient to induce cervical remodeling prematurely as well as actually induce preterm birth. Inflammatory mediators, such as IL-1β, upregulate the expression of HAS type 2 in the cervix of pregnant mice, suggesting a role of inflammation in cervical ripening.[157] Likewise, in a mouse model of intrauterine inflammation, before delivery, there is a potent immune response in the cervix.[151,158]

Despite knowledge that inflammation can promote cervical remodeling in mice, it remains unclear regarding how inflammation or infection may trigger changes in the cervix and, more importantly, what are the processes that govern these molecular events and how target therapies might be targeted to reduce these changes. New animal data suggest that the cervical epithelium may play a critical role in inflammation-induced cervical remodeling and perhaps contribute to prematurity. The cervical epithelium is an important protective barrier during pregnancy against infection and mechanical trauma.[159] Genes involved in epithelial cell differentiation pathway in mice models are progressively upregulated during cervical ripening with greater expression during cervical dilatation at term and post partum.[151,160] In addition, progestational agents are able to change the expression of genes involved in the epithelial barrier in cervical tissues, suggesting that alterations in these pathways may predispose to premature cervical remodeling.[161]

Although it is known that proinflammatory cytokines can elicit an inflammatory response in the pregnant uterus, there is limited knowledge regarding how expression of myometrial cytokines correlates to uterine activity. Experiments in mice have shown that when one uterine horn is ligated, the expression of inflammatory mediators after injection of bacterial products in the myometrium is greater in the exposed horn (direct contact) compared with the free horn; nevertheless, uterine contractions and preterm delivery can be induced in both the ligated and free horn,[162] suggesting that the degree of immune activation (once a threshold is met) is sufficient to induce preterm birth.

Growing evidence suggests that TNF-α and IL-1 induce uterine contractions and PTL in mice and rabbits.[35,163] In rhesus nonhuman primates, increased levels of TNF-α, IL-1β, IL-6, PGE2, and PGF2α, which correlate with uterine contractions, are seen after exposure to group B streptococcus.[138] Nevertheless, it seems that among all inflammatory cytokines induced after bacterial exposure in pregnant rhesus monkeys, only IL-1β and TNF-α are capable of provoking intense uterine contractions resulting ultimately in PTL.[141]

Morbidity Associated with Inflammation-Induced Preterm Birth in the Fetus and Neonate

Preterm birth complicated by infection and/or inflammation is associated with poor respiratory (bronchopulmonary dysplasia and chronic lung disease), neurologic (cerebral palsy, periventricular leukomalacia, and intraventricular hemorrhage), and neurobehavioral outcomes.[121,164–167] Mouse models of localized (uterine or cervical) injection of live microorganisms or LPS have been proposed to assess the effects of inflammation-induced preterm birth in the fetal brain.[168] Intrauterine inflammation associated with preterm birth leads to increased cytokine response in the fetal brain, white matter damage, and neuronal injury in fetal mice.[168–170] To elucidate if fetal brain injury is the consequence of preterm delivery or whether inflammatory processes were necessary for this injury, Burd and colleagues[171] compared the fetal effects of a mouse model of intrauterine inflammation-induced preterm birth (intrauterine LPS injection) to a noninfectious preterm birth model induced with exposure to mifepristone. The investigators observed that the expression of proinflammatory cytokine (IL-1β, IL-6, and TNF-α) in fetal brain was increased only in fetuses exposed to inflammation; furthermore, fetal neuronal injury was only apparent in fetuses exposed to prematurity and inflammation. Meanwhile, exposure to the process of preterm parturition in the absence of an inflammatory response did not evoke brain injury. These findings suggest that it is the inflammatory processes rather than the preterm birth process, which is responsible for poor fetal outcomes.[171]

What Has Been Learned from Animal Models: Potential Therapeutic Interventions

Antimicrobial agents have failed to prevent spontaneous PTL in women with intact membranes.[78] This lack of success of antimicrobial treatment to prevent preterm birth has reinforced the search of potential targets identified within the inflammatory process surrounding PTL. Data from animal models suggest that immunomodulatory agents, such as IL-10 and glucocorticoids, are effective in suppressing cytokine-induced contractions and inflammation-induced preterm birth.[34,172]

Glucocorticoids display well-recognized anti-inflammatory activity when used in chronic diseases characterized by inflammation.[173] Despite their wide use to induce fetal maturation, glucocorticoids have not yet been used to decrease the inflammatory maternal response. Recent data have demonstrated the beneficial effect of 17P in decreasing the recurrence of preterm birth.[117] In addition to the proposed uterine relaxation mechanism for this agent, 17P may interfere with the host immune response. Progestogen modulate the immunologic response[174,175]; however, the immunomodulating effect of progestational agents is divergent depending on the drug used, the cell activated, and the type of immune response.[176] The use of dexamethasone or MPA (progestogen with glucocorticoid activity) in a localized intra-uterine inflammation mouse model was successful in reducing the rate of preterm birth.[158] Similar reductions of preterm birth in mice after the injection of LPS were observed when MPA was compared with 17P, although MPA seemed superior to 17P because there was less maternal and fetal morbidity.[131] The anti-inflammatory properties of these progestational agents hold promise but caution is recommended until further studies can explore this type of interventions.

Based on proposed pathogenesis that LPS activating its cognate receptor TLR4 contributes to preterm birth, work has investigated the use of a TLR4 antagonist in nonhuman primates. These data from pregnant rhesus monkeys have shown that pretreatment with TLR4 antagonist decreased uterine contractions and the expression of inflammatory cytokines after intra-amniotic infusion with LPS.[177] This work has not yet been extrapolated to other animal models or to humans.

The increase in proinflammatory cytokines induced by LPS is mediated by the pleiotropic transcription factor, NF-κB.[178] Meanwhile, NF-κB is activated by a variety of agents, such as cytokines and reactive oxidative species.[179] Because the antioxidant N-acetylcysteine (NAC) inhibits NF-κB activation,[180] the use of NAC has been proposed to ameliorate LPS effects because it might inhibit cytokine production by inhibiting oxidant-mediated activation of transcription factors.[181–183] Pretreatment with NAC (before LPS administration) has been shown to suppress the inflammatory response and leukocyte infiltration seen in the placenta with LPS-induced PTL in a mice model,[184,185] suggesting a potential therapeutic role for NAC pretreatment in the prevention of neurologic damage associated with inflammation-induced preterm birth. Post-treatment administration of NAC after systemic exposure to LPS in mice and ovine, however, could aggravate PTL, enhance the inflammatory pro-oxidant effects on the brain, and induce fetal hypoxemia and hypotension, leading to a serious compromise of the fetal physiologic status.[185,186] Because clinically most inflamed/infected pregnancies are not detected antenatally—at least until better biomarkers are discovered—NAC treatment of pregnancy may not hold clinical promise at the present time.

FINAL REMARKS

Inflammation alone or as a consequence of infection is implicated in spontaneous PTL and preterm birth. It is worthy of continued investigation to determine if these inflammatory processes are causative of preterm birth or surrogates of other biologic pathways. Successful interventions are not likely to occur until the pathogenesis of preterm birth and the role of inflammation in causing not only parturition but also fetal and neonatal injury is fully elucidated. Likely targets for therapy may be the maternal immune response and/or premature cervical remodeling. It will be a challenge to detect changes in the maternal immune response because it likely occurs locally in the uterus, cervix, and placenta and may not be detectable systemically in the mother. Detecting cervical remodeling, triggered by inflammation, may also be problematic unless accurate biomarkers of this process can be identified. The road to preventing prematurity may be long but is one that must be traveled.

REFERENCES

1. Hamilton BE, Minino AM, Martin JA, et al. Annual summary of vital statistics: 2005. Pediatrics 2007;119(2):345–60.
2. Goldenberg RL, Culhane JF, Iams JD, et al. Epidemiology and causes of preterm birth. Lancet 2008;371(9606):75–84.
3. Elovitz MA. Anti-inflammatory interventions in pregnancy: now and the future. Semin Fetal Neonatal Med 2006;11(5):327–32.
4. Elovitz MA, Mrinalini C. Animal models of preterm birth. Trends Endocrinol Metab 2004;15(10):479–87.
5. Romero R, Brody DT, Oyarzun E, et al. Infection and labor. III. Interleukin-1: a signal for the onset of parturition. Am J Obstet Gynecol 1989;160(5 Pt 1):1117–23.
6. Cherouny PH, Pankuch GA, Romero R, et al. Neutrophil attractant/activating peptide-1/interleukin-8: association with histologic chorioamnionitis, preterm delivery, and bioactive amniotic fluid leukoattractants. Am J Obstet Gynecol 1993;169(5):1299–303.
7. Romero R, Manogue KR, Mitchell MD, et al. Infection and labor. IV. Cachectin-tumor necrosis factor in the amniotic fluid of women with intraamniotic infection and preterm labor. Am J Obstet Gynecol 1989;161(2):336–41.
8. Goldenberg RL, Hauth JC, Andrews WW. Intrauterine infection and preterm delivery. N Engl J Med 2000;342(20):1500–7.
9. Knox IC Jr, Hoerner JK. The role of infection in premature rupture of the membranes. Am J Obstet Gynecol 1950;59(1):190–4.
10. Gilles HM, Lawson JB, Sibelas M, et al. Malaria, anaemia and pregnancy. Ann Trop Med Parasitol 1969;63(2):245–63.
11. Heard N, Jordan T. An investigation of malaria during pregnancy in Zimbabwe. Cent Afr J Med 1981;27(4):62–3, 66–8.

12. Patrick MJ. Influence of maternal renal infection on the foetus and infant. Arch Dis Child 1967;42(222):208–13.
13. Wren BG. Subclinical renal infection and prematurity. Med J Aust 1969;2(12): 596–600.
14. Goldenberg RL, Culhane JF, Johnson DC. Maternal infection and adverse fetal and neonatal outcomes. Clin Perinatol 2005;32(3):523–59.
15. Romero R, Oyarzun E, Mazor M, et al. Meta-analysis of the relationship between asymptomatic bacteriuria and preterm delivery/low birth weight. Obstet Gynecol 1989;73(4):576–82.
16. Goepfert AR, Jeffcoat MK, Andrews WW, et al. Periodontal disease and upper genital tract inflammation in early spontaneous preterm birth. Obstet Gynecol 2004;104(4):777–83.
17. Srinivas SK, Sammel MD, Stamilio DM, et al. Periodontal disease and adverse pregnancy outcomes: is there an association? Am J Obstet Gynecol 2009; 200(5):497, e1–8.
18. Offenbacher S, Beck JD, Jared HL, et al. Effects of periodontal therapy on rate of preterm delivery: a randomized controlled trial. Obstet Gynecol 2009;114(3):551–9.
19. Newnham JP, Newnham IA, Ball CM, et al. Treatment of periodontal disease during pregnancy: a randomized controlled trial. Obstet Gynecol 2009;114(6): 1239–48.
20. Macones GA, Parry S, Nelson DB, et al. Treatment of localized periodontal disease in pregnancy does not reduce the occurrence of preterm birth: results from the Periodontal Infections and Prematurity Study (PIPS). Am J Obstet Gynecol 2010;202(2):147, e1–8.
21. Goncalves LF, Chaiworapongsa T, Romero R. Intrauterine infection and prematurity. Ment Retard Dev Disabil Res Rev 2002;8(1):3–13.
22. Romero R, Salafia CM, Athanassiadis AP, et al. The relationship between acute inflammatory lesions of the preterm placenta and amniotic fluid microbiology. Am J Obstet Gynecol 1992;166(5):1382–8.
23. Russell P. Inflammatory lesions of the human placenta. III. The histopathology of villitis of unknown aetiology. Placenta 1980;1(3):227–44.
24. Mueller-Heubach E, Rubinstein DN, Schwarz SS. Histologic chorioamnionitis and preterm delivery in different patient populations. Obstet Gynecol 1990; 75(4):622–6.
25. Yoon BH, Romero R, Park JS, et al. The relationship among inflammatory lesions of the umbilical cord (funisitis), umbilical cord plasma interleukin 6 concentration, amniotic fluid infection, and neonatal sepsis. Am J Obstet Gynecol 2000; 183(5):1124–9.
26. Romero R, Mazor M. Infection and preterm labor. Clin Obstet Gynecol 1988; 31(3):553–84.
27. Blumenfeld YJ, Lee HC, Gould JB, et al. The effect of preterm premature rupture of membranes on neonatal mortality rates. Obstet Gynecol 2010;116(6):1381–6.
28. Hargreaves DC, Medzhitov R. Innate sensors of microbial infection. J Clin Immunol 2005;25(6):503–10.
29. Youssef RE, Ledingham MA, Bollapragada SS, et al. The role of toll-like receptors (TLR-2 and -4) and triggering receptor expressed on myeloid cells 1 (TREM-1) in human term and preterm labor. Reprod Sci 2009;16(9):843–56.
30. Kim YM, Romero R, Chaiworapongsa T, et al. Toll-like receptor-2 and -4 in the chorioamniotic membranes in spontaneous labor at term and in preterm parturition that are associated with chorioamnionitis. Am J Obstet Gynecol 2004; 191(4):1346–55.

31. Krikun G, Lockwood CJ, Abrahams VM, et al. Expression of Toll-like receptors in the human decidua. Histol Histopathol 2007;22(8):847–54.

32. Romero R, Wu YK, Brody DT, et al. Human decidua: a source of interleukin-1. Obstet Gynecol 1989;73(1):31–4.

33. Romero R, Durum S, Dinarello CA, et al. Interleukin-1 stimulates prostaglandin biosynthesis by human amnion. Prostaglandins 1989;37(1):13–22.

34. Sadowsky DW, Novy MJ, Witkin SS, et al. Dexamethasone or interleukin-10 blocks interleukin-1beta-induced uterine contractions in pregnant rhesus monkeys. Am J Obstet Gynecol 2003;188(1):252–63.

35. Romero R, Mazor M, Tartakovsky B. Systemic administration of interleukin-1 induces preterm parturition in mice. Am J Obstet Gynecol 1991;165(4 Pt 1):969–71.

36. Andrews WW, Hauth JC, Goldenberg RL, et al. Amniotic fluid interleukin-6: correlation with upper genital tract microbial colonization and gestational age in women delivered after spontaneous labor versus indicated delivery. Am J Obstet Gynecol 1995;173(2):606–12.

37. Cox SM, King MR, Casey ML, et al. Interleukin-1 beta, -1 alpha, and -6 and prostaglandins in vaginal/cervical fluids of pregnant women before and during labor. J Clin Endocrinol Metab 1993;77(3):805–15.

38. Gomez R, Romero R, Galasso M, et al. The value of amniotic fluid interleukin-6, white blood cell count, and gram stain in the diagnosis of microbial invasion of the amniotic cavity in patients at term. Am J Reprod Immunol 1994;32(3):200–10.

39. Hillier SL, Witkin SS, Krohn MA, et al. The relationship of amniotic fluid cytokines and preterm delivery, amniotic fluid infection, histologic chorioamnionitis, and chorioamnion infection. Obstet Gynecol 1993;81(6):941–8.

40. Messer J, Eyer D, Donato L, et al. Evaluation of interleukin-6 and soluble receptors of tumor necrosis factor for early diagnosis of neonatal infection. J Pediatr 1996;129(4):574–80.

41. Romero R, Avila C, Santhanam U, et al. Amniotic fluid interleukin 6 in preterm labor. Association with infection. J Clin Invest 1990;85(5):1392–400.

42. Saito S, Kasahara T, Kato Y, et al. Elevation of amniotic fluid interleukin 6 (IL-6), IL-8 and granulocyte colony stimulating factor (G-CSF) in term and preterm parturition. Cytokine 1993;5(1):81–8.

43. Ghezzi F, Gomez R, Romero R, et al. Elevated interleukin-8 concentrations in amniotic fluid of mothers whose neonates subsequently develop bronchopulmonary dysplasia. Eur J Obstet Gynecol Reprod Biol 1998;78(1):5–10.

44. Romero R, Ceska M, Avila C, et al. Neutrophil attractant/activating peptide-1/interleukin-8 in term and preterm parturition. Am J Obstet Gynecol 1991;165(4 Pt 1):813–20.

45. Yoon BH, Romero R, Jun JK, et al. Amniotic fluid cytokines (interleukin-6, tumor necrosis factor-alpha, interleukin-1 beta, and interleukin-8) and the risk for the development of bronchopulmonary dysplasia. Am J Obstet Gynecol 1997;177(4):825–30.

46. Gonzalez C, Cava F, Ayllon A, et al. Biological variation of interleukin-1beta, interleukin-8 and tumor necrosis factor-alpha in serum of healthy individuals. Clin Chem Lab Med 2001;39(9):836–41.

47. Romero R, Mazor M, Wu YK, et al. Infection in the pathogenesis of preterm labor. Semin Perinatol 1988;12(4):262–79.

48. Casey ML, Cox SM, Beutler B, et al. Cachectin/tumor necrosis factor-alpha formation in human decidua. Potential role of cytokines in infection-induced preterm labor. J Clin Invest 1989;83(2):430–6.

49. Romero R, Mazor M, Manogue K, et al. Human decidua: a source of cachectin-tumor necrosis factor. Eur J Obstet Gynecol Reprod Biol 1991;41(2):123–7.

50. Fortunato SJ, Menon R, Lombardi SJ. Role of tumor necrosis factor-alpha in the premature rupture of membranes and preterm labor pathways. Am J Obstet Gynecol 2002;187(5):1159–62.

51. Watari K, Nakao S, Fotovati A, et al. Role of macrophages in inflammatory lymphangiogenesis: enhanced production of vascular endothelial growth factor C and D through NF-kappaB activation. Biochem Biophys Res Commun 2008;377(3):826–31.

52. Maymon E, Romero R, Pacora P, et al. Evidence of in vivo differential bioavailability of the active forms of matrix metalloproteinases 9 and 2 in parturition, spontaneous rupture of membranes, and intra-amniotic infection. Am J Obstet Gynecol 2000;183(4):887–94.

53. Romero R, Chaiworapongsa T, Espinoza J, et al. Fetal plasma MMP-9 concentrations are elevated in preterm premature rupture of the membranes. Am J Obstet Gynecol 2002;187(5):1125–30.

54. Chwalisz K, Benson M, Scholz P, et al. Cervical ripening with the cytokines interleukin 8, interleukin 1 beta and tumour necrosis factor alpha in guinea-pigs. Hum Reprod 1994;9(11):2173–81.

55. Kajikawa S, Kaga N, Futamura Y, et al. Lipoteichoic acid induces preterm delivery in mice. J Pharmacol Toxicol Methods 1998;39(3):147–54.

56. Hirsch E, Filipovich Y, Mahendroo M. Signaling via the type I IL-1 and TNF receptors is necessary for bacterially induced preterm labor in a murine model. Am J Obstet Gynecol 2006;194(5):1334–40.

57. Klein LL, Gibbs RS. Infection and preterm birth. Obstet Gynecol Clin North Am 2005;32(3):397–410.

58. Keelan JA, Blumenstein M, Helliwell RJ, et al. Cytokines, prostaglandins and parturition–a review. Placenta 2003;24(Suppl A):S33–46.

59. Romero R, Espinoza J, Kusanovic JP, et al. The preterm parturition syndrome. BJOG 2006;113(Suppl 3):17–42.

60. Mays JK, Figueroa R, Shah J, et al. Amniocentesis for selection before rescue cerclage. Obstet Gynecol 2000;95(5):652–5.

61. Romero R, Gonzalez R, Sepulveda W, et al. Infection and labor. VIII. Microbial invasion of the amniotic cavity in patients with suspected cervical incompetence: prevalence and clinical significance. Am J Obstet Gynecol 1992;167(4 Pt 1):1086–91.

62. Guzick DS, Winn K. The association of chorioamnionitis with preterm delivery. Obstet Gynecol 1985;65(1):11–6.

63. Markenson GR, Martin RK, Tillotson-Criss M, et al. The use of the polymerase chain reaction to detect bacteria in amniotic fluid in pregnancies complicated by preterm labor. Am J Obstet Gynecol 1997;177(6):1471–7.

64. Harger JH, Meyer MP, Amortegui A, et al. Low incidence of positive amnionic fluid cultures in preterm labor at 27–32 weeks in the absence of clinical evidence of chorioamnionitis. Obstet Gynecol 1991;77(2):228–34.

65. Perni SC, Vardhana S, Korneeva I, et al. Mycoplasma hominis and Ureaplasma urealyticum in midtrimester amniotic fluid: association with amniotic fluid cytokine levels and pregnancy outcome. Am J Obstet Gynecol 2004;191(4):1382–6.

66. Oh KJ, Lee SE, Jung H, et al. Detection of ureaplasmas by the polymerase chain reaction in the amniotic fluid of patients with cervical insufficiency. J Perinat Med 2010;38(3):261–8.

67. Tsekoura EA, Konstantinidou A, Papadopoulou S, et al. Adenovirus genome in the placenta: association with histological chorioamnionitis and preterm birth. J Med Virol 2010;82(8):1379–83.

68. Oyarzun E, Yamamoto M, Kato S, et al. Specific detection of 16 micro-organisms in amniotic fluid by polymerase chain reaction and its correlation with preterm delivery occurrence. Am J Obstet Gynecol 1998;179(5):1115–9.
69. Steel JH, Malatos S, Kennea N, et al. Bacteria and inflammatory cells in fetal membranes do not always cause preterm labor. Pediatr Res 2005;57(3):404–11.
70. McDonald HM, Brocklehurst P, Gordon A. Antibiotics for treating bacterial vaginosis in pregnancy. Cochrane Database Syst Rev 2007;1:CD000262.
71. Okun N, Gronau KA, Hannah ME. Antibiotics for bacterial vaginosis or Trichomonas vaginalis in pregnancy: a systematic review. Obstet Gynecol 2005;105(4): 857–68.
72. Goldenberg RL, Culhane JF. Infection as a cause of preterm birth. Clin Perinatol 2003;30(4):677–700.
73. Romero R, Espinoza J, Goncalves LF, et al. The role of inflammation and infection in preterm birth. Semin Reprod Med 2007;25(1):21–39.
74. Galask RP, Varner MW, Petzold CR, et al. Bacterial attachment to the chorioamniotic membranes. Am J Obstet Gynecol 1984;148(7):915–28.
75. Cassell GH, Davis RO, Waites KB, et al. Isolation of Mycoplasma hominis and Ureaplasma urealyticum from amniotic fluid at 16–20 weeks of gestation: potential effect on outcome of pregnancy. Sex Transm Dis 1983;10(Suppl 4): 294–302.
76. Horowitz S, Mazor M, Romero R, et al. Infection of the amniotic cavity with Ureaplasma urealyticum in the midtrimester of pregnancy. J Reprod Med 1995; 40(5):375–9.
77. Gray DJ, Robinson HB, Malone J, et al. Adverse outcome in pregnancy following amniotic fluid isolation of Ureaplasma urealyticum. Prenat Diagn 1992;12(2): 111–7.
78. King J, Flenady V. Prophylactic antibiotics for inhibiting preterm labour with intact membranes. Cochrane Database Syst Rev 2002;4:CD000246.
79. Debillon T, Gras-Leguen C, Verielle V, et al. Intrauterine infection induces programmed cell death in rabbit periventricular white matter. Pediatr Res 2000; 47(6):736–42.
80. Gibbs RS, Davies JK, McDuffie RS Jr, et al. Chronic intrauterine infection and inflammation in the preterm rabbit, despite antibiotic therapy. Am J Obstet Gynecol 2002;186(2):234–9.
81. Goldenberg RL, Mercer BM, Meis PJ, et al. The preterm prediction study: fetal fibronectin testing and spontaneous preterm birth. NICHD Maternal Fetal Medicine Units Network. Obstet Gynecol 1996;87(5 Pt 1):643–8.
82. Goldenberg RL, Klebanoff M, Carey JC, et al. Vaginal fetal fibronectin measurements from 8 to 22 weeks' gestation and subsequent spontaneous preterm birth. Am J Obstet Gynecol 2000;183(2):469–75.
83. Goldenberg RL, Thom E, Moawad AH, et al. The preterm prediction study: fetal fibronectin, bacterial vaginosis, and peripartum infection. NICHD Maternal Fetal Medicine Units Network. Obstet Gynecol 1996;87(5 Pt 1):656–60.
84. Andrews WW, Sibai BM, Thom EA, et al. Randomized clinical trial of metronidazole plus erythromycin to prevent spontaneous preterm delivery in fetal fibronectin-positive women. Obstet Gynecol 2003;101(5 Pt 1):847–55.
85. Khoury MJ, Bertram L, Boffetta P, et al. Genome-wide association studies, field synopses, and the development of the knowledge base on genetic variation and human diseases. Am J Epidemiol 2009;170(3):269–79.
86. Winkvist A, Mogren I, Hogberg U. Familial patterns in birth characteristics: impact on individual and population risks. Int J Epidemiol 1998;27(2):248–54.

87. Macones GA, Parry S, Elkousy M, et al. A polymorphism in the promoter region of TNF and bacterial vaginosis: preliminary evidence of gene-environment interaction in the etiology of spontaneous preterm birth. Am J Obstet Gynecol 2004; 190(6):1504–8 [discussion: 1503A].

88. Gomez LM, Sammel MD, Appleby DH, et al. Evidence of a gene-environment interaction that predisposes to spontaneous preterm birth: a role for asymptomatic bacterial vaginosis and DNA variants in genes that control the inflammatory response. Am J Obstet Gynecol 2010;202(4):386, e381–6.

89. Engel SA, Erichsen HC, Savitz DA, et al. Risk of spontaneous preterm birth is associated with common proinflammatory cytokine polymorphisms. Epidemiology 2005;16(4):469–77.

90. Carroll SG, Nicolaides KH. Fetal haematological response to intra-uterine infection in preterm prelabour amniorrhexis. Fetal Diagn Ther 1995;10(5): 279–85.

91. Alexander JM, Gilstrap LC, Cox SM, et al. Clinical chorioamnionitis and the prognosis for very low birth weight infants. Obstet Gynecol 1998;91(5 Pt 1): 725–9.

92. Hitti J, Tarczy-Hornoch P, Murphy J, et al. Amniotic fluid infection, cytokines, and adverse outcome among infants at 34 weeks' gestation or less. Obstet Gynecol 2001;98(6):1080–8.

93. Wu YW, Colford JM Jr. Chorioamnionitis as a risk factor for cerebral palsy: a meta-analysis. JAMA 2000;284(11):1417–24.

94. Leviton A, Paneth N. White matter damage in preterm newborns–an epidemiologic perspective. Early Hum Dev 1990;24(1):1–22.

95. Yoon BH, Romero R, Park JS, et al. Fetal exposure to an intra-amniotic inflammation and the development of cerebral palsy at the age of three years. Am J Obstet Gynecol 2000;182(3):675–81.

96. Johnson S, Hollis C, Kochhar P, et al. Psychiatric disorders in extremely preterm children: longitudinal finding at age 11 years in the EPICure study. J Am Acad Child Adolesc Psychiatry 2010;49(5):453–63, e451.

97. Schieve LA, Baio J, Rice CE, et al. Risk for cognitive deficit in a population-based sample of U.S. children with autism spectrum disorders: variation by perinatal health factors. Disabil Health J 2010;3(3):202–12.

98. Indredavik MS. Extremely preterm children at increased risk of autism spectrum disorders. Evid Based Ment Health 2010;13(3):92.

99. Johnson S, Hollis C, Kochhar P, et al. Autism spectrum disorders in extremely preterm children. J Pediatr 2010;156(4):525–31, e522.

100. Gomez R, Romero R, Ghezzi F, et al. The fetal inflammatory response syndrome. Am J Obstet Gynecol 1998;179(1):194–202.

101. Pacora P, Chaiworapongsa T, Maymon E, et al. Funisitis and chorionic vasculitis: the histological counterpart of the fetal inflammatory response syndrome. J Matern Fetal Neonatal Med 2002;11(1):18–25.

102. Romero R, Gomez R, Ghezzi F, et al. A fetal systemic inflammatory response is followed by the spontaneous onset of preterm parturition. Am J Obstet Gynecol 1998;179(1):186–93.

103. Wenstrom KD, Andrews WW, Tamura T, et al. Elevated amniotic fluid interleukin-6 levels at genetic amniocentesis predict subsequent pregnancy loss. Am J Obstet Gynecol 1996;175(4 Pt 1):830–3.

104. Arntzen KJ, Kjollesdal AM, Halgunset J, et al. IL-1, IL-6, IL-8 and soluble TNF receptors in relation to chorioamnionitis and premature labor. J Perinat Med 1998;26(1):17–26.

105. Steinborn A, Kuhnert M, Halberstadt E. Immunmodulating cytokines induce term and preterm parturition. J Perinat Med 1996;24(4):381–90.
106. Maeda K, Matsuzaki N, Fuke S, et al. Value of the maternal interleukin 6 level for determination of histologic chorioamnionitis in preterm delivery. Gynecol Obstet Invest 1997;43(4):225–31.
107. Tu FF, Goldenberg RL, Tamura T, et al. Prenatal plasma matrix metalloproteinase-9 levels to predict spontaneous preterm birth. Obstet Gynecol 1998;92(3):446–9.
108. Wei SQ, Fraser W, Luo ZC. Inflammatory cytokines and spontaneous preterm birth in asymptomatic women: a systematic review. Obstet Gynecol 2010;116(2 Pt 1): 393–401.
109. Thomakos N, Daskalakis G, Papapanagiotou A, et al. Amniotic fluid interleukin-6 and tumor necrosis factor-alpha at mid-trimester genetic amniocentesis: relationship to intra-amniotic microbial invasion and preterm delivery. Eur J Obstet Gynecol Reprod Biol 2010;148(2):147–51.
110. Daskalakis G, Thomakos N, Papapanagiotou A, et al. Amniotic fluid interleukin-18 at mid-trimester genetic amniocentesis: relationship to intraamniotic microbial invasion and preterm delivery. BJOG 2009;116(13):1743–8.
111. Kusanovic JP, Romero R, Jodicke C, et al. Amniotic fluid soluble human leukocyte antigen-G in term and preterm parturition, and intra-amniotic infection/inflammation. J Matern Fetal Neonatal Med 2009;22(12):1151–66.
112. Soto E, Romero R, Richani K, et al. Evidence for complement activation in the amniotic fluid of women with spontaneous preterm labor and intra-amniotic infection. J Matern Fetal Neonatal Med 2009;22(11):983–92.
113. Bastek JA, Brown AG, Anton L, et al. Biomarkers of inflammation and placental dysfunction are associated with subsequent preterm birth. J Matern Fetal Neonatal Med 2011;24(4):600–5.
114. Lockwood CJ, Senyei AE, Dische MR, et al. Fetal fibronectin in cervical and vaginal secretions as a predictor of preterm delivery. N Engl J Med 1991;325(10):669–74.
115. Feinberg RF, Kliman HJ, Lockwood CJ. Is oncofetal fibronectin a trophoblast glue for human implantation? Am J Pathol 1991;138(3):537–43.
116. Lu GC, Goldenberg RL, Cliver SP, et al. Vaginal fetal fibronectin levels and spontaneous preterm birth in symptomatic women. Obstet Gynecol 2001;97(2):225–8.
117. Meis PJ, Klebanoff M, Thom E, et al. Prevention of recurrent preterm delivery by 17 alpha-hydroxyprogesterone caproate. N Engl J Med 2003;348(24):2379–85.
118. Beck P, Adler P, Szlachter N, et al. Synergistic effect of human relaxin and progesterone on human myometrial contractions. Int J Gynaecol Obstet 1982;20(2): 141–4.
119. Astle S, Slater DM, Thornton S. The involvement of progesterone in the onset of human labour. Eur J Obstet Gynecol Reprod Biol 2003;108(2):177–81.
120. Buhimschi IA, Buhimschi CS, Weiner CP. Protective effect of N-acetylcysteine against fetal death and preterm labor induced by maternal inflammation. Am J Obstet Gynecol 2003;188(1):203–8.
121. Vrachnis N, Vitoratos N, Iliodromiti Z, et al. Intrauterine inflammation and preterm delivery. Ann N Y Acad Sci 2010;1205:118–22.
122. Cowchock S. Prevention of fetal death in the antiphospholipid antibody syndrome. Lupus 1996;5(5):467–72.
123. Kramer BW, Moss TJ, Willet KE, et al. Dose and time response after intraamniotic endotoxin in preterm lambs. Am J Respir Crit Care Med 2001;164(6):982–8.
124. Newnham JP, Moss TJ, Kramer BW, et al. The fetal maturational and inflammatory responses to different routes of endotoxin infusion in sheep. Am J Obstet Gynecol 2002;186(5):1062–8.

125. Mitchell BF, Taggart MJ. Are animal models relevant to key aspects of human parturition? Am J Physiol Regul Integr Comp Physiol 2009;297(3):R525–45.

126. Gravett MG, Adams KM, Sadowsky DW, et al. Immunomodulators plus antibiotics delay preterm delivery after experimental intraamniotic infection in a nonhuman primate model. Am J Obstet Gynecol 2007;197(5):518, e511–8.

127. Hirsch E, Saotome I, Hirsh D. A model of intrauterine infection and preterm delivery in mice. Am J Obstet Gynecol 1995;172(5):1598–603.

128. Elovitz MA, Wang Z, Chien EK, et al. A new model for inflammation-induced preterm birth: the role of platelet-activating factor and Toll-like receptor-4. Am J Pathol 2003;163(5):2103–11.

129. Warburton D, Schwarz M, Tefft D, et al. The molecular basis of lung morphogenesis. Mech Dev 2000;92(1):55–81.

130. Elovitz MA, Mrinalini C. Can medroxyprogesterone acetate alter Toll-like receptor expression in a mouse model of intrauterine inflammation? Am J Obstet Gynecol 2005;193(3 Pt 2):1149–55.

131. Elovitz MA, Mrinalini C. The use of progestational agents for preterm birth: lessons from a mouse model. Am J Obstet Gynecol 2006;195(4):1004–10.

132. Schlafer DH, Yuh B, Foley GL, et al. Effect of Salmonella endotoxin administered to the pregnant sheep at 133–142 days gestation on fetal oxygenation, maternal and fetal adrenocorticotropic hormone and cortisol, and maternal plasma tumor necrosis factor alpha concentrations. Biol Reprod 1994;50(6):1297–302.

133. Grigsby PL, Hirst JJ, Scheerlinck JP, et al. Fetal responses to maternal and intraamniotic lipopolysaccharide administration in sheep. Biol Reprod 2003;68(5):1695–702.

134. Dombroski RA, Woodard DS, Harper MJ, et al. A rabbit model for bacteria-induced preterm pregnancy loss. Am J Obstet Gynecol 1990;163(6 Pt 1):1938–43.

135. Heddleston L, McDuffie RS Jr, Gibbs RS. A rabbit model for ascending infection in pregnancy: intervention with indomethacin and delayed ampicillin-sulbactam therapy. Am J Obstet Gynecol 1993;169(3):708–12.

136. Davies JK, Shikes RH, Sze CI, et al. Histologic inflammation in the maternal and fetal compartments in a rabbit model of acute intra-amniotic infection. Am J Obstet Gynecol 2000;183(5):1088–93.

137. Grigsby PL, Novy MJ, Waldorf KM, et al. Choriodecidual inflammation: a harbinger of the preterm labor syndrome. Reprod Sci 2010;17(1):85–94.

138. Gravett MG, Witkin SS, Haluska GJ, et al. An experimental model for intraamniotic infection and preterm labor in rhesus monkeys. Am J Obstet Gynecol 1994;171(6):1660–7.

139. Novy MJ, Duffy L, Axthelm MK, et al. Ureaplasma parvum or Mycoplasma hominis as sole pathogens cause chorioamnionitis, preterm delivery, and fetal pneumonia in rhesus macaques. Reprod Sci 2009;16(1):56–70.

140. Sadowsky DW, Haluska GJ, Gravett MG, et al. Indomethacin blocks interleukin 1beta-induced myometrial contractions in pregnant rhesus monkeys. Am J Obstet Gynecol 2000;183(1):173–80.

141. Sadowsky DW, Adams KM, Gravett MG, et al. Preterm labor is induced by intraamniotic infusions of interleukin-1beta and tumor necrosis factor-alpha but not by interleukin-6 or interleukin-8 in a nonhuman primate model. Am J Obstet Gynecol 2006;195(6):1578–89.

142. Fidel PL Jr, Romero R, Wolf N, et al. Systemic and local cytokine profiles in endotoxin-induced preterm parturition in mice. Am J Obstet Gynecol 1994;170(5 Pt 1):1467–75.

143. Kaga N, Katsuki Y, Obata M, et al. Repeated administration of low-dose lipo-polysaccharide induces preterm delivery in mice: a model for human preterm parturition and for assessment of the therapeutic ability of drugs against preterm delivery. Am J Obstet Gynecol 1996;174(2):754–9.

144. Hirsch E, Muhle RA, Mussalli GM, et al. Bacterially induced preterm labor in the mouse does not require maternal interleukin-1 signaling. Am J Obstet Gynecol 2002;186(3):523–30.

145. Wang H, Hirsch E. Bacterially-induced preterm labor and regulation of prostaglandin-metabolizing enzyme expression in mice: the role of toll-like receptor 4. Biol Reprod 2003;69(6):1957–63.

146. Liu H, Redline RW, Han YW. Fusobacterium nucleatum induces fetal death in mice via stimulation of TLR4-mediated placental inflammatory response. J Immunol 2007;179(4):2501–8.

147. Alexopoulou L, Holt AC, Medzhitov R, et al. Recognition of double-stranded RNA and activation of NF-kappaB by Toll-like receptor 3. Nature 2001; 413(6857):732–8.

148. Kawai T, Adachi O, Ogawa T, et al. Unresponsiveness of MyD88-deficient mice to endotoxin. Immunity 1999;11(1):115–22.

149. Filipovich Y, Lu SJ, Akira S, et al. The adaptor protein MyD88 is essential for E coli-induced preterm delivery in mice. Am J Obstet Gynecol 2009;200(1): 93.e91–8.

150. Word RA, Li XH, Hnat M, et al. Dynamics of cervical remodeling during pregnancy and parturition: mechanisms and current concepts. Semin Reprod Med 2007;25(1):69–79.

151. Gonzalez JM, Xu H, Chai J, et al. Preterm and term cervical ripening in CD1 Mice (Mus musculus): similar or divergent molecular mechanisms? Biol Reprod 2009;81(6):1226–32.

152. Straach KJ, Shelton JM, Richardson JA, et al. Regulation of hyaluronan expression during cervical ripening. Glycobiology 2005;15(1):55–65.

153. Liggins GC. Ripening of the cervix. Semin Perinatol 1978;2(3):261–71.

154. Kelly RW. Inflammatory mediators and cervical ripening. J Reprod Immunol 2002;57(1/2):217–24.

155. Hassan SS, Romero R, Haddad R, et al. The transcriptome of the uterine cervix before and after spontaneous term parturition. Am J Obstet Gynecol 2006; 195(3):778–86.

156. Timmons BC, Fairhurst AM, Mahendroo MS. Temporal changes in myeloid cells in the cervix during pregnancy and parturition. J Immunol 2009;182(5):2700–7.

157. Uchiyama T, Sakuta T, Kanayama T. Regulation of hyaluronan synthases in mouse uterine cervix. Biochem Biophys Res Commun 2005;327(3):927–32.

158. Elovitz M, Wang Z. Medroxyprogesterone acetate, but not progesterone, protects against inflammation-induced parturition and intrauterine fetal demise. Am J Obstet Gynecol 2004;190(3):693–701.

159. Timmons B, Akins M, Mahendroo M. Cervical remodeling during pregnancy and parturition. Trends Endocrinol Metab 2010;21(6):353–61.

160. Timmons BC, Mahendroo M. Processes regulating cervical ripening differ from cervical dilation and postpartum repair: insights from gene expression studies. Reprod Sci 2007;14(Suppl 8):53–62.

161. Xu H, Gonzalez JM, Ofori E, et al. Preventing cervical ripening: the primary mechanism by which progestational agents prevent preterm birth? Am J Obstet Gynecol 2008;198(3):314, e311–8.

162. Hirsch E, Wang H. The molecular pathophysiology of bacterially induced preterm labor: insights from the murine model. J Soc Gynecol Investig 2005; 12(3):145–55.

163. Bry K, Hallman M. Transforming growth factor-beta opposes the stimulatory effects of interleukin-1 and tumor necrosis factor on amnion cell prostaglandin E2 production: implication for preterm labor. Am J Obstet Gynecol 1992;167(1): 222–6.

164. Grether JK, Nelson KB. Maternal infection and cerebral palsy in infants of normal birth weight. JAMA 1997;278(3):207–11.

165. Dammann O, Leviton A. Infection remote from the brain, neonatal white matter damage, and cerebral palsy in the preterm infant. Semin Pediatr Neurol 1998; 5(3):190–201.

166. Limperopoulos C, Bassan H, Sullivan NR, et al. Positive screening for autism in ex-preterm infants: prevalence and risk factors. Pediatrics 2008;121(4):758–65.

167. Lindstrom K, Lindblad F, Hjern A. Psychiatric morbidity in adolescents and young adults born preterm: a Swedish national cohort study. Pediatrics 2009; 123(1):e47–53.

168. Elovitz MA, Mrinalini C, Sammel MD. Elucidating the early signal transduction pathways leading to fetal brain injury in preterm birth. Pediatr Res 2006;59(1): 50–5.

169. Burd I, Chai J, Gonzalez J, et al. Beyond white matter damage: fetal neuronal injury in a mouse model of preterm birth. Am J Obstet Gynecol 2009;201(3): 279, e271–8.

170. Bell MJ, Hallenbeck JM. Effects of intrauterine inflammation on developing rat brain. J Neurosci Res 2002;70(4):570–9.

171. Burd I, Bentz AI, Chai J, et al. Inflammation-induced preterm birth alters neuronal morphology in the mouse fetal brain. J Neurosci Res 2010;88(9): 1872–81.

172. Terrone DA, Rinehart BK, Granger JP, et al. Interleukin-10 administration and bacterial endotoxin-induced preterm birth in a rat model. Obstet Gynecol 2001;98(3):476–80.

173. Scott DL, Wolfe F, Huizinga TW. Rheumatoid arthritis. Lancet 2010;376(9746): 1094–108.

174. Szekeres-Bartho J, Barakonyi A, Par G, et al. Progesterone as an immunomodulatory molecule. Int Immunopharmacol 2001;1(6):1037–48.

175. Bamberger CM, Else T, Bamberger AM, et al. Dissociative glucocorticoid activity of medroxyprogesterone acetate in normal human lymphocytes. J Clin Endocrinol Metab 1999;84(11):4055–61.

176. Simoncini T, Mannella P, Fornari L, et al. Differential signal transduction of progesterone and medroxyprogesterone acetate in human endothelial cells. Endocrinology 2004;145(12):5745–56.

177. Adams Waldorf KM, Persing D, Novy MJ, et al. Pretreatment with toll-like receptor 4 antagonist inhibits lipopolysaccharide-induced preterm uterine contractility, cytokines, and prostaglandins in rhesus monkeys. Reprod Sci 2008;15(2):121–7.

178. Lappas M, Permezel M, Georgiou HM, et al. Regulation of phospholipase isozymes by nuclear factor-kappaB in human gestational tissues in vitro. J Clin Endocrinol Metab 2004;89(5):2365–72.

179. Barnes PJ, Karin M. Nuclear factor-kappaB: a pivotal transcription factor in chronic inflammatory diseases. N Engl J Med 1997;336(15):1066–71.

180. Schenk H, Klein M, Erdbrugger W, et al. Distinct effects of thioredoxin and anti-oxidants on the activation of transcription factors NF-kappa B and AP-1. Proc Natl Acad Sci U S A 1994;91(5):1672–6.
181. Kim H, Seo JY, Roh KH, et al. Suppression of NF-kappaB activation and cytokine production by N-acetylcysteine in pancreatic acinar cells. Free Radic Biol Med 2000;29(7):674–83.
182. Verhasselt V, Vanden Berghe W, Vanderheyde N, et al. N-acetyl-L-cysteine inhibits primary human T cell responses at the dendritic cell level: association with NF-kappaB inhibition. J Immunol 1999;162(5):2569–74.
183. Pahan K, Sheikh FG, Namboodiri AM, et al. N-acetyl cysteine inhibits induction of no production by endotoxin or cytokine stimulated rat peritoneal macro-phages, C6 glial cells and astrocytes. Free Radic Biol Med 1998;24(1):39–48.
184. Paintlia MK, Paintlia AS, Singh AK, et al. Attenuation of lipopolysaccharide-induced inflammatory response and phospholipids metabolism at the feto-maternal interface by N-acetyl cysteine. Pediatr Res 2008;64(4):334–9.
185. Xu DX, Chen YH, Wang H, et al. Effect of N-acetylcysteine on lipopolysaccharide-induced intra-uterine fetal death and intra-uterine growth retardation in mice. Toxicol Sci 2005;88(2):525–33.
186. Probyn ME, Cock ML, Duncan JR, et al. The anti-inflammatory agent N-acetyl cysteine exacerbates endotoxin-induced hypoxemia and hypotension and induces polycythemia in the ovine fetus. Neonatology 2010;98(2):118–27.

Abruption-Associated Prematurity

Christina S. Han, MD*, Frederick Schatz, PhD,
Charles J. Lockwood, MD

KEYWORDS

- Decidua • Hemorrhage • Prematurity • Abruption
- Inflammation • Cytokines

Despite intense investigations into its pathogenesis and prevention, preterm delivery (PTD) remains a major public health concern. In 2008, the preterm birth rate in United States was 12.3%, with PTD a major worldwide contributor of perinatal morbidity and mortality.[1] Long-term sequelae of prematurity include pulmonary dysfunction, blindness, hearing loss, gastrointestinal malfunction, intraventricular hemorrhage, mental retardation, and cerebral palsy. Health care costs associated with these acute and chronic complications of prematurity exceed $26 billion per year.[2]

An increasing body of evidence now links decidual hemorrhage (DH) to PTD, with approximately 10% of all PTD attributed to bleeding-related events.[3] While vaginal bleeding can rarely arise from cervical polyps, most cases originate from the decidua basalis (placental abruption) or the decidua parietalis (retrochorionic hematoma). The occurrence of vaginal bleeding in the first trimester and in more than one trimester is respectively associated with two- and seven-fold increased risks of PTD compared with no bleeding.[4–8] The occurrence of a clinically evident abruption, together with occult DH and retrochorionic hematoma formation, complicates almost 40% of PTDs due to preterm labor with intact membrane and preterm premature rupture of the fetal membranes (PPROM) between 22 and 38 weeks, versus 0.8% after term delivery ($P<.01$).[7]

Beyond inducing prematurity, pregnancies complicated by placental abruption display an increase in perinatal mortality beginning at about 28 weeks of gestation (**Fig. 1**). The resulting neonates exhibit increased rates of perinatal asphyxia, intraventricular hemorrhage, periventricular leukomalacia, cerebral palsy, and mortality, compared with age-matched controls.[9,10] The demographic profile of DH-associated PTD differs from infection-associated PTD, with the former occurring more frequently in patients who are married, older, white, parous, college-educated and tobacco users.[11] Other risk factors for DH include PPROM (thus, DH is both a cause and

---

The authors have nothing to disclose.
Department of Obstetrics, Gynecology & Reproductive Sciences, Yale University School of Medicine, 333 Cedar Street, New Haven, CT 06520-8063, USA
* Corresponding author.
E-mail address: christina.han@yale.edu

Clin Perinatol 38 (2011) 407–421
doi:10.1016/j.clp.2011.06.001
0095-5108/11/$ – see front matter © 2011 Elsevier Inc. All rights reserved.

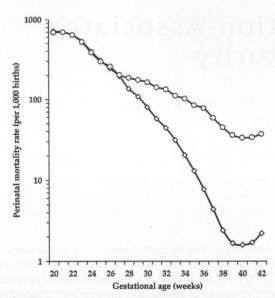

Fig. 1. Perinatal mortality in pregnancies with and without abruption across gestation, 2000–2002. Circles, pregnancies with abruption; Diamonds, pregnancies without abruption. (*From* Oyelese Y, Ananth CV. Placental abruption. Obstet Gynecol 2006;108(4):1007; with permission.)

consequence of this condition), as well as trauma, substance use, hypertensive disorders, renal disorders, multiple gestations, rapid uterine decompression, and history of abruption in a prior pregnancy (**Table 1**).[12–15]

DECIDUALIZATION

Each menstrual cycle begins with hypoxia-induced angiogenesis and estradiol (E_2)-induced proliferation of epithelium and stromal cells, which had been sloughed off at the end of the previous infertile cycle. Coincident with the occurrence of ovulation is an elevation in plasma progesterone (P_4) levels, which blocks further mitotic activity and initiates differentiation of the E_2-primed cells. In the luteal phase of the human menstrual cycle, P_4 stimulates E_2-primed human endometrial stromal cells to decidualize.[16,17]

The process of decidualization begins around blood vessels and beneath the glands. It involves changes in differentiation that transform the interstitial extracellular matrix (ECM) of the follicular phase endometrium to an ECM enriched with basal laminar-type proteins and proteins that promote hemostasis. Under continued P_4 stimulation, decidualization spreads wave-like throughout the late luteal phase endometrium.[18]

After implantation, blastocyst-derived extravillous trophoblasts (EVTs) traverse the decidua and enter the inner third of the myometrium. This stepwise process begins with attachment of EVT-expressed adhesion molecules to specific basal laminar proteins in the decidual ECM.[19] Trophoblasts then breach decidual capillaries to provide the embryo with a rich source of oxygen and nutrients, and eventually remodel maternal spiral arteries to form high-capacitance, low-resistance vessels that increase blood flow to the fetal–placental unit.[20] Invasion of decidual capillaries and arteries occurs within a matrix of decidual cells that express tissue factor (TF) under continued

Table 1
Risk factors for decidual hemorrhage

Risk Factor	OR or RR
Trauma	4.3–15.0
Cocaine use	5.0–10.0
Oligohydramnios	2.5–10
Chorioamnionitis	2.0–2.5
Maternal age and parity	1.1–3.7
Hypertensive disorders	
Eclampsia	3.3–3.9
Chronic hypertension with preeclampsia	7.8
Chronic hypertension	1.8–5.1
Mild and severe preeclampsia	0.4–4.5
PPROM	1.8–5.1
Multiple gestations	1.5–3.0
Alcohol use	1.5–1.7
Renal disorders	1.4–1.8
Tobacco use	1.4–2.5
Dietary or nutritional deficiency	0.9–2.0
Male fetus	0.9–1.3

Abbreviations: OR, odds ratio; PPROM, preterm premature rupture of membranes; RR, relative risk.
Data from Refs.[12–14]

stimulation by P_4. Elevated decidual cell expression of TF is temporally and spatially positioned to promote hemostasis during this invasive process.[21]

ROLE OF TISSUE FACTOR

TF is a transmembrane 45-kDa glycoprotein member of the class 2 cytokine receptor family.[21–23] Unlike endothelial cells, which do not normally express TF, tissues that are highly vulnerable to bleeding such as the brain and placental villi constitutively express high levels of TF.[24,25] Expression of TF may provide an evolutionary advantage in prevention of fatal hemorrhage. In human endometrial stromal cells, P_4 uniquely induces high levels of TF to prevent hemorrhage during placentation, but in the absence of a conception, P_4 withdrawal promotes inhibition of TF expression to facilitate menstruation.[22]

In response to vascular injury, the clotting cascade is initiated by binding of extravasated circulating factor VII to the hydrophilic extracellular domain of perivascular cell membrane-bound TF. Factor VII auto-activates upon binding to TF to form the TF/VIIa complex, and triggers a greater than 100-fold increase in catalytic activity.[26] The TF/VIIa complex cleaves prothrombin to thrombin, which then ultimately converts fibrinogen to fibrin. The final hemostatic plug is formed when fibrin monomers self-polymerize and are cross-linked by thrombin-activated factor XIIIa.[27,28] Simultaneously, thrombin induces platelet plug formation. The clotting cascade (**Fig. 2**) meets maternal hemostatic demands, beginning at the initial breach of decidual capillaries by syncytiotrophoblast, through EVT remodeling of spiral arteries,[20,29] and finally during physiologic placental detachment at the third stage of labor.[29]

The maternal–fetal interface at term displays prominent immunostaining for TF in decidual cells while cytotrophoblasts are virtually devoid of TF immunostaining.[30]

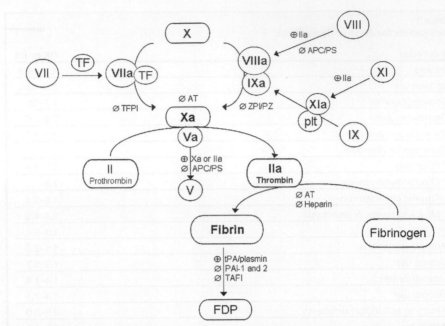

Fig. 2. Hemostatic, thrombotic, and fibrinolytic pathways. Ø, inhibitory effect; ⊕, stimulatory effect. (*From* Han CS, Paidas MJ, Lockwood CJ. Clotting disorders. In: James DK, Steer PJ, Weiner CP, et al, editors. High-risk pregnancy: management options. New York: Saunders; 2010. p. 740; with permission.)

That abruption-induced thrombin formation is promoted by decidual cell-expressed TF and linked to PTD as indicated by:

- The standard use of fibrinogen consumption to measure abruption severity
- Enhanced fibrin deposition in the decidua
- The high sensitivity and specificity with which elevated circulating thrombin–antithrombin (TAT) complex levels predict the subsequent occurrence of PTD associated with PTL or PPROM.[31–34]

DIRECT AND INDIRECT ROLES FOR THROMBIN IN PTD AND PPROM

Through this protective cascade, abruption results in an intense local generation of thrombin, which paradoxically predisposes to PPROM and PTD. In addition to promoting hemostasis via its extracellular actions, thrombin induces several biologic effects via decidual cell membrane-bound protease-activated receptors (PARs), a family of four distinct 7-membrane G protein-coupled receptors. As is the case for thrombin, each PAR ligand is a serine protease that binds to and cleaves its receptor to expose an N-terminal tethered ligand domain that autoactivates the cleaved receptor.[34]

Among its protean cellular effects, thrombin induces proliferation and chemotaxis of pro-inflammatory immune and mesenchymal cells and activates endothelial cells via PAR-1, 3, and 4. In contrast, PAR-2 is primarily a receptor for trypsin and trypsin-like enzymes, which include the TF/VIIa complex.[35–37] Binding to PARs can directly induce production of matrix metalloproteinases (MMPs), which degrade various ECM components.[38–40] Bioengineering measurements taken together with comprehensive histologic and biochemical observations indicate that the fibrillar collagen-rich amnion and choriodecidua ECM provide greater than additive tensile strength and structural integrity that withstand disruptive forces derived from the human fetus and myometrium.[41] The weakest membrane component, the choriodecidua, was observed to rupture first, followed by its amnion support structure. Proteases secreted by neighboring cell types degrade collagens I and IV in the ECM of choriodecidua and amnion, thereby impairing the integrity and strength of these ECMs.[42]

The MMPs are the primary mediators of ECM degradation. Specifically, the collagenases, exemplified by MMP-1, effectively degrade fibrillar collagens; additionally, the stromelysins, exemplified by MMP-3, degrade a broad array of ECM components, as well as activate the secreted zymogenic forms of pro-MMP-1 and pro-MMP-9 to promote an ECM-degrading cascade. Finally, the gelatinases, exemplified by MMP-9 and MMP-2, preferentially degrade basal laminar proteins such as collagen IV.[38–45] In cultured human term decidual cells, thrombin markedly augments MMP-1 and MMP-3.[46,47] Third trimester human decidua contains abundant, constitutively expressed MMP-2, as well as the key regulators of MMP activity, tissue inhibitors of MMPs (TIMP-1 and TIMP-2).[19] A rich decidual infiltrate of neutrophils, which express high levels of such ECM-degrading proteases as elastase, collagenase, and MMP-9, accompanies abruption-induced PPROM even in the absence of infection.[48–50]

The association between PPROM and intra-amniotic infections is well-established, and strong evidence now links PPROM with placental abruption in the absence of infection.[5] In the amniotic fluid of women with PTD and coexisting chorioamnionitis, levels of interleukin-8 (IL-8), the primary neutrophil chemoattractant and activator,[51,52] and IL-6, a decisive mediator of chronic inflammation, are elevated.[53,54] Similarly, the authors observed that thrombin elicited a dose-dependent elevation in IL-8 secretion by decidual cells compared with untreated cultures ($P<.05$), with 2.5 U/mL of thrombin increasing IL-8 levels by greater than 14-fold.[55] The decidua of placental sections of abruption-induced PPROM in the absence of infection showed colocalization of the immunoreactive IL-8 with fibrin deposits consistent with thrombin induction of IL-8 production by decidual cells. Furthermore, immunostaining for the neutrophil marker CD15 in placentas after overt abruption, with or without PPROM, showed marked decidual neutrophil infiltration that peaked after PPROM, whereas decidua from gestational age-matched controls were virtually devoid of neutrophils. Neutrophil infiltrates also colocalized with fibrin deposition. As a rich source of proteases, neutrophils contribute to degradation of ECM and abruption-mediated PPROM.[52]

Additionally, thrombin has been shown to be a potent direct uterotonic agent both in vitro and in vivo.[56] Using a rat model, thrombin was shown to increase frequency, intensity, and tone of myometrial contractions in a dose-dependent manner. Pretreatment of thrombin with hirudin, a thrombin inactivator, or heparin suppressed the uterotonic effects of thrombin.

Therefore, during DH, thrombin generated from TF localized on the cell membranes of decidual cells is positioned to induce PPROM and PTD directly via enhanced decidual cell-expressed MMP expression, and indirectly by promoting neutrophil trafficking and uterine contractility, as summarized in **Fig. 3**. These pathologic mechanisms together contribute to a 7-fold increase in risk of PPROM when vaginal bleeding is seen in more than one trimester.[6–8]

CLINICAL MANIFESTATIONS OF DECIDUAL HEMORRHAGE

Abruptions associated with preterm labor and PPROM usually reflect subacute, chronic processes. However, acute, clinically evident abruptions can lead to both

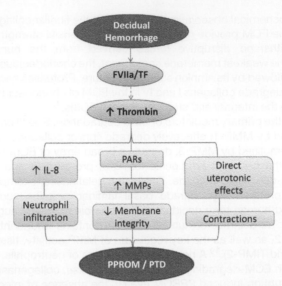

Fig. 3. Pathway to prematurity from decidual hemorrhage. *Abbreviations:* ECM, extracellular matrix; FVIIa, activated factor VII; MMP, matrix metalloproteinases; PAR, protease-activated receptors; TF, tissue factor. (*Courtesy of* Charles J. Lockwood, MD, New Haven, Connecticut.)

maternal and fetal death. Abruptions are defined as the partial or complete separation of a normally implanted placenta from the placental implantation site before delivery. Abruption occurs in 0.48% to 1.8% of pregnancies, and its incidence may be increasing.[57,58] In recent decades, a disproportionate increase has been seen in African American women.[59] The incidence of abruption is highest between 24 and 28 weeks of gestation and decreases as gestation advances (**Fig. 4**).[9,10]

Diagnosis of placental abruption is based on classical clinical findings of vaginal bleeding, abdominal pain, and increased uterine contractions. Differential diagnoses include placenta previa, vasa previa, cervical lesions, infection (cervicitis), trauma, urinary source, and others.[60] Approximately, 10% to 35% of abruptions may be concealed within the uterus, and therefore result in clinical underestimation of blood loss.[61,62]

Physical examination may reveal a rigid abdomen secondary to tetanic contractions or Couvelaire uterus, vaginal bleeding, and evidence of maternal hypoperfusion or fetal distress. Cardiotocography may display uterine tachysystole with or without a National Institute of Child Health and Human Development (NICHD) category 3 fetal heart rate tracing. Although ultrasound evaluation of the placenta can sometimes show presence of a retroplacental or retrochorionic hematoma, approximately 50% of placental abruptions produce no distinct ultrasound findings.[10] Clinical sequelae include fetal manifestations of uteroplacental insufficiency, maternal complications of hemorrhage, or as previously described, premature birth.

The severity of DH ranges from subclinical separation of the placenta, incidentally detected on ultrasound or on gross examination of placenta after delivery, to major abruption with associated clinical sequelae. The grading of placental abruptions is seen in **Table 2**. Grade 3 placental abruption occurs in approximately 0.2% of pregnancies.[61] Formation of a hematoma in the decidua may result in compression

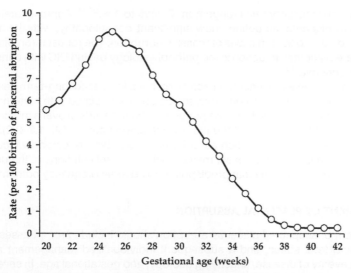

Fig. 4. Rates of abruption across gestation, United States, 2000–2002. (*From* Oyelese Y, Ananth CV. Placental abruption. Obstet Gynecol 2006;108(4):1007; with permission.)

of the overlying intervillous space, local destruction of the placental parenchyma, and fetal hypoxia. Therefore, chronic placental abruption often manifests as uteroplacental insufficiency, fetal growth restriction, or oligohydramnios. Most pregnancies complicated by abruption result in the delivery of an infant weighing less than the 10th percentile for gestational age.[62]

In severe cases, placental abruption involving greater than 50% separation can result in intrauterine fetal demise.[10] With a perinatal mortality rate of approximately 12%, placental abruption carries a 15-fold increase in risk of intrauterine and neonatal demise compared with controls. At the optimal gestational age of 40 weeks (when overall perinatal mortality normally nadirs), perinatal mortality was 19-fold greater for abruption complicated than for nonabruption-associated births (34.6 vs 1.8 per 1000 births, respectively). Mortality with abruption was more likely to occur antepartum than after delivery (relative risk for stillbirth was 18 compared with 10 for neonatal death).[63]

Maternal sequelae of placental abruption include complications of severe hemorrhage, such as hypotension, hysterectomy, disseminated intravascular coagulation (DIC), massive transfusions, intensive care unit admission, and multisystem organ

Table 2					
Grading of placental abruption					
Grade	Vaginal Bleeding	Uterine Tetany	Fetal Distress	Maternal Shock	Ultrasound Finding
0	−	−	−	−	Small retroplacental clot
1	+	+/−	−	−	+/−
2	+/−	+/−	+	−	+/−
3	+/−	+	Fetal demise	+ with possible coagulopathy	+/−

Data from Bernischke K, Kaufmann P. Pathology of the human placenta. New York: Springer; 2000.

failure. Maternal mortality rates range from 0.04% to 1%.[64,65] Approximately 10% of patients with placental abruption show significant coagulopathy, with the incidence increasing to 20% to 30% in cases of massive abruption. The robust thrombin production in severe placental abruption is the pathophysiology behind DIC with consumptive hypofibrinogenemia.[10]

Women who have experienced an abruption have increased long-term health risks. Placental abruption with fetal compromise has been associated with maternal cardiovascular sequelae later in life in a large population-based study of over a million women, with an adjusted hazard ratio of 2.0 (95% confidence interval [CI]: 1.7–2.2).[66] These future cardiovascular events, such as ischemic heart disease, cerebrovascular accident, and peripheral artery disease, may be delayed manifestations of the underlying maternal vascular pathology that predisposed to adverse pregnancy outcomes.

MANAGEMENT OF PLACENTAL ABRUPTION

Management of suspected placental abruption should include prompt assessment of maternal and fetal status, and a subsequent individualized management algorithm based on severity of disease, underlying etiology, and gestational age. In severe cases of placental abruption with life-threatening hemorrhage, maternal hemodynamic stabilization is the priority. As previously mentioned, most maternal complications result from hypovolemic shock secondary to massive blood loss, whether concealed or clinically visible. Maternal vital signs, including blood pressure, heart rate, and urine output should be closely monitored. Hypovolemia may be masked in cases of abruption in which severe hypertension is the etiology.

Crystalloid, colloid, and blood product resuscitation may be initiated through 2 wide-bore intravenous lines, if necessary. Identification and correction of underlying risk factors, such as trauma, or a hypertensive crisis, also play an important role in the management of placental abruption. A multidisciplinary approach should be undertaken, if available, with appropriate consultations with perinatologists, neonatologists, anesthesiologists, operating room staff, blood bank personnel, and intensive care specialists.

Laboratory evaluation should include blood type and Rhesus-D status, complete blood counts, coagulation studies, and cross-matching of blood products. Hypofibrinogenemia is a result of the intense thrombin response and is the most sensitive indicator of coagulopathy. Prothrombin time and partial thromboplastin time may be elevated in cases of severe abruption. Kleihauer-Betke, an acid elution test employed to assess the presence of fetal hemoglobin in maternal circulation, may be useful in calculation of Rhesus-D immunoglobulin dosage in patients who are Rhesus-D negative.

If the fetus is at a gestational age deemed to be potentially viable, continuous fetal cardiotocography should be initiated to determine fetal well-being. Antenatal corticosteroids may be administered between 24 + 0/7 to 33 + 6/7 weeks of gestation for promotion of fetal lung maturity and prevention of prematurity-associated complications. If fetal decompensation unresponsive to intrauterine resuscitation occurs or the fetus is above 34 + 0/7 weeks of gestation, delivery should be expeditiously effected. Vaginal delivery can be attempted if the fetal heart rate tracing remains reassuring and the maternal status remains stable. Given the intense uterotonic effects of thrombin, patients may often undergo spontaneous labor without need for induction or augmentation. Cesarean delivery should be performed if the patient is remote from delivery with evidence of fetal distress, intolerance of labor, or for routine obstetric indications.

In the case of an intrauterine fetal demise secondary to a massive abruption, the mode of delivery is dependent on maternal status, severity of hemorrhage, and other obstetric complicating factors, such as prior classical hysterotomy incision. Vaginal delivery is the preferred modality in most cases, unless urgent delivery is necessary for maternal stabilization.

If the mother and fetus are both stable, such as in a mild, subacute, or chronic abruption, ultrasound evaluation of the intrauterine environment may be undertaken, including assessment of the placental location, placental appearance, amniotic fluid index, and fetal growth. Placenta previa may be present in 10% of placental abruptions.

Ultrasonographic appearance of a hematoma evolves over time. In the acute phase, the blood is hyperechoic to isoechoic when compared with the placenta. (**Figs. 5** and **6**) As the hematoma organizes and resolves, the insult appears hypoechoic within a week and may be anechoic within 2 weeks.[67] (**Figs. 7** and **8**) Exclusion of a retroplacental hematoma, however, does not exclude the presence of placental abruption.

The use of tocolytics in placental abruption has classically been discouraged; however, a few small nonrandomized studies have shown possible benefit to administration of tocolytic agents to prolong gestation.[68,69] Further studies are needed to elucidate the risks and benefits of tocolysis.

Careful management of a patient with placental abruption should continue into the postpartum period, given the risks of DIC and postpartum uterine atony. Uterotonic agents, such as oxytocin, carboprost, misoprostol, and methyl-ergonovine, should be readily available.

PLACENTAL EVALUATION

Gross examination of a placenta may reveal a fresh clot attached to the maternal surface of the placenta in cases of recent placental abruption. Chronic or remote abruption may be seen as fibrin deposition at the site of abruption with infarcts or depression of the overlying placental parenchyma. Microscopic examination reveals hemosiderin-laden macrophages and evidence of villous hemorrhage.[70]

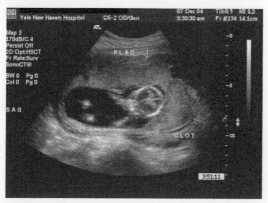

Fig. 5. A large retroplacental hematoma is seen extending from the lateral aspect of the placenta. A fluid collection that is hyperechoic compared to the placenta is likely a hematoma in the acute phase.

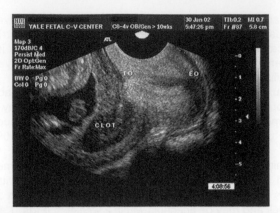

Fig. 6. A retroplacental hematoma is seen overlying the cervical os, resulting in symptomatic vaginal bleeding. EO, external cervical os; IO, internal cervical os.

Histologic etiologies for DH include ischemic placental diseases, poor spiral artery remodeling, spiral artery thrombosis, and sclerotic lesions in myometrial arteries.[6,8,57] It is important to note, however, that evidence of abruption can be seen in up to 4.5% of placentas examined routinely, suggesting that small episodes of placental abruption are more common than those diagnosed clinically.[71]

RECURRENCE, PREDICTION, AND PREVENTION

The recurrence rate of placental abruption ranges from 6% to 17% after a first episode, similar to the recurrence risk of PTD, and increases to 25% after 2 episodes. Approximately 7% to 15% of massive abruptions resulting in intrauterine fetal demise have the same outcome in a subsequent pregnancy.[10,72,73] Thirty percent of all future pregnancies in women who have had a prior placental abruption do not carry to viability.[72]

Although multiple trials exist for various treatments in the prevention of pre-eclampsia, no randomized–controlled trials exist for prevention of placental abruption. Prevention of recurrent abruption begins with correction of underlying modifiable risk

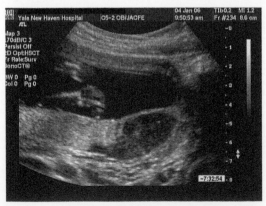

Fig. 7. A hypoechoic retrochorionic hematoma is seen at the lateral edge of a placenta, likely indicating resolution of the hematoma. Echogenicity may fade within two weeks of clot formation.

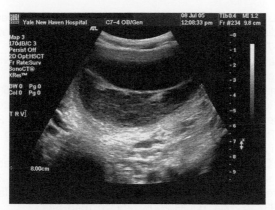

Fig. 8. Large 8 cm retromembranous hematoma with hypoechoic appearance, indicative of clot organization.

factors. Consideration should be given to interval resection of a uterine septum or submucous myoma. Other established risk factors for placental abruption, such as cigarette smoking, drug use, chronic hypertension, pregnancy-induced hypertension, and preeclampsia, should be addressed. Preconceptional and prenatal counseling on the harmful effects of smoking and drug abuse during pregnancy can help to reduce the incidence of placental abruption and other adverse outcomes of pregnancy.[3]

SUMMARY

DH is an important contributor to PTD and associated health care costs. Management of abruption should be individualized, and the patient should be counseled on risks of recurrence. Recent translational investigations on the role of TF and thrombin have helped to shed light on the complex disease process. Additional future research is imperative to development of targeted therapies in the treatment and prevention of placental abruption and PTD.

REFERENCES

1. Martin JA, Osterman MJ, Sutton PD. Are preterm births on the decline in the United States? Recent data from the National Vital Statistics System. NCHS Data Brief 2010;(39):1–8.
2. Behrman RE, Butler AS. Societal costs of prematurity. In: Behrman RE, Butler AS, editors. Preterm birth: causes, consequences, and prevention. Washington, DC: National Academies Press; 2007. p. 398–429.
3. Ananth CV, Berkowitz GS, Savitz DA, et al. Placental abruption and adverse perinatal outcomes. JAMA 1999;282(17):1646–51.
4. Williams MA, Mittendorf R, Lieberman E, et al. Adverse infant outcomes associated with first-trimester vaginal bleeding. Obstet Gynecol 1991;78(1):14–8.
5. Harger JH, Hsing AW, Tuomala RE, et al. Risk factors for preterm premature rupture of fetal membranes: a multicenter case–control study. Am J Obstet Gynecol 1990;163:130–7.
6. Ananth CV, Peltier MR, Chavez MR, et al. Recurrence of ischemic placental disease. Obstet Gynecol 2007;110(1):128–33.

7. Salafia CM, Lopez-Zeno JA, Sherer DM, et al. Histologic evidence of old intra-uterine bleeding is more frequent in prematurity. Am J Obstet Gynecol 1995; 173(4):1065–70.

8. Naeye RL. Maternal age, obstetric complications, and the outcome of pregnancy. Obstet Gynecol 1983;61(2):210–6.

9. Oyelese Y, Ananth CV. Placental abruption. Obstet Gynecol 2006;108(4):1005–16.

10. Creasy RK, Resnik R, Iams JD, et al. Creasy and Resnik's maternal–fetal medicine: principles and practice. Philadelphia: Saunders Elsevier; 2009.

11. Strobino B, Pantel-Silverman J. Gestational vaginal bleeding and pregnancy outcome. Am J Epidemiol 1989;129(4):806–15.

12. Yeo L, Ananth CV, Vintzileos AM. Placental abruption. In: Sciarra J, editor. Gynecology and Obstetrics. Hagerstown (MD): Lippincott, Williams & Wilkins; 2003. p. 1–25.

13. Schiff MA. Pregnancy outcomes following hospitalisation for a fall in Washington State from 1987 to 2004. BJOG 2008;115(13):1648–54.

14. Ananth CV, Smulian JC, Demissie K, et al. Placental abruption among singleton and twin births in the United States: risk factor profiles. Am J Epidemiol 2001; 153(8):771–8.

15. Roque H, Paidas MJ, Funai EF, et al. Maternal thrombophilias are not associated with early pregnancy loss. Thromb Haemost 2004;91(2):290–5.

16. Lockwood CJ, Krikun G, Hickey M, et al. Decidualized human endometrial stromal cells mediate hemostasis, angiogenesis, and abnormal uterine bleeding. Reprod Sci 2009;16(2):162–70.

17. Tabanelli S, Tang B, Gurpide E. In vitro decidualization of human endometrial stromal cells. J Steroid Biochem Mol Biol 1992;42:337–44.

18. Kearns M, Lala PK. Life history of decidual cells: a review. Am J Reprod Immunol 1983;3(2):78–82.

19. Lockwood CJ, Oner C, Uz YH, et al. Matrix metalloproteinase 9 (MMP9) expression in preeclamptic decidua and MMP9 induction by tumor necrosis factor alpha and interleukin 1 beta in human first trimester decidual cells. Biol Reprod 2008; 78(6):1064–72.

20. Moore KL. The developing human. Philadelphia: W. B. Saunders Company; 1998.

21. Lockwood CJ, Nemerson Y, Guller S, et al. Progestational regulation of human endometrial stromal cell tissue factor expression during decidualization. J Clin Endocrinol Metab 1993;76(1):231–6.

22. Lockwood CJ, Krikun G, Papp C, et al. The role of progestationally regulated stromal cell tissue factor and type-1 plasminogen activator inhibitor (PAI-1) in endometrial hemostasis and menstruation. Ann N Y Acad Sci 1994;734:57–79.

23. Runic R, Schatz F, Krey L, et al. Alterations in endometrial stromal cell tissue factor protein and messenger ribonucleic acid expression in patients experiencing abnormal uterine bleeding while using Norplant-2 contraception. J Clin Endocrinol Metab 1997;82(6):1983–8.

24. Drake TA, Morrissey JH, Edgington TS. Selective cellular expression of tissue factor in human tissues. Implications for disorders of hemostasis and thrombosis. Am J Pathol 1989;134(5):1087–97.

25. Mackman N. Role of tissue factor in hemostasis, thrombosis, and vascular development. Arterioscler Thromb Vasc Biol 2004;24(6):1015–22.

26. Neuenschwander PF, Fiore MM, Morrissey JH. Factor VII autoactivation proceeds via interaction of distinct protease-cofactor and zymogen-cofactor complexes. Implications of a two-dimensional enzyme kinetic mechanism. J Biol Chem 1993;268(29):21489–92.

27. Nemerson Y. Tissue factor and hemostasis. Blood 1988;71(1):1–8.

28. Bach RR. Initiation of coagulation by tissue factor. CRC Crit Rev Biochem 1988; 23(4):339–68.
29. Pijnenborg R, Vercruysse L, Hanssens M. The uterine spiral arteries in human pregnancy: facts and controversies. Placenta 2006;27:939–58.
30. Lockwood CJ, Murk W, Kayisli UA, et al. Progestin and thrombin regulate tissue factor expression in human term decidual cells. J Clin Endocrinol Metab 2009; 94(6):2164–70.
31. Chaiworapongsa T, Espinoza J, Yoshimatsu J, et al. Activation of coagulation system in preterm labor and preterm premature rupture of membranes. J Matern Fetal Neonatal Med 2002;11(6):368–73.
32. Elovitz MA, Baron J, Phillippe M. The role of thrombin in preterm parturition. Am J Obstet Gynecol 2001;185(5):1059–63.
33. Rosen T, Kuczynski E, O'Neill LM, et al. Plasma levels of thrombin–antithrombin complexes predict preterm premature rupture of the fetal membranes. J Matern Fetal Med 2001;10(5):297–300.
34. Macfarlane SR, Seatter MJ, Kanke T, et al. Proteinase-activated receptors. Pharmacol Rev 2001;53(2):245–82.
35. Gabazza EC, Taguchi O, Kamada H, et al. Progress in the understanding of protease-activated receptors. Int J Hematol 2004;79(2):117–22.
36. Cottrell GS, Amadesi S, Schmidlin F, et al. Protease-activated receptor 2: activation, signaling and function. Biochem Soc Trans 2003;31:1191–7.
37. Riewald M, Ruf W. Orchestration of coagulation protease signaling by tissue factor. Trends Cardiovasc Med 2002;12(4):149–54.
38. Bohm SK, McConalogue K, Kong W, et al. Proteinase-activated receptors: new functions for old enzymes. News Physiol Sci 1998;13:231–40.
39. Grand RJ, Turnell AS, Grabham PW. Cellular consequences of thrombin receptor activation. Biochem J 1996;313:353–68.
40. Lockwood CJ, Paidas M, Murk WK, et al. Involvement of human decidual cell-expressed tissue factor in uterine hemostasis and abruption. Thromb Res 2009;124(5):516–20.
41. Westermarck J, Kahari VM. Regulation of matrix metalloproteinase expression in tumor invasion. FASEB J 1999;13(8):781–92.
42. Cohen M, Meisser A, Bischof P. Metalloproteinases and human placental invasiveness. Placenta 2006;27(8):783–93.
43. Nagase H, Visse R, Murphy G. Structure and function of matrix metalloproteinases and TIMPs. Cardiovasc Res 2006;69(3):562–73.
44. Moore RM, Mansour JM, Redline RW, et al. The physiology of fetal membrane rupture: insight gained from the determination of physical properties. Placenta 2006;27:1037–51.
45. Parry S, Strauss JF 3rd. Premature rupture of the fetal membranes. N Engl J Med 1998;338(10):663–70.
46. Rosen T, Schatz F, Kuczynski E, et al. Thrombin-enhanced matrix metalloproteinase-1 expression: a mechanism linking placental abruption with premature rupture of the membranes. J Matern Fetal Neonatal Med 2002;11(1):11–7.
47. Mackenzie AP, Schatz F, Krikun G, et al. Mechanisms of abruption-induced premature rupture of the fetal membranes: thrombin enhanced decidual matrix metalloproteinase-3 (stromelysin-1) expression. Am J Obstet Gynecol 2004; 191(6):1996–2001.
48. Helmig BR, Romero R, Espinoza J, et al. Neutrophil elastase and secretory leukocyte protease inhibitor in prelabor rupture of membranes, parturition and intra-amniotic infection. J Matern Fetal Neonatal Med 2002;12(4):237–46.

49. Maymon E, Romero R, Pacora P, et al. Human neutrophil collagenase (matrix metalloproteinase 8) in parturition, premature rupture of the membranes, and intrauterine infection. Am J Obstet Gynecol 2000;183(1):94–9.
50. Van den Steen PE, Proost P, Wuyts A, et al. Neutrophil gelatinase B potentiates interleukin-8 tenfold by aminoterminal processing, whereas it degrades CTAP-III, PF-4, and GRO-alpha and leaves RANTES and MCP-2 intact. Blood 2000;96(8):2673–81.
51. Baggiolini M, Dewald B, Moser B. Human chemokines: an update. Annu Rev Immunol 1997;15:675–705.
52. Zeilhofer HU, Schorr W. Role of interleukin-8 in neutrophil signaling. Curr Opin Hematol 2000;7(3):178–82.
53. Scheller J, Ohnesorge N, Rose-John S. Interleukin-6 trans-signaling in chronic inflammation and cancer. Scand J Immunol 2006;63(5):321–9.
54. Saji F, Samejima Y, Kamiura S, et al. Cytokine production in chorioamnionitis. J Reprod Immunol 2000;47(2):185–96.
55. Lockwood CJ, Toti P, Arcuri F, et al. Mechanisms of abruption-induced premature rupture of the fetal membranes: thrombin-enhanced interleukin-8 expression in term decidua. Am J Pathol 2005;167(5):1443–9.
56. Elovitz MA, Saunders T, Ascher-Landsberg J, et al. Effects of thrombin on myometrial contractions in vitro and in vivo. Am J Obstet Gynecol 2000;183(4): 799–804.
57. Hall DR. Abruptio placentae and disseminated intravascular coagulopathy. Semin Perinatol 2009;33(3):189–95.
58. Rasmussen S, Irgens LM, Bergsjo P, et al. The occurrence of placental abruption in Norway 1967–1991. Acta Obstet Gynecol Scand 1996;75(3): 222–8.
59. Ananth CV, Oyelese Y, Yeo L, et al. Placental abruption in the United States, 1979 through 2001: temporal trends and potential determinants. Am J Obstet Gynecol 2005;192(1):191–8.
60. Han CS, Paidas MJ, Lockwood CJ. Clotting disorders. In: James DK, Steer PJ, Weiner CP, et al, editors. High-risk pregnancy: management options. New York: Saunders; 2010. p. 739–52.
61. Knuppel AR, Drukker JE. Bleeding in late pregnancy: antepartum bleeding. In: Hayashi RH, Castillo MS, editors. High-risk pregnancy: a team approach. Philadelphia: Saunders; 1986. p. 547.
62. Fraser R, Watson R. Bleeding during the latter half of pregnancy. In: Chalmers I, editor. High-risk pregnancy: a team approach. London: Oxford University Press; 1989. p. 89.
63. Ananth CV, Wilcox AJ. Placental abruption and perinatal mortality in the United States. Am J Epidemiol 2001;153(4):332–7.
64. Tikkanen M, Gissler M, Metsaranta M, et al. Maternal deaths in Finland: focus on placental abruption. Acta Obstet Gynecol Scand 2009;88(10):1124–7.
65. Egley C, Cefalo R. Abruptio placenta. In: Studd J, editor. Progress in Obstetrics and Gynecology. London: Churchill Livingstone; 1985. p. 108.
66. Ray JG, Vermeulen MJ, Schull MJ, et al. Cardiovascular health after maternal placental syndromes (CHAMPS): population-based retrospective cohort study. Lancet 2005;366(9499):1797–803.
67. Nyberg DA, Cyr DR, Mack LA, et al. Sonographic spectrum of placental abruption. AJR Am J Roentgenol 1987;148(1):161–4.
68. Saller DN Jr, Nagey DA, Pupkin MJ, et al. Tocolysis in the management of third trimester bleeding. J Perinatol 1990;10(2):125–8.

69. Towers CV, Pircon RA, Heppard M. Is tocolysis safe in the management of third-trimester bleeding? Am J Obstet Gynecol 1999;180:1572–8.
70. Bernischke K, Kaufmann P. Pathology of the human placenta. New York: Springer; 2000.
71. Fox H, Sebire N. Pathology of the placenta (major problems in pathology). London: Saunders; 2007.
72. Hibbard BM, Jeffcoate TN. Abruptio placentae. Obstet Gynecol 1966;27(2): 155–67.
73. Sher G, Statland BE. Abruptio placentae with coagulopathy: a rational basis for management. Clin Obstet Gynecol 1985;28(1):15–23.

Medically Indicated—Iatrogenic Prematurity

Amy E. Wong, MD, William A. Grobman, MD, MBA*

KEYWORDS

- Prematurity • Preterm delivery • Medical indications
- Iatrogenic

Significant attention has been recently devoted to the continued high rate of preterm deliveries, and in particular to the increase in late preterm births.[1] Although the goal of obstetric practice has been to decrease the rate of preterm birth and its associated morbidity and mortality, some guidelines still recommend delivery before 37 weeks of gestation in certain circumstances when continued gestation could lead to maternal or fetal compromise. Indeed, iatrogenic preterm deliveries owing to medical indications comprise 28% to 40% of all preterm births.[2,3] Moreover, the frequency of these iatrogenic preterm deliveries has markedly increased in recent years. From 1998 to 2000, the incidence of medically indicated preterm birth increased by 55% in singleton pregnancies and 50% in twin pregnancies.[4,5] At least one reason for this rise is the increasing prevalence of high-risk pregnancies, associated with changes in the obstetric population, such as older age of childbearing and increased frequency of multiple gestations. Whether there are other factors that have contributed to the rise, such as a changing threshold for recommending delivery at a preterm gestation, remains uncertain. This article reviews the common medical indications for which a fetus may be delivered before 37 weeks of gestation. In each case, obstetric providers must weigh the risks of pregnancy prolongation with those of iatrogenic premature delivery to determine the optimal plan of management.

MATERNAL INDICATIONS: PREGNANCY-RELATED
Hypertensive Disorders

Hypertensive disorders, which include gestational hypertension and preeclampsia, are the most common medical complications of pregnancy.[6] They affect 6% to

The authors have no disclosures.

Division of Maternal-Fetal Medicine, Department of Obstetrics and Gynecology, Northwestern University, Feinberg School of Medicine, 250 East Superior Street, Suite 05-2175, Chicago, IL 60611, USA

* Corresponding author.

E-mail address: w-grobman@northwestern.edu

Clin Perinatol 38 (2011) 423–439
doi:10.1016/j.clp.2011.06.002
0095-5108/11/$ – see front matter

10% of pregnancies,[7] and have been reported to be responsible for 15% to 43% of preterm births.[2,6] Gestational hypertension is defined as a systolic blood pressure of 140 mm Hg or higher or diastolic blood pressure of 90 mm Hg or higher on at least 2 occasions at least 6 hours apart after 20 weeks of gestation in a previously normotensive patient. Preeclampsia, which can develop in a previously normotensive patient or in a patient with known chronic hypertension, is diagnosed by the presence of hypertension and new-onset proteinuria. Severe preeclampsia occurs if systolic blood pressure is 160 mm Hg or higher or diastolic blood pressure is 110 mm Hg or higher, and/or when end-organ damage occurs as evidenced by renal function abnormalities, including large proteinuria, liver function abnormalities, and neurologic symptoms.[8]

As preeclampsia is a leading cause of maternal mortality, contributing to 16% of maternal deaths in the United States,[9] and delivery is the only definitive treatment, timing of delivery is an important consideration in every case. Maternal morbidities associated with hypertensive disease include placental abruption; a central nervous system event, such as stroke or seizure; end-organ dysfunction, particularly involving the kidney; and coagulopathy. Data are insufficient to determine the optimal gestational age to deliver patients affected by preeclampsia, but many perform expectant management of mild preeclampsia until 37 weeks, at which time delivery is warranted because of the risk of maternal adverse outcomes outweighing the risk of prematurity-related morbidity. However, delivery as early as 34 weeks, even without evidence of maternal decompensation or fetal distress, has been considered and performed, given the unpredictable nature of preeclampsia progression and complications associated with the disease.

Women with gestational hypertension, in contrast, more typically have been managed expectantly until at least 37 weeks, if not further.[7] One recent trial, however, grouped women with gestational hypertension and mild preeclampsia together in an attempt to determine the best course of management.[10] This multicenter trial (HYPITAT) randomly assigned 756 women with mild preeclampsia or gestational hypertension who were at least 36 weeks of gestation to delivery or expectant management, and found a decreased risk in adverse maternal outcome without increased neonatal morbidity when delivery was performed at presentation. However, the subgroup of women who presented between 36 and 37 weeks was relatively small, and it remains uncertain as to whether delivery during the preterm period truly optimizes maternal and/or perinatal outcomes for this population.

In cases of severe preeclampsia, in which the likelihood of maternal morbidity is even further increased, delivery at any gestational age may be considered, and delivery during the preterm period is always indicated. There is evidence from randomized trials that women with particular presentations of severe preeclampsia may be expectantly managed until 32 to 34 weeks of gestation.[11,12] Odendaal and colleagues[11] randomized 38 women between 28 and 34 weeks with severe preeclampsia to immediate delivery or to expectant management until 34 weeks, with delivery in the latter group if there was worsening of preeclampsia, HELLP (hemolysis, elevated liver enzymes, low platelet count), or fetal compromise. Those who received expectant management delivered an average of 7 days later and had neonates with fewer neonatal complications. In the study by Sibai and colleagues,[12] 95 women between 28 and 32 weeks with severe preeclampsia similarly were randomized to immediate delivery or expectant management. The latter approach prolonged pregnancy by a mean of 15.4 days, and was associated with reduced neonatal morbidity and increased birth weight.

Intrahepatic Cholestasis of Pregnancy

Intrahepatic cholestasis of pregnancy (IHCP) has been described to occur in 0.32% of women in the United States,[13] although it has been reported to vary with geography and race. For example, rates as high as 5.6% have been noted in a Latina-American population.[14] It is a condition characterized by pruritis and biochemical evidence of liver dysfunction, particularly elevated serum bile acids in the absence of other liver disease. IHCP occurs only in pregnancy, with onset usually in the third trimester. Eighty percent of cases occur after 30 weeks of gestation.[15] The pruritis that is described typically involves the entire body, does not have a corresponding rash, and frequently localizes to the palms of the hands and soles of the feet.

One major concern associated with IHCP is the increased risk of stillbirth.[16–18] The etiology of fetal complications is poorly understood, but is thought to relate to the increase in bile acid concentration in the fetal circulation. The reported frequency of perinatal mortality has ranged widely, with some rates described as high as 10% to 15%.[19,20] Some have noted a predominance of stillbirth at approximately 37 to 39 weeks of gestation.[21,22] Significant maternal complications from IHCP are rare, as medications such as ursodeoxycholic acid often are effective at alleviating maternal symptoms and improving biochemical abnormalities, and symptoms resolve soon after delivery.

Multiple reports of fetal demise despite antenatal monitoring with nonstress testing[16,23] have led to the consensus that fetal surveillance does not prevent fetal demise. Therefore, experts have suggested delivery in the later preterm period.[24] Some have suggested that this active intervention at an early gestational age has led to a reduction in the perinatal mortality rate.[25] There is no consensus on the optimal timing of delivery, but some experts have advocated delivery at 36 to 37 weeks, even without amniocentesis to assess fetal lung maturity, as the risk of fetal death is considered to outweigh the risk of prematurity at this gestational age.[26–29] Correspondingly, most preterm deliveries in pregnancies affected by IHCP are iatrogenic.[17,27]

Maternal Indications: Preexisting Maternal Conditions

Pregnancy has the potential to adversely affect the course and severity of conditions that the mother already has before pregnancy. Given the physiologic changes of pregnancy, many chronic conditions can be exacerbated, thereby placing maternal health in jeopardy for the benefit of pregnancy prolongation and the corresponding reduction of neonatal morbidity because of prematurity. In each case, the decision to perform delivery rests on defining the point at which continuing with pregnancy poses excessive risk to the health of the mother.

One of the more common maternal indications for preterm delivery is cardiac disease, which occurs in 1% to 4% of pregnancies and has been reported to account for up to 10% to 25% of maternal mortality,[30,31] with congenital disease as the most common condition. It appears that the severity of chronic heart disease, as indicated by rate of complications and hospitalizations, is increasing with time.[32] Maternal death may occur as a result of pulmonary hypertension, cardiomyopathy, coronary artery disease, and sudden arrhythmia.[33] Data documenting the optimal timing of delivery in pregnancies complicated by cardiac disease are extremely limited and primarily consist of retrospective cohort studies and case series. A 2008 study examining outcomes of pregnancies complicated by maternal congenital cardiac disease reported a preterm birth rate of 17.7%.[34] Given the extreme heterogeneity of type and severity of cardiac conditions, antenatal management, including antepartum surveillance and timing of delivery, must be tailored to the individual.

Management of women with preexisting renal disease is similarly challenging owing to the increase in renal plasma flow and glomerular filtration rate that occurs in pregnancy. The incidence of renal disease in the pregnant population is 0.02% to 0.12%.[35–37] The likelihood of both maternal and fetal adverse outcomes is directly related to the degree of renal impairment.[37–40] During the pregnancy course, a woman with preexisting renal disease is at greater risk of developing preeclampsia, worsening hypertension, or deterioration of renal function, which may prompt preterm delivery. The risk of disease progression is greatest when serum creatinine is higher than 2.0 mg/dL at the beginning of pregnancy.[39] For example, in patients with mild renal dysfunction, but creatinine that remains lower than 1.4 mg/dL, the incidence of preeclampsia is 11% and rate of preterm delivery is 20%. These frequencies compare favorably with patients on dialysis who have a rate of preeclampsia of up to 80% and preterm delivery rate of up to 85%.[41]

Pregnancy also has the potential to burden the respiratory system because of the anatomic and physiologic changes that occur. The obstetric population is particularly susceptible to respiratory failure; respiratory illness and the need for mechanical ventilation have been shown to be higher in pregnant patients who are admitted to the intensive care unit than in nonpregnant patients.[42] Although acute respiratory failure is rare, occurring in fewer than 0.1% of pregnancies,[43] patients who have underlying pulmonary conditions, such as asthma, and an additional insult, such as influenza or pneumonia, experience higher morbidity and mortality of the mother and the fetus.[44–46] Rarely, restrictive or interstitial lung disease, cystic fibrosis, or sarcoidosis may cause severe chronic respiratory compromise such that the patient is unable tolerate the additional respiratory stress caused by pregnancy, and a preterm delivery may be warranted for maternal benefit.

One of the most challenging complications of pregnancy is maternal malignancy. Cancer complicates approximately 0.02% to 0.10% of all pregnancies,[47] and is expected to occur with an increasing incidence because of the rising age of childbearing. The most common malignancies experienced during pregnancy include cervical cancer, breast cancer, malignant melanoma, and Hodgkin lymphoma. Management of these patients requires the perinatologist, in conjunction with an oncology team, to weigh the maternal benefit of optimal diagnostic workup and treatment with chemotherapy, radiotherapy, or surgery with the risks of malformation or death that these interventions may pose to the fetuses. Additionally, in some cases, such as when chemotherapy will lead to bone marrow suppression that would make the patient susceptible to infection and postpartum hemorrhage at the time of delivery,[48] iatrogenic delivery also aids in the avoidance of maternal risks. This cumulative balance of risks and benefits to both the mother and fetus may lead to the choice of preterm delivery.

FETAL INDICATIONS
Fetal Anemia

Severe fetal anemia results in a compromised fetus that may require preterm delivery to optimize perinatal outcome. Important causes of fetal anemia include alloimmunization, parvovirus B19 infection, and fetomaternal hemorrhage. Although these etiologies are managed differently, all share the risk of fetal demise and require close surveillance and careful decision-making to determine optimal timing of delivery.

Alloimmunization

The placental transfer of maternal immunoglobulin G that is targeted against an antigen on the fetal erythrocyte causes fetal red cell hemolysis and hemolytic disease of the fetus/newborn. The goal of management is to identify fetuses that suffer an anemia to such a degree that there is an imminent risk of fetal hydrops and/or death, and to perform intrauterine transfusion (IUT) and/or delivery before these develop. However, IUTs have been associated with a major complication rate of 1% to 2%

per procedure,[49] which includes the possibility of requiring an emergent preterm delivery. Also, because one of the major complications of IUTs is fetal demise, this procedure is not typically performed after 34 weeks of gestation. Thus, fetuses with severe anemia after this gestational age typically require delivery, even if still preterm.[50]

Parvovirus B19

Maternal infection by parvovirus B19 during pregnancy is another major etiology of fetal anemia. Although approximately 50% of pregnant women are immune to the virus because of prior infection,[51] the incidence of seroconversion in the pregnant population has been described as 2.4%[52] with an estimated vertical transplacental transmission rate of 33%.[53] In a series of 1018 cases of maternal parvovirus infection, 6.3% experienced fetal demise, all of which occurred when maternal infection occurred before 20 weeks of gestation. The overall risk of hydrops fetalis, which generally occurs within 8 weeks of maternal infection, was 3.9% with a peak incidence of hydrops between 17 and 24 weeks.[54] Unlike immune-mediated anemia, however, anemia caused by parvovirus may resolve spontaneously with response by the fetal immune system.[55] Nevertheless, because this will not always occur, many women who have a severely anemic fetus associated with parvovirus infection are recommended to undergo an IUT.[56] As with alloimmunization to fetal red blood cells, the development of severe anemia and performing an IUT may lead to emergent scenarios that require preterm delivery.

Fetomaternal hemorrhage

Although the introduction of fetal blood into maternal circulation is believed to occur to some degree in all pregnancies,[57] clinically significant fetomaternal hemorrhage may occur after abdominal trauma, placental abruption, invasive diagnostic procedures (chorionic villous sampling or amniocentesis), or spontaneously. The volume of fetal blood that is transfused that is considered clinically significant has not been conclusively established, but a hemorrhage of more than 20 mL per kilogram of estimated fetal weight has been associated with poor outcomes, including preterm delivery, transfer to the neonatal intensive care unit, and neonatal transfusion.[58] Suspicion for significant fetomaternal hemorrhage should occur in the context of persistent maternal perception of decreased fetal movement, unexplained hydrops, or unexplained elevation of middle cerebral artery Doppler studies consistent with anemia.[59] Evaluation should include the Kleihauer-Betke test or flow cytometry to attempt identification of fetal red blood cells in maternal blood, and assessment of fetal status with nonstress testing, which may demonstrate late decelerations or a sinusoidal pattern if the fetus is anemic.[60] When assessment does not demand urgent delivery, IUT can be considered as a treatment option to delay delivery of a premature infant. As noted previously, however, this procedure typically is not undertaken after 34 weeks of gestation and may itself be associated with complications that lead to the need for preterm delivery. Moreover, in some cases, fetal decompensation in the setting of a significant acute hemorrhage may be so great that premature delivery is required to avoid an intrauterine fetal demise. Timing of delivery must be made on an individual case basis, as severity and timing of fetomaternal hemorrhage and its impact on fetal well-being differs in each patient.

Intrauterine Growth Restriction

The suspicion of fetal growth restriction (IUGR), typically defined as an estimated fetal weight less than the tenth percentile for gestational age, is a concerning finding because it suggests that the in utero environment may be suboptimal for fetal growth. The corollary is that delivery may be advantageous, and lead to better overall perinatal outcome, despite the potential morbidity associated with prematurity. Delivery for suspected IUGR contributes to 2% to 4% of preterm births.[61] A population-based study of more than 1.4 million deliveries in California reported an increased frequency of IUGR in pregnancies complicated by prematurity, with as many as 12.3% of infants born at 30 weeks affected by IUGR.[62]

Whether the risks of preterm delivery are outweighed by the risks of pregnancy prolongation depends on multiple factors, including gestational age, degree of growth restriction, and antenatal surveillance results. Surveillance of fetuses with IUGR includes monitoring with ultrasonography to assess growth velocity, antenatal testing with nonstress testing or biophysical profiles, and umbilical artery Doppler studies. As gestational age and birth weight are the primary determinants of neonatal outcome, close monitoring of progression of fetal compromise of early-onset IUGR is particularly important to balance the risk of fetal demise with the risks of prematurity.[63] Particularly at fewer than 28 weeks of gestation, each day gained in utero is associated with an increased intact survival by 1% to 2%.[64]

In some scenarios (eg, IUGR at 36 weeks of gestation with reverse end-diastolic flow on umbilical artery Doppler), there is consensus that delivery is the optimal approach. In others, however, the combination of factors provides less certain direction. Two recent randomized trials have addressed optimal timing of delivery in 2 such scenarios. The multicenter Growth Restriction Intervention Trial (GRIT) assigned 548 women with 588 fetuses between 24 and 36 weeks with growth restriction and compromise as evidenced by abnormal umbilical artery Doppler studies to immediate delivery or expectant management until the need for delivery was clearly indicated.[65] Expectant management delayed delivery by an average of only 4 days and was associated with more stillbirths, but this was offset by a higher incidence in neonatal deaths in the immediate delivery group, yielding a similar incidence of perinatal death (10% with immediate delivery vs 9% with delayed delivery).

The Disproportionate Intrauterine Growth Intervention Trial at Term (DIGITAT) trial randomized 650 women with suspected IUGR to expectant management with intensive fetal surveillance or to immediate delivery.[66] In contrast to the GRIT trial, the earliest gestational age eligible for enrollment was 36 weeks. Although expectant management led to a prolongation of pregnancy of an average of 9.6 days and delivery of infants weighing an average of 130 g more, there was no difference in the composite neonatal outcome. Data such as these suggest that delivery of a growth-restricted fetus at 36 weeks, even in the setting of reassuring antepartum testing, may be a reasonable management approach. There is not, however, consensus about this conclusion.

Multiple Gestation: Discordant Twins

The rate of multiple gestation during the past few decades has been increasing, largely because of the increased use of assisted reproductive technology. In the United States, the rate of multiple pregnancy has increased from 1.9% in 1980 to 3.2% in 2006.[67] Approximately 60% of twins deliver preterm, accounting for up to 18% of preterm births.[68] Prematurity is often a result of spontaneous preterm labor or preterm premature rupture of membranes, but iatrogenic preterm deliveries of multiple gestation contributes up to 30% of preterm birth in twin gestations.[69] This high rate of iatrogenic deliveries is related to the higher risk of complications with multiple gestation, including the higher risk of hypertensive disorders and gestational diabetes mellitus.[70]

Twins are generally considered to have discordant growth when there is at least a 20% difference in estimated fetal weight between the smaller twin and the larger twin.[71] The cause of discordant fetal growth has been attributed to different genetic potential of dizygotic twins, crowding in utero, unequal sharing of placental mass, and umbilical cord abnormalities.[72–74] Perinatal mortality has been demonstrated to correlate closely with degree of growth discordance; 5.6 deaths per 1000 live births occur in twins that are 15% to 19% discordant, whereas 43.4 deaths per 1000 live births occur in pairs that are greater than 30% discordant.[75] In a series of 1370 twin pregnancies, greater birth weight discordance was associated not only with intra-uterine fetal demise, but also with preterm delivery. As in the setting of growth restriction, the decision to proceed with delivery in the setting of twin discordance depends on multiple factors, including the degree of discordance, whether there is one twin affected by IUGR, and antenatal surveillance.

Multiple Gestation: Monochorionic Twins and Twin-Twin Transfusion Syndrome

Monochorionic twin pregnancies are associated with greater perinatal morbidity and mortality compared with dichorionic twins and have a greater frequency of preterm delivery.[73,76–78] A large Dutch cohort of 1407 twin pregnancies demonstrated that monochorionic twins, compared with dichorionic twins, have a higher perinatal mortality rate (11.6% vs 5.9%) and deliver an average of 8 days earlier (35 + 4 vs 36 + 5 weeks).[78] A unique complication of monochorionic gestations is twin-twin transfusion syndrome (TTTS), which occurs in 10% to 15% of cases,[79,80] and is associated with a mortality rate of up to 80%.[81] In this condition, unbalanced placental arteriovenous anastomoses lead to shunting of blood from one fetus to its co-twin, causing a polyhydramnios/oligohydramnios sequence that may ultimately lead to fetal death. Treatment of TTTS may include amnioreduction, fetoscopic laser coagulation of placental anastomoses, or selective fetocide. Even with these modalities, and certainly without them, the risk of fetal physiologic decompensation and intrauterine demise exists. Correspondingly, the need for iatrogenic delivery to avoid in utero demise may be needed, and may result in preterm birth.

Even without the development of TTTS, the stillbirth rate in monochorionic twins after 32 weeks of gestation has been reported to range from 1.2% to 4.3%.[77,82] Some experts have used these data to argue for routine preterm delivery of monochorionic twins. Recommendations of timing of delivery have been as early 34 to 35 weeks after administration of antenatal corticosteroids.[83] Other experts, however, have recommended awaiting delivery until 37 to 38 weeks.[84,85]

Multiple Gestation: Monoamniotic Twins

Monochorionic-monoamniotic twins, which compose 1% to 5% of monozygotic twin pregnancies, have been associated with a perinatal mortality rate of 30% to 70%.[86] With the advent of more accurate diagnosis on sonography, intensive fetal surveillance, and earlier delivery, recent series have report a lower loss rate of 8% to 20%.[84,87–89] Regardless, many of the fetal deaths that do occur are attributed to cord entanglement owing to the shared amniotic sac. Recommendations regarding fetal surveillance and optimal timing of delivery remain unclear and management protocols vary widely among centers. A retrospective multicenter observational study of 96 sets of monoamniotic twins found improved perinatal survival in pregnancies that were admitted electively to the hospital (median gestational age 26 + 5 weeks) for fetal monitoring (continuously or 2–3 times daily) compared with pregnancies that were managed as outpatients with fetal monitoring performed 1 to 3 times weekly, and did not find an increase in iatrogenic prematurity with more intensive inpatient fetal monitoring.[89] There is also no consensus on timing of delivery; some experts recommend delivery at 32 weeks after corticosteroid administration, whereas others propose expectant management until 35 weeks with or without amniocentesis to demonstrate fetal lung maturity.[84,87,90] Following either of these schemes, however, will result in the large majority of monoamntiotic twins being prematurely delivered. Delivery is generally recommended to be performed via cesarean section to avoid complications from cord entanglement.[91]

PREGNANCY COMPLICATIONS
Preterm Premature Rupture of Membranes

Preterm premature rupture of membranes (PPROM), spontaneous rupture of membranes before 37 weeks, occurs in 3% of pregnancies and is associated with 30% of preterm deliveries.[92] In a study of 21,771 late preterm births between 34 and 36 weeks of gestation, 80% were attributed to idiopathic preterm labor or premature rupture of membranes.[93]

Expectant management of rupture of membranes after 34 weeks has been associated with increased risk of intrauterine infection, increased risk of prolonged maternal hospital stay, and decreased umbilical cord pH at delivery,[94] as well as neonatal sepsis.[95] As such, delivery is generally indicated if rupture occurs at or after 34 weeks.[96] Some experts have suggested that testing for fetal lung maturity can be considered between 32 and 34 weeks of gestation, with iatrogenically initiated delivery if result demonstrates maturity.[97,98]

As obstetricians continue to work toward decreasing the neonatal morbidity associated with prematurity, the potential benefit of continuing pregnancy beyond 34 weeks is being revisited. A Dutch prospective randomized trial is under way to assess the outcomes of induction of labor compared with those of expectant management after PPROM between 34 and 37 weeks' gestation.[99]

Placenta Previa, Placenta Accreta, and Vasa Previa

Placenta previa, the condition in which the placenta overlies the internal cervical os, occurs in approximately 4 per 1000 pregnancies.[100] The risk of placenta previa increases with the number of prior cesarean deliveries, with a rate of 0.65% in women with 1 prior cesarean delivery, 1.80% in those with 2 prior cesarean deliveries, 3.00% in those with 3 prior cesarean deliveries, and 10.00% with 4 or more prior cesarean deliveries.[101] This condition is associated with significant fetal and maternal morbidity because of the risk of hemorrhage from the placenta in response to uterine contractions or cervical change.[102] When vaginal bleeding occurs before 34 weeks, expectant management to allow administration of antenatal corticosteroids may be considered, although severe bleeding, particularly in the setting of maternal or fetal compromise, is an indication for immediate delivery. In the absence of vaginal bleeding, there is no consensus regarding the optimal gestational for delivery of asymptomatic patients with placenta previa, although many experts would recommend delivery at approximately 37 weeks' gestation. This iatrogenic delivery would preclude continued pregnancy and the risks to the mother and the fetus from an emergent hemorrhage. The results of a recent decision analysis, on the other hand, have suggested that 36 weeks is the preferable gestational age for delivery of these patients.[103]

Placenta accreta, a placental implantation abnormality, occurs when the placental trophoblastic tissue is abnormally invasive. The incidence of this condition has been described as 1 in 533 pregnancies in a large series.[104] Major risk factors include prior cesarean section and placenta previa; the risk of accreta for women with both placenta previa and one prior cesarean is 24%.[101] Owing to the abnormal adherence of the placenta, the patient is at high risk of severe hemorrhage and its associated complications, such as need for hysterectomy, disseminated intravascular coagulopathy, and death.[105]

Because placenta accreta and its poor associated outcomes are rare, there are few data to guide the decision of optimal timing of delivery. One concern, particularly in the setting of a suspected placenta accreta in a woman with a placenta previa and a prior cesarean, is the possibility of emergent hemorrhage and unscheduled delivery. This is of such concern given that the invasive placentation may be associated with a much more morbid operation, including the occurrence of visceral injury and major transfusion. In cases of placenta percreta with bladder invasion, for example, maternal death rates as high as 10% have been reported.[106] Thus, a scheduled delivery, even if premature, allows a better maternal outcome. There are some retrospective data to support this position.[107,108] Correspondingly, experts have suggested that delivery at 36 to 37 weeks is a reasonable option to balance maternal and perinatal risks. However, a recent decision analysis suggests delivery as early as 34 weeks after administration of antenatal corticosteroids, without the need for demonstration of fetal lung maturity, may be a reasonable approach under certain circumstances.[109]

Vasa previa, which is characterized by the presence of fetal vessels coursing through placental membranes directly over the internal cervical os, can also have catastrophic consequences, specifically for the fetus. With an estimated incidence of 1 in 1500 births,[110] it is associated with a high perinatal mortality of 56% in the absence of prenatal diagnosis[111] because of the risk of rupture of the fetal vessels with rupture of the membranes, and subsequent rapid fetal exsanguination. With prenatal sonographic diagnosis, however, perinatal mortality has been reported to be significantly lower. There is no evidence from randomized trials as to the optimal timing of delivery. Because of the risk of unpredictable bleeding with rapid fetal death, experts have recommended delivery at 35 to 36 weeks, after administration of antenatal corticosteroids, and without amniocentesis for fetal lung maturity.[112]

Placental Abruption

Placental abruption, the premature separation of the placenta from the uterus, complicates about 1% of pregnancies and contributes to up to 5% to 10% of preterm births.[113,114] It occurs more frequently in pregnancies also complicated by hypertension, rupture of membranes, intra-amniotic infection, ischemic placental disease, trauma, and cocaine and cigarette use and is associated with significant perinatal morbidity and mortality.[115]

Although mild cases of placental abruption can have few, if any, fetal or maternal consequences, severe abruption can cause fetal death and maternal obstetric hemorrhage, hemodynamic instability and hypovolemic shock, and development of disseminated intravascular coagulation. Chronic placental abruption, in which patients experience intermittent episodes of light vaginal bleeding, are associated with the subsequent development of fetal growth restriction, oligohydramnios, and premature rupture of membranes. A population-based cohort study of 7.5 million pregnancies in the United States reported a perinatal death rate in the setting of abruption of 12%.[116]

Pregnancy outcome depends on severity of the abruption and the gestational age at which it occurs. Therefore, management must be individualized. When abruption occurs at term or near-term, prompt delivery is indicated with close intrapartum monitoring of both the mother and the fetus.[115] At gestational ages before 34 weeks, if both maternal and fetal statuses are reassuring, expectant management can be considered to delay delivery to avoid unnecessary prematurity and to allow for the administration of antenatal corticosteroids. Nevertheless, the clinical severity of some abruptions may be such that iatrogenic preterm delivery is warranted. In contrast, timing of delivery in the setting of chronic abruption with continued reassuring maternal and fetal status has been recommended by experts to be performed at 37 to 38 weeks.[115]

Prior Uterine Surgery

Patients who have had prior cesarean delivery via a classical hysterotomy have a 6% to 12% risk of uterine rupture during labor in a subsequent pregnancy.[117,118] Because uterine rupture of a classical cesarean scar is a potentially catastrophic event, with a significantly increased risk of fetal mortality, and has been reported to occur before or early in labor,[119,120] delivery before 39 weeks to minimize risk of spontaneous labor and its potential sequelae is commonly performed. Moreover, given the risks, some experts have advocated for delivery as early as 36 weeks, particularly if fetal lung maturity has been confirmed.

There remains no clear consensus on the optimal timing of delivery. A decision-analysis attempted to address the issue of delivery timing after a previous classical hysterotomy and compared 4 strategies: (1) delivery at 39 weeks; (2) delivery at 36 weeks without amniocentesis; (3) amniocentesis at 36 weeks with delivery if evidence of fetal lung maturity, or 48 hours after antenatal corticosteroids if immature; and (4) weekly amniocentesis starting at 36 weeks with delivery upon fetal lung maturity.[121] The model demonstrated that delivery at 36 weeks without amniocentesis for fetal lung maturity was associated with the lowest risk of severe adverse maternal-neonatal catastrophic outcomes.

Similarly, prior transmural myomectomy or transfundal uterine surgery has been associated with uterine rupture in labor. However, the true incidence of uterine rupture is difficult to quantify from the existing literature, as most reports describe case series with a small number of patients. Some series of women with prior abdominal myomectomy have not reported an increased risk of rupture, whereas others have reported a rate of up to 4%.[122] With the introduction of a laparoscopic approach to myomectomy, it has been suggested that there is a greater risk of uterine rupture because of the technical challenge of properly closing the myometrial defect[123]; investigators have reported uterine rupture rates that range from 0.26% to 3.00%.[124,125] It has been postulated that the degree of risk after myomectomy varies with surgical approach (abdominal vs laparoscopic), method of myometrial closure, whether the endometrial cavity is involved, and how significantly the myometrium has been disturbed (ie, number, size, and location of fibroids removed).[126,127] Very few data exist to guide recommendations on optimal timing of delivery to decrease the risk of rupture. In many circumstances, delivery, even if iatrogenic, is not initiated until after 37 weeks. However, because some circumstances may be considered to mimic the setting of a classical cesarean scar, some women have been delivered before 37 weeks to avoid the chance of labor and the attendant risks of uterine rupture and perinatal morbidity and mortality.

SUMMARY

The important issue of preterm birth and associated perinatal and infant morbidity and mortality has become a national priority.[128] In the effort to decrease the preterm delivery rate, however, it must be remembered that there are complications of pregnancy for which a delivery before 37 weeks' gestation is indicated because of deterioration of maternal and/or fetal status with pregnancy prolongation. Complications that may lead to iatrogenic preterm birth include pregnancy-related maternal complications and preexisting maternal conditions; fetal complications, including anemia, growth restriction, growth discordance in a multiple gestation, twin-twin transfusion syndrome, or a monoamniotic multiple gestation; and pregnancy complications such as PPROM, abnormal placental implantation and vasa previa, placental abruption, and uterine scar from prior surgery.

In most of these clinical situations, there is little trial-based evidence to guide the decision of delivery timing. An additional factor that limits the ability to establish guidelines is the heterogeneity of patients' situations. Therefore, each case must be evaluated on an individual basis to weigh the risks associated with prematurity with the risks to both the mother and the fetus of pregnancy prolongation.

REFERENCES

1. Damus K. Prevention of preterm birth: a renewed national priority. Curr Opin Obstet Gynecol 2008;20:590–6.
2. Meis PJ, Goldenberg RL, Mercer BM, et al. The preterm prediction study: risk factors for indicated preterm births. Maternal-fetal medicine units network of the National Institute of Child Health and Human Development. Am J Obstet Gynecol 1998;178:562–7.
3. Ananth CV, Vintzileos AM. Medically indicated preterm birth: recognizing the importance of the problem. Clin Perinatol 2008;35:53–67.
4. Ananth CV, Joseph KS, Oyelese Y, et al. Trends in preterm birth and perinatal mortality among singletons: United States, 1989 through 2000. Obstet Gynecol 2005;105:1084–91.
5. Ananth CV, Joseph KS, Demissie K, et al. Trends in twin preterm birth subtypes in the United States, 1989 through 2000: impact on perinatal mortality. Am J Obstet Gynecol 2005;193:1076–82.
6. Roberts JM, Pearson G, Cutler J, et al. Summary of the NHLBI working group on research on hypertension during pregnancy. Hypertension 2003;41:437–45.
7. Sibai BM. Diagnosis and management of gestational hypertension and preeclampsia. Obstet Gynecol 2003;102:181–92.
8. American College of Obstetricians and Gynecologists. Diagnosis and management of preeclampsia and eclampsia. ACOG Practice Bulletin 33. Washington, DC: American College of Obstetricians and Gynecologists; 2002.
9. Kahn KS, Wojdyla D, Say L, et al. WHO analysis of causes of maternal death: a systematic review. Lancet 2006;367:1066–74.
10. Koopmans CM, Bijlenga D, Groen H, et al. Induction of labour versus expectant monitoring for gestational hypertension or mild pre-eclampsia after 36 weeks' gestation (HYPITAT): a multicentre, open-label randomised controlled trial. Lancet 2009;374:979–88.
11. Odendaal HJ, Pattinson RC, Bam R, et al. Aggressive or expectant management for patients with severe preeclampsia between 28–34 weeks' gestation: a randomized controlled trial. Obstet Gynecol 1990;76:1070–5.
12. Sibai BM, Mercer BM, Schiff E, et al. Aggressive versus expectant management of severe preeclampsia at 28 to 32 weeks' gestation: a randomized controlled trial. Am J Obstet Gynecol 1994;171:818–22.
13. Laifer SA, Stiller RJ, Siddiqui DS, et al. Ursodeoxycholic acid for the treatment of intrahepatic cholestasis of pregnancy. J Matern Fetal Med 2001;10:131–5.
14. Lee RH, Goodwin TM, Greenspoon J, et al. The prevalence of intrahepatic cholestasis of pregnancy in a primarily Latina Los Angeles population. J Perinatol 2006;26:527–32.

15. Kenyon AP, Piercy CN, Girling J, et al. Obstetric cholestasis, outcome with active management: a series of 70 cases. Br J Obstet Gynaecol 2002;109:282–8.

16. Rioseco AJ, Ivankovic MB, Manzur A, et al. Intrahepatic cholestasis of pregnancy: a retrospective case-control study of perinatal outcome. Am J Obstet Gynecol 1994;170:890–5.

17. Bacq Y, Sapey T, Brechot MC, et al. Intrahepatic cholestasis of pregnancy: a French prospective study. Hepatology 1997;26:358–64.

18. Zecca E, De Luca D, Marras M, et al. Intrahepatic cholestasis of pregnancy and neonatal respiratory distress syndrome. Pediatrics 2006;117:1669–72.

19. Reid R, Ivey KJ, Rencoret RH, et al. Fetal complications of obstetric complications. Br Med J 1976;1:870–2.

20. Fisk NM, Bye WB, Storey BS. Maternal features of obstetric cholestasis: 20 years experience at King George V Hospital. Aust N Z J Obstet Gynaecol 1988;28:172–6.

21. Williamson C, Hems LM, Goulis DG, et al. Clinical outcome in a series of cases of obstetric cholestasis identified via a patient support group. Br J Obstet Gynaecol 2004;111:676–81.

22. Geenes V, Williamson C. Intrahepatic cholestasis of pregnancy. World J Gastroenterol 2009;15:2049–66.

23. Alsulyman OM, Ouzounian JG, Ames-Castro M, et al. Intrahepatic cholestasis of pregnancy: perinatal outcome associated with expectant management. Am J Obstet Gynecol 1996;175:957–60.

24. Williamson C, Mackillop L. Diseases of the liver, biliary system, and pancreas. In: Creasy RK, Resnik R, Iams JD, et al, editors. Creasy & Resnik's maternal-fetal medicine: principles and practice. 6th edition. Philadelphia: Saunders Elsevier; 2009. p. 1059–77.

25. Fisk NM, Storey GN. Fetal outcome in obstetric cholestasis. Br J Obstet Gynaecol 1988;95:1137–43.

26. Roncaglia N, Arreghini A, Locatelli A, et al. Obstetric cholestasis: outcome with active management. Eur J Obstet Gynecol Reprod Biol 2002;100:167–70.

27. Lee RH, Kwok KM, Ingles S, et al. Pregnancy outcomes during an era of aggressive management for intrahepatic cholestasis of pregnancy. Am J Perinatol 2008;225:341–5.

28. Mays JK. The active management of intrahepatic cholestasis of pregnancy. Curr Opin Obstet Gynecol 2010;22:100–3.

29. Pathak B, Sheibani L, Lee RH. Cholestasis of pregnancy. Obstet Gynecol Clin North Am 2010;37:269–82.

30. Chang J, Elam-Evans LD, Berg CJ, et al. Pregnancy-related mortality surveillance—United States, 1991–1999. MMWR Surveill Summ 2003;52:1–8.

31. Klein LL, Galan HL. Cardiac disease in pregnancy. Obstet Gynecol Clin North Am 2004;31:429–59.

32. Kuklina EV, Callaghan WM. Chronic heart disease and severe obstetric morbidity among hospitalizations for pregnancy in the USA: 1995–2006. BJOG 2011;118(3):345–52.

33. Foley MR, Rokey R, Belfort MA. Cardiac disease. In: Belfort MA, Saade GR, Foley MR, et al, editors. Critical care obstetrics. 5th edition. Molden (MA): Blackwell Publishing Company; 2010. p. 256–82.

34. Ford AA, Wylie BJ, Waksmonski CA, et al. Maternal congenital cardiac disease: outcomes of pregnancy in a single tertiary care center. Obstet Gynecol 2008;112:828–33.

35. Cunningham FG, Cox SM, Harstad TW, et al. Chronic renal disease and pregnancy outcome. Am J Obstet Gynecol 1990;163:453–9.

36. Fink JC, Schwartz SM, Benedetti TJ, et al. Increased risk of adverse maternal and infant outcomes among women with renal disease. Paediatr Perinat Epidemiol 1998;12:277–87.

37. Fischer MJ, Lehnerz SD, Hebert JR, et al. Kidney disease is an independent risk factor for adverse fetal and maternal outcomes in pregnancy. Am J Kidney Dis 2004;43:415–23.

38. Hou SH. Frequency and outcome of pregnancy in women on dialysis. Am J Kidney Dis 1994;23:60–3.

39. Jones DC, Hayslett JP. Outcome of pregnancy in women with moderate or severe renal insufficiency. N Engl J Med 1996;335:226–32.

40. Bar J, Orvieto R, Shalev Y, et al. Pregnancy outcome in women with primary renal disease. Isr Med Assoc J 2000;2:178–81.

41. Okundaye I, Abrinko P, Hou S. Registry of pregnancy in dialysis patients. Am J Kidney Dis 1998;31:766–73.

42. El-Solh AA, Grant BJ. A comparison of severity of illness scoring systems for critically ill obstetric patients. Chest 1996;110:1299–304.

43. Chen CY, Chen CP, Wang KG, et al. Factors implicated in the outcome of pregnancies complicated by acute respiratory failure. J Reprod Med 2003;48: 641–8.

44. Goodnight WH, Soper DE. Pneumonia in pregnancy. Crit Care Med 2005;33: S390–7.

45. Murphy VE, Clifton VL, Gibson PG. Asthma exacerbations during pregnancy: incidence and association with adverse pregnancy outcomes. Thorax 2006; 61:169–76.

46. Brown CM. Severe influenza A virus (H1N1) infection in pregnancy. Obstet Gynecol 2010;115:412–4.

47. Kennedy S, Yudkin P, Greenall M. Cancer in pregnancy. Eur J Surg Oncol 1993; 19:405–7.

48. Weisz B, Meirow D, Schiff E, et al. Impact and treatment of cancer during pregnancy. Expert Rev Anticancer Ther 2004;4:889–902.

49. Van Kamp IL, Klumper FJ, Oepkes D, et al. Complications of intrauterine intravascular transfusion for fetal anemia due to maternal red-cell alloimmunization. Am J Obstet Gynecol 2005;192:171–7.

50. Moise KJ. Management of rhesus alloimmunization in pregnancy. Obstet Gynecol 2008;112:164–76.

51. Harger JH, Adler SP, Koch WC, et al. Prospective evaluation of 618 pregnant women exposed to parvovirus B19: risks and symptoms. Obstet Gynecol 1998;91:413–20.

52. van Gessel PH, Gaytant MA, Vossen AC, et al. Incidence of parvovirus B19 infection among an unselected population of pregnant women in the Netherlands: a prospective study. Eur J Obstet Gynecol Reprod Biol 2006;128: 46–9.

53. Public Health Laboratory Service Working Party on Fifth Disease. Prospective study of human parvovirus B19 infection in pregnancy. Br Med J 1990;30: 1166–70.

54. Enders M, Weidner A, Zoellner I. Fetal morbidity and mortality after acute human parvovirus B19 infection in pregnancy: prospective evaluation of 1018 cases. Prenat Diagn 2004;24:513–8.

55. Brennand J, Cameron A. Fetal anaemia: diagnosis and management. Best Pract Res Clin Obstet Gynaecol 2008;22:15–29.

56. Rodis JF, Borgida AF, Wilson M, et al. Management of parvovirus in pregnancy and outcomes of hydrops: a survey of the members of the Society of Perinatal Obstetricians. Am J Obstet Gynecol 1998;179:985–8.

57. Sebring ES, Polesky HF. Fetomaternal hemorrhage: incidence, risk factors, time of occurrence, and clinical effects. Transfusion 1990;30:344–57.

58. Rubod C, Deruelle P, Le Goueff F, et al. Long-term prognosis for infants after massive fetomaternal hemorrhage. Obstet Gynecol 2007;110:256–60.

59. Wylie BJ, D'Alton ME. Fetomaternal hemorrhage. Obstet Gynecol 2010;1115: 1039–51.

60. Modanlou HD, Freeman RK, Ortiz O, et al. Sinusoidal fetal heart rate pattern and severe fetal anemia. Obstet Gynecol 1977;49:537–41.

61. Slattery MM, Morrison JJ. Preterm delivery. Lancet 2002;360:1489–97.

62. Gilbert WM, Danielsen B. Pregnancy outcomes associated with intrauterine growth restriction. Am J Obstet Gynecol 2003;188:1596–601.

63. Baschat AA. Fetal growth restriction—from observation to intervention. J Perinat Med 2010;38:239–46.

64. Baschat AA, Cosmi E, Bilardo CM, et al. Predictors of neonatal outcome in early-onset placental dysfunction. Obstet Gynecol 2007;109:253–61.

65. GRIT Study Group. A randomized trial of timed delivery for the compromised preterm fetus: short term outcomes and Bayesian interpretation. BJOG 2003; 110:27–32.

66. Boers KE, Vijgen SM, Bijlenga D, et al. Induction versus expectant monitoring for intrauterine growth restriction at term: randomized equivalence trial (DIGITAT). BMJ 2010;341:c7087.

67. Martin JA, Park MM. Trends in twin and triplet births: 1980–97. Natl Vital Stat Rep 1999;47:1–17 (National Center for Health Statistics).

68. Moutquin JM. Classification and heterogeneity of preterm birth. Br J Obstet Gynaecol 2003;110:30–3.

69. Kogan MD, Alexander GR, Kotelchuck M, et al. Trends in twin birth outcomes and prenatal care utilization in the United States, 1981–1997. JAMA 2000;284: 335–41.

70. Chauhan SP, Scardo JA, Hayes E, et al. Twins: prevalence, problems, and preterm births. Am J Obstet Gynecol 2010;203:305–15.

71. Talbot GT, Goldstein RF, Nesbitt T. Is size discordance an indication for delivery of preterm twins? Am J Obstet Gynecol 1997;177:1050–4.

72. Eberle AM, Levesque D, Vintzileos AM, et al. Placental pathology in discordant twins. Am J Obstet Gynecol 1993;169:931–5.

73. Victoria A, Mora G, Arias F. Perinatal outcome, placental pathology, and severity of discordance in monochorionic and dichorionic twins. Obstet Gynecol 2001; 97:310–5.

74. Fick AL, Feldstein VA, Norton ME, et al. Unequal placental sharing and birth weight discordance in monochorionic diamniotic twins. Am J Obstet Gynecol 2006;195:178–83.

75. Branum AM, Schoendorf KC. The effect of birth weight discordance on twin neonatal mortality. Obstet Gynecol 2003;101:570–4.

76. Roque H, Gillen-Goldstein J, Funai E, et al. Perinatal outcomes in monoamniotic gestations. J Matern Fetal Neonatal Med 2003;13:414–21.

77. Barigye O, Pasquini L, Galea P, et al. High risk of unexpected late fetal death in monochorionic twins despite intensive ultrasound surveillance: a cohort study. PLoS Med 2005;2:521–7.

78. Hack KE, Derks JB, Elias SG, et al. Increased perinatal mortality and morbidity in monochorionic versus dichorionic twin pregnancies: clinical implications of a large Dutch cohort study. Br J Obstet Gynaecol 2008;115:58–67.

79. Sebire NJ, Snijders RJ, Hughes K, et al. The hidden mortality of monochorionic twin pregnancies. Br J Obstet Gynaecol 1997;104:1203–7.

80. Bermudez C, Becerra CH, Bornick PW, et al. Placental types and twin-twin transfusion syndrome. Am J Obstet Gynecol 2002;187:489–94.

81. Gonsoulin W, Moise KJ, Kirshon B, et al. Outcome of twin-twin transfusion diagnosed before 28 weeks of gestation. Obstet Gynecol 1990;75:214–6.

82. Simoes T, Amaral N, Lerman R, et al. Prospective risk of intrauterine death of monochorionic-diamniotic twins. Am J Obstet Gynecol 2006;195:134–9.

83. Cleary-Goldman J, D'Alton ME. Prospective risk of intrauterine death of monochorionic-diamniotic twins. Am J Obstet Gynecol 2007;196:e11.

84. Hack KE, Derks JB, Schaap AH, et al. Perinatal outcome of monoamniotic twin pregnancies. Obstet Gynecol 2009;113:353–60.

85. Smith NA, Wilkins-Haug L, Santolaya-Forgas J, et al. Contemporary management of monochorionic diamniotic twins: outcomes and delivery recommendations revisited. Am J Obstet Gynecol 2010;203:133,e1–6

86. Beasley E, Megerian G, Gerson A, et al. Monoamniotic twins: case series and proposal for antenatal management. Obstet Gynecol 1999;93:130–4.

87. Rodis JF, McIlveen PF, Egan JF, et al. Monoamniotic twins: improved perinatal survival with accurate prenatal diagnosis and antenatal fetal surveillance. Am J Obstet Gynecol 1997;177:1046–9.

88. Allen VM, Windrim R, Barrett J, et al. Management of monoamniotic twin pregnancies: a case series and systematic review of the literature. Br J Obstet Gynaecol 2001;108:931–6.

89. Heyborne KD, Porreco RP, Garite TJ, et al. Improved perinatal survival of monoamniotic twins with intensive inpatient monitoring. Am J Obstet Gynecol 2005;192:96–101.

90. Ezra Y, Shveiky D, Ophir E, et al. Intensive management and early delivery reduce antenatal mortality in monoamniotic twin pregnancies. Acta Obstet Gynecol Scand 2005;84:432–5.

91. Cruikshank DP. Intrapartum management of twin gestations. Obstet Gynecol 2007;109:1167–76.

92. Mercer BM. Preterm premature rupture of the membranes. Obstet Gynecol 2003;101:178–93.

93. McIntire DD, Leveno KJ. Neonatal mortality and morbidity rates in late preterm births compared with births at term. Obstet Gynecol 2008;111:35–41.

94. Naef RW, Albert JR, Ross EL, et al. Premature rupture of membranes at 34 to 37 weeks' gestation: aggressive versus conservative management. Am J Obstet Gynecol 1998;178:126–30.

95. van der Ham DP, van der Heijden J, Ravelli AC, et al. Neonatal outcome of pregnancies complicated by PPROM between 34 and 37 weeks of gestation. Am J Obstet Gynecol 2010;201:S182.

96. American College of Obstetricians and Gynecologists. Premature rupture of membranes. ACOG Practice Bulletin #80. Washington, DC: American College of Obstetricians and Gynecologists; 2007.

97. Mercer BM, Crocker LG, Boe NM, et al. Induction versus expectant management in premature rupture of the membranes with mature amniotic fluid at 32 to 36 weeks: a randomized trial. Am J Obstet Gynecol 1993;169:775–82.

98. American College of Obstetricians and Gynecologists. Fetal lung maturity. ACOG Practice Bulletin #97. Washington, DC: American College of Obstetricians and Gynecologists; 2008.

99. van der Ham DP, Nijhuis JG, Mol BW, et al. Induction of labour versus expectant management in women with preterm prelabour rupture of membranes between 34 and 37 weeks (the PPROMEXIL-trial). BMC Pregnancy Childbirth 2007;7:11.

100. Faiz AS, Ananth CV. Etiology and risk factors for placenta previa: an overview and meta-analysis of observational studies. J Matern Fetal Neonatal Med 2003;13:175–90.

101. Clark SL, Koonings PP, Pheland JP. Placenta previa/accreta and prior cesarean section. Obstet Gynecol 1985;66:89–92.

102. Grobman WA, Gersnoviez R, Landon MB, et al. Pregnancy outcomes for women with placenta previa in relation to the number of prior cesarean deliveries. Obstet Gynecol 2007;110:1249–55.

103. Zlatnik MG, Little SE, Kohli P, et al. When should women with placenta previa be delivered? A decision analysis. J Reprod Med 2010;55:373–81.

104. Wu S, Kocherginsky M, Hibbard JU. Abnormal placentation: twenty-year analysis. Am J Obstet Gynecol 2005;192:1458–61.

105. SMFM Clinical Opinion. Placenta accreta. Am J Obstet Gynecol 2010;203:430–9.

106. Hudon L, Belfort MA, Broome DR. Diagnosis and management of placenta percreta: a review. Obstet Gynecol Surv 1998;53:509–17.

107. O'Brien JM, Barton JR, Donaldson ES. The management of placenta percreta: conservative and operative strategies. Am J Obstet Gynecol 1996;175:1632–8.

108. Warshak CR, Ramos GA, Eskander R, et al. Effect of predelivery diagnosis in 99 consecutive cases of placenta accreta. Obstet Gynecol 2010;115:65–9.

109. Robinson BK, Grobman WA. Effectiveness of timing strategies for delivery of individuals with placenta previa and accreta. Obstet Gynecol 2010;116:835–42.

110. Oyelese KO, Turner M, Lees C, et al. Vasa previa: an avoidable obstetric tragedy. Obstet Gynecol Surv 1999;54:138–45.

111. Oyelese Y, Catanzarite V, Prefumo F, et al. Vasa previa: the impact of prenatal diagnosis on outcomes. Obstet Gynecol 2004;103:937–42.

112. Oyelese Y, Smulian JC. Placenta previa, placenta accreta, and vasa previa. Obstet Gynecol 2006;107:927–41.

113. Ananth CV, Berkowitz GS, Savitz DA, et al. Placental abruption and adverse perinatal outcomes. JAMA 1999;282:1646–51.

114. Sheiner E, Shoham-Vardi I, Hadar A, et al. Incidence, obstetric risk factors and pregnancy outcome of preterm placental abruption: a retrospective analysis. J Matern Fetal Neonatal Med 2002;11:34–9.

115. Oyelese Y, Ananth CV. Placental abruption. Obstet Gynecol 2006;108:1005–16.

116. Ananth CV, Wilcox AJ. Placental abruption and perinatal mortality in the United States. Am J Epidemiol 2001;153:332–7.

117. Wilson AL. Labor and delivery after cesarean section. Am J Obstet Gynecol 1951;62:1225–33.

118. Halperin ME, Moore DC, Hannah WJ. Classical versus low-segment transverse incision for preterm caesarean section: maternal complications and outcome of subsequent pregnancies. Br J Obstet Gynaecol 1988;95:990–6.

119. Rahman J, Al-Sibai MH, Rahman MS. Rupture of the uterus in labor: a review of 96 cases. Acta Obstet Gynecol Scand 1985;64:311–5.

120. Hofmeyr GJ, Say L, Gulmezoglu AM. WHO systematic review of maternal mortality and morbidity: the prevalence of uterine rupture. Br J Obstet Gynaecol 2005;112:1221–8.

121. Stotland N, Lipschitz LS, Caughey AB. Delivery strategies for women with a previous classic cesarean delivery: a decision analysis. Am J Obstet Gynecol 2002;187:1203–8.

122. Gamet JD. Uterine rupture during pregnancy. An analysis of 133 patients. Obstet Gynecol 1964;23:898–905.

123. Nezhat C. The "cons" of laparoscopic myomectomy in women who may reproduce in the future. Int J Fertil Menopausal Stud 1996;41:280–3.

124. Dubuisson JB, Fauconnier A, Deffarges JV, et al. Pregnancy outcome and deliveries following laparoscopic myomectomy. Hum Reprod 2000;15:869–73.

125. Sizzi O, Rosetti A, Malzoni M, et al. Italian multicenter study on complications of laparoscopic myomectomy. J Minim Invasive Gynecol 2007;14:453–62.

126. Koh C, Janik G. Laparoscopic myomectomy: the current status. Curr Opin Obstet Gynecol 2003;15:295–310.

127. Parker WH, Einarsson J, Istre O, et al. Risk factors for uterine rupture after laparoscopic myomectomy. J Minim Invasive Gynecol 2010;17:51–4.

128. Ashton DM, Lawrence HC, Adams NL, et al. Surgeon General's conference on the prevention of preterm birth. Obstet Gynecol 2009;113:925–30.

Outcomes of Preterm Infants: Morbidity Replaces Mortality

Marilee C. Allen, MD[a,b],*, Elizabeth A. Cristofalo, MD[a,b],
Christina Kim[a]

KEYWORDS

- Infant • Premature • Neonatal mortality • Cerebral palsy
- Disability • Intellectual • Learning disabilities

Over the last 50 years in the United States a rising preterm birth rate, a progressive decrease in preterm mortality, and a lowering of the limit of viability have made preterm birth a significant public health problem.[1] Recent data suggest a leveling of these trends. The preterm birth rate actually decreased from 12.8% in 2006 to 12.3% in 2008.[2] There have been only small annual variations in the preterm-related infant mortality rates, which were 2.38 and 2.42 per 1000 live births in 2000 and 2006, respectively.[3] Despite increasingly aggressive obstetric and neonatal care for the most extremely preterm infants in the last decade, there has been no lowering of the limit of viability below 23 weeks.[4–6] Preterm survival is the lowest for those infants, and increases to more than 80% survival for infants born at 26 weeks, and more than 90% survival for infants born after 27 weeks' gestation.[1,7] Survival is greater than 99% for infants born at 34 to 36 weeks' gestation (late preterm infants), but nonetheless their mortality rate is more than 3 to 5 times higher than the rate for infants born at full term.[8,9]

Preterm birth is associated with injuries to many organ systems (eg, pulmonary, gastrointestinal, visual) that are due to: (1) factors that precipitate preterm delivery (eg, infection and inflammation), (2) physiologic instability on transition to extrauterine life, (3) insufficient endogenous protective factors (eg, thyroxin, cortisol), (4) the required use of these immature organ systems to support extrauterine life, and (5) side effects, known and mostly unknown, of treatment.[1] Organ system injury results in the many complications of prematurity, including chronic lung disease, necrotizing enterocolitis, central nervous system (CNS) injury, and retinopathy of prematurity (ROP). Neonatal morbidities occur most frequently in the most immature survivors,

[a] Division of Neonatology, Department of Pediatrics, Nelson 2-133, 600 North Wolfe Street, Baltimore, MD 21287, USA
[b] NICU Developmental Followup Clinic, The Kennedy Krieger Institute, Baltimore, MD, USA
* Corresponding author. Division of Neonatology, Department of Pediatrics, The Johns Hopkins Hospital, Nelson 2-133, 600 North Wolfe Street, Baltimore, MD 21287.
E-mail address: mallen2@jhmi.edu

Clin Perinatol 38 (2011) 441–454
doi:10.1016/j.clp.2011.06.011
0095-5108/11/$ – see front matter © 2011 Elsevier Inc. All rights reserved.

born at the lower limit of viability, and are associated with high mortality rates and later adverse health, growth, and neurodevelopmental outcomes.[1,4,10,11]

Improving preterm outcomes is no longer about saving more preterm babies; the major challenges, prevention and improved outcomes of preterm survivors, are more difficult to solve.[1] Neonatal intensive care is an imperfect substitute for a mother's womb. Although a focus on survival is important, improving preterm outcomes requires a better understanding of how to promote organ growth and maturation. Neuromaturation, the functional development of the CNS, is a dynamic process that promotes and shapes CNS structural development.[12] In this article the authors review preterm outcomes with the recognition that multiple factors influence neuromaturation, leading to a range of neurodevelopmental disabilities, dysfunctions, and altered CNS processing. These factors include (but are not limited to): causes of and trauma from preterm delivery; the imperfect attempts by the neonatal intensive care unit (NICU) to provide physiologic stability, respiratory support, and nutrition; insufficient endogenous neuroprotective agents; infection and multiple other promoters of inflammation; preterm exposure to medications with adverse side effects and unrecognized toxins; increased and sometimes overwhelming sensory stimulation; loss of unfettered movement; and the increased resistance of gravity when no longer surrounded by amniotic fluid.

NEUROMOTOR OUTCOMES

The earliest recognized signs of CNS dysfunction are neuromotor abnormalities on examination and infant motor delay. Many neuromotor abnormalities, including asymmetries, hypotonia, and extensor hypertonia, can be evident while an infant is still in the NICU, before 40 weeks' postmenstrual age (gestational age plus chronologic age).[13,14] Preterm neuromaturation after term includes acquisition of infant motor milestones, according to age adjusted for degree of prematurity.[15,16] Cerebral palsy (CP) and minor neuromotor dysfunction (MND, or developmental coordination disorder, DCD) are diagnosed clinically, based on persistence of neuromotor abnormalities on examination and severity of motor delay. Children born preterm exhibit a spectrum of motor disability, from severe quadriplegia (more common in those born extremely preterm), to the milder spastic diplegias and hemiplegias, to mild motor dysfunction characterized by mild neuromotor abnormalities (MND/DCD), to normal motor function.[17–20]

Cerebral Palsy

As with mortality rates, the prevalence of CP increases with decreasing gestational age and birth weight (BW) categories, with the greatest increase at the lower limit of viability.[21–23] Large regional population studies report CP prevalence in terms of live births, whereas multicenter and single-center studies generally use preterm survivors as the denominator. This distinction is most important in extremely preterm infants who have the highest mortality rates. By gestational age categories, the preterm CP prevalence per 1000 live births, compared with 0.9 to 1.43 for those born at term, is 6.1 for 32 to 36 weeks; 21.6 for 28 to 36 weeks; 43.7 for 28 to 31 weeks; and 55.6 to 114.6 for birth before 28 weeks' gestation.[20,24] By gestational age categories, ranges for CP prevalence among preterm survivors are 0.9% to 1% for birth between 32 and 36 weeks' gestation; 3% to 8% for birth before 30 to 32 weeks; 8% to 19% for birth before 28 weeks; 15% for birth before 27 weeks' gestation; and 15% to 21% for birth before 25 or 26 weeks' gestation.[4,7,22,24–31] Two European studies have reported increasing CP prevalence by decreasing week of gestation, from 1% at 34 weeks to 19% at 26 weeks.[22,23]

Most preterm infants who develop CP have the spastic type, characterized by increased muscle tone and reflexes, limitation of voluntary motor control, and a propensity to develop contractures. Among preterm children with CP, 48% to 58% develop spastic diplegia (involving both lower extremities), 14% to 29% develop hemiplegia (involving unilateral upper and lower extremity), and up to 7% develop the much more severe quadriplegia.[20,31] As many as 50% to 70% of preterm children with CP have mild to moderate CP and are able to walk independently or with aides; severe motor disability occurs in 7% to 10%, and up to 55% of children born before 25 or 26 weeks' gestation who develop CP.[19,21,22,24] Children who have CP often have accompanying higher rates of cognitive impairment, sensory impairment, epilepsy, and learning disability.

Minor Neuromotor Dysfunction

Preterm survivors who do not develop CP are at increased risk for mild motor impairments (ie, MND, DCD) which may include early and marked hand preference, overflow movements, fine motor dysfunction, motor planning difficulties, graphomotor impairment (including poor handwriting), poor visual spatial abilities, and sensorimotor integration or processing problems. A systematic review pooled data from 14 studies of children born before 33 weeks' gestation or with BW below 1501 g (none included children with CP) for a meta-analysis: the preterm group had statistically significantly poorer performance than controls on each of 3 standardized tests of age-appropriate motor function.[32] Another systematic review of preterm children who did not have CP pooled data from 11 studies for a random-effects meta-analysis.[18] The study found a pooled prevalence estimate of 40.5% (95% confidence interval [CI] 32.1%, 48.9%) for mild motor impairment (motor scores between 1 and 2 standard deviations [SD] below the mean) and 19.0% (95% CI 14.2%, 23.8%) for moderate motor impairment (motor score at or more than 2 SD below the mean). MND or DCD and their associated problems can adversely influence a child's self-help skills (eg, dressing), play (eg, on playground equipment), school performance (eg, handwriting), peer relationships, and self-esteem.

Brain Injury and Motor Impairments

Among the many risk factors for CP in preterm infants are male gender, intrauterine growth restriction, sepsis, surgery, high-frequency ventilation, and postnatal steroids; the strongest predictors are abnormalities on neonatal neuroimaging, including intraventricular hemorrhage (IVH), intraparenchymal hemorrhage (IPH), hemorrhagic infarction, posthemorrhagic hydrocephalus, ventricular dilation, white matter injury (WMI), and periventricular leukomalacia (PVL).[4,22,31,33–36] One multicenter study (the ELGAN study) of 1053 infants born before 28 weeks' gestation in 2002–2004 found that those with focal and/or diffuse WMI with late ventriculomegaly on neonatal head ultrasonography had the highest rates of CP at 2 years (52% and 44%, respectively), especially spastic quadriplegia.[33]

Magnetic resonance imaging (MRI) studies of children and adolescents born preterm provide some insight into brain injury and motor impairment. A volumetric MRI study of children who had PVL as neonates found statistically significant correlations between severity of motor dysfunction and the extent of pyramidal tract injury and total white matter volume.[37] Minor neuromotor dysfunction has been associated with thinning of the posterior corpus callosum and cerebral white matter abnormalities on MRI at age 7 years.[38,39] Difficulty with eye-hand coordination was associated with fractional anisotropy values in the cingulum, fornix, anterior commissure, corpus callosum, and right uncinate fasciculus on diffusion tensor imaging (DTI) in 2-year-olds born before 34 weeks' gestation.[40]

A DTI study of 28 preterm children with CP who had periventricular WMI compared with 35 full-term controls demonstrates the close relationship between the development of motor control and sensory input pathways.[41] On DTI with color maps of 26 central white matter tracts, the preterm children with CP had more severe injury to the posterior thalamic radiation pathways than to the descending corticospinal tract. Injury to the thalamic radiation pathways correlated with the preterm children's touch threshold, proprioception, and severity of motor impairment. No significant correlations with either sensory or motor outcomes were seen with corticospinal tract injury. These findings suggest that disruption of sensory tract pathways occurred independently from injury to the motor control pathways, and influenced motor function.

SENSORY OUTCOMES

Children and adolescents born preterm have higher rates of hearing impairment and visual impairment than controls.[1] Children born before 25 to 26 weeks' gestation have the highest rates of bilateral severe hearing impairment, 2% to 6%.[4,19,42,43] Identification of hearing impairment early in infancy is critical for early language development. Children with severe bilateral hearing impairment generally require amplification. When hearing aids do not improve hearing, cochlear implants may be indicated. Universal neonatal hearing screening has improved the early diagnosis of moderate to severe hearing impairments.

Severe visual impairment occurs in 1% of children born before 30 weeks' gestation, 1% to 2% born before 27 weeks' gestation, and as many as 9% to 12% born before 25 to 26 weeks' gestation.[19,25,30,42,43] Studies of 10- to 12-year-olds with BW below 1500 g or 1701 g have reported statistically significant reduction of near and distant visual acuity, contrast sensitivity, and stereopsis, as well as higher rates of strabismus.[44,45] As many as 44% of 11-year-olds born before 26 weeks' gestation had visual problems, including myopia and strabismus, compared with 19% of full-term controls. Late sequelae of ROP include retinal detachments, glaucoma, and cataracts in adults.[46] Although current and future treatments for ROP improve visual outcomes for preterm children with ROP, life-long ophthalmologic follow-up is indicated for those with severe ROP.

COGNITIVE OUTCOMES

Intelligence tests in children, adolescents, and adults are standardized psychometric measures of various aspects of intelligence; an average of subtest scores yields an intelligence quotient (IQ). Dimensions of intelligence include reasoning, understanding complex language, problem solving, visual motor, visual perception, visual and auditory processing, abstract thinking, and memory. Intellectual disability (ID), formerly called mental retardation, is defined as performance less than 2 SD below the mean on both intelligence and adaptive function tests. Assessment of intellectual abilities is most accurate in adolescents and adults, and in those without significant motor or sensory impairments.

IQ Scores and Intellectual Disability

Populations of children, adolescents, and young adults born preterm generally demonstrate a normal range of IQ scores, as well as mean IQ scores within the normal range of intelligence.[1,47–50] When compared with full-term controls, however, the mean IQ score is statistically significantly lower in the preterm group, with the lowest mean IQ scores in those born before 25 to 26 weeks' gestation. A meta-analysis that pooled data from 15 studies found statistically significant lower IQ scores in the preterm group, with a mean weighted difference of 10.8 IQ points (95% CI 9.2, 12.5).[47] For children born before 33 weeks' gestation at birth, IQ scores decrease by 1.3 to 1.7 IQ points for every week of gestational age.[47,48,50] Longitudinal preterm outcome studies have found that statistically significantly lower mean IQ scores than controls persist into young adulthood.[51–53] Even in adults, IQ scores are strongly associated with parental education and socioeconomic status.[48,53,54] Using multiple regression models, one study of young adults born before 32 weeks' gestation or with BW below 1500 g found that those with highly educated parents had a 14-point difference in mean IQ scores compared with those with less well educated parents.[48]

In a study of 11-year-olds who were born before 26 weeks' gestation in 1995, their mean IQ score was 84 ± 18, compared with the control mean of 104 ± 11; the mean difference was −20 points (95% CI −17, −23).[19] Excluding 16 children with severe ID changed the mean difference between the preterm and control group to −17 points (95% CI −19, −14). Preterm boys scored 8 points lower than preterm girls (95% CI 3, 13). The mean difference in IQ scores was not significantly changed when results were adjusted for socioeconomic status. Concerned about obsolete test norms, the investigators instead used the IQ score distribution from the full-term control group, and as many as 40% (95% CI 33%, 47%) had IQ scores more than 2 SD below the control group's mean, and 25% had IQ scores between 1 and 2 SD below the control group's mean. When they used multiple imputation to correct for loss to follow-up, the estimate for IQ scores more than 2 SD below the mean was 45% (95% CI 38%, 52%). A recent study of 1.8- to 2-year-olds born before 25 weeks' gestation in 2002–2004 reported that 51% had a Mental Developmental Index more than 2 SD below the test mean.[4]

Higher rates of ID and lower mean IQ scores than full-term controls are strongly associated with abnormalities on neonatal head ultrasonography, including severe IVH and IPH, posthemorrhagic hydrocephalus requiring a shunt, periventricular hemorrhagic infarction, and WMI.[34,55–58] Although not a universal finding, a study of 1.5- to 2-year-olds with BW below 1000 g found a statistically significant lower mean IQ score and higher rates of cognitive scores more than 2 SD below the mean in children with germinal matrix hemorrhage or IVH without ventriculomegaly (odds ratio [OR] 2.0, 95% CI 1.2, 3.3) compared with infants with no ultrasound abnormalities.[59] Neonatal MRI studies have found correlations between WMI and cognitive delay.[36,60] Among preterm children with normal neonatal neuroimaging studies, however, up to 25% to 27% have cognitive scores more than 2 SD below the mean.[36,55,59,61] When MRI was performed at school age, lower IQ scores correlated with reduced volumes of sensorimotor and midtemporal cortices, caudate, gray matter, and white matter.[38,62–64]

Cognitive Impairments

In preterm outcome studies that excluded children with CP, ID, and/or severe sensory impairment, the preterm group had statistically significantly lower mean IQ scores than the control group.[47,50,56,58,65–75] In many of these studies, preterm children with no CP or severe sensory impairment and IQ scores in the normal range demonstrate statistically significant lower mean test scores than full-term controls in vocabulary, language processing, verbal memory, visual motor, visual perceptual, visual spatial memory, perceptual organizing, and/or problem solving. These deficits may be initially subtle and unrecognized, but can interfere with a child's ability to learn and to function as they progress through elementary, middle, and high school.

MRI studies of children and adolescents born preterm have reported significant associations between specific neuropsychological impairments and MRI findings. Deficits in memory and numeracy were associated with smaller hippocampal volumes.[76] A visuospatial deficit in judging the orientation of a line was associated with decreased gray matter and increased white matter volumes of the right ventral extrastriatal cortex.[76] Poor visual navigation skills were associated with volumetric extent of WMI of the right parieto-occipital cortex.[77] A series of MRI studies in a subset of children with BW below 1250 g has demonstrated differences in language processing compared with full-term controls. On functional MRI, preterm 8-year-olds had a different pattern of brain activity while performing a semantic processing task; it was more like the pattern seen when control children performed phonological processing tasks.[78] The more the brain activity pattern with semantic processing resembled the pattern seen with phonological processing in controls, the poorer were the child's language comprehension abilities. Connectivity analysis with functional MRI revealed that, unlike in full-term controls, auditory language function in preterm children involved more connections between both cerebral hemispheres: preterm children had statistically significantly stronger neural circuits between Wernicke's area and the right frontal gyrus (Broca) and both left and right supramarginal gyri of the inferior parietal lobes.[79] One can speculate that this alternative pattern may result in less efficient auditory language processing.

Executive Dysfunction

Executive function is an important cognitive function used to plan and organize one's approach to a task, control impulses, monitor progress, assess situations, and formulate a response to changing conditions. Tests of working memory, divided attention, response inhibition, verbal fluency, information processing speed, concept generation, and mental flexibility have been used to evaluate executive function in preterm children and adolescents.[75,80–86]

Two systematic reviews report that preterm children and adolescents have statistically significantly greater problems with executive function than do full-term controls.[81,82] One study pooled data from 12 studies for meta-analyses, and found statistically significantly lower scores in the preterm group on tests of verbal fluency, working memory, and cognitive flexibility, but with small combined effect sizes of 0.57 SD, 0.36 SD, and 0.49 SD, respectively.[81] Meta-analyses of pooled data from 5 to 13 studies for 8 executive function skills found statistically significantly lower mean scores in the preterm group for selective attention, sustained attention, response inhibition, phonemic fluency, and planning, but not for semantic fluency, shifting between tasks, or sorting.[82] Effect sizes for tests of response inhibition, selective attention, and sustained attention were significantly influenced by gestational age at birth. Phonemic fluency was significantly influenced by chronologic age at the time of testing (ie, performance improved with age).

Problems with executive function extend into adulthood. In a study of 20- to 25-year-olds who had no impairments and were born before 33 weeks' gestation, the preterm group had statistically significantly lower scores than controls on tests of response inhibition and mental flexibility.[86] A study of 18- to 27-year-olds with no impairments and BW below 1500 g found statistically significantly slower reaction times in tests of simple reaction time, choice, working memory, divided attention, and learning reaction times.[84]

Executive dysfunction in preterm children and adolescents has been associated with findings on neuroimaging studies. A longitudinal follow-up study of 16-year-olds with BW below 1250 g who had no CP, ID, or severe sensory impairments reported statistically significantly lower mean scores than controls on tests of phonological fluency, verbal inhibition, and immediate and delayed verbal memory and visuospatial memory.[73] These scores strongly correlated with severe brain injury on neonatal ultrasonography and maternal education. In an MRI study of 15-year-olds with BW below 1501 g, 9 had impaired problem solving and cognitive flexibility.[87] MRI studies revealed ventricular dilation in all 9 adolescents with executive dysfunction, 8 had significantly reduced white matter volume (OR 18.0, 95% CI 1.9, 169.0) and 7 had thinning of the corpus callosum (OR 9.5, 95% CI 1.6, 37). In studies of adolescents born before 33 weeks' gestation, semantic fluency impairments were associated with decreased volumes of white matter in the thalamus and the corpus callosum.[88,89]

Specific Learning Disability

Despite normal IQ scores, variability in cognitive abilities increases the risk of specific learning disabilities, and academic and school problems. Studies of children and adolescents born preterm who did not have CP, ID, or sensory impairments have reported lower scores than full-term controls on tests of reading, writing, spelling, and arithmetic.[69,81,83,90,91] A large study of 970 elementary school children born preterm reported statistically significantly lower scores in tests of reading and math than full-term controls, especially in the early grades.[91] A systematic review of achievement scores in preterm and full-term control children pooled data from 14 studies for meta-analyses; the preterm group had statistically significantly lower scores on tests in the preterm group on tests of math, reading, and spelling.[81] Combined effect sizes were greatest for math (−0.60 SD, 95% CI −0.74, −0.46) and spelling (−0.76 SD, 95% CI −1.13, −0.40) than for reading (−0.48 SD, 95% CI −0.60, −0.34).

The diagnosis of a specific learning disability entails low scores on a test of reading, writing, spelling, or arithmetic/mathematics; a normal IQ score; and adequate exposure to teaching of that subject. In an international comparison of children with BW below 1000 g with normal intelligence, low test scores (1 or more SD below the mean) were reported in 19% to 54% for reading, 24% to 69% for math, and 34% to 61% for spelling.[92] A study of 11-year-olds reported a higher rate of specific learning disability for reading and/or math in children with BW below 750 g (67%) compared with full-term controls (34%).[66] One study found that the best predictors of academic achievement in 9- to 10-year-olds born before 31 weeks' gestation were preterm birth, processing speed, and working memory.[83]

Academic problems associated with preterm birth are reflected in school problems. Children and adolescents born preterm had statistically significantly higher rates of suspension from kindergarten, use of special education resources, failing and repeating one or more grades in school, and low teacher ratings.[58,66,71,83,91,93] Even children born between 32 and 34 weeks' gestation and 34 and 36 weeks' gestation had a statistically significant increase in these school problems compared with full-term children.[91,93] Many preterm outcome studies of young adults born preterm have found statistically significant differences in lower academic achievement, high school graduation rates, and college/university attendance compared with full-term controls.[51,53,94–97] A large Norwegian study that linked multiple national databases demonstrated that educational level attained by adulthood decreased with decreasing gestational age.[98]

BEHAVIOR AND SOCIAL-EMOTIONAL ADJUSTMENT

Attention-deficit disorders (ADD), behavior problems, and social-emotional difficulties are associated with prematurity. Meta-analyses have found statistically increased rates of ADD, internalizing behaviors (eg, anxiety, depression, withdrawn behavior), and externalizing behaviors (eg, delinquency, aggression, oppositional behavior) in children and adolescents born preterm compared with full-term controls.[47,70,81] Two systematic reviews have found statistically significantly higher rates of ADD in the preterm group than in full-term controls.[47,81] A random effects meta-analysis of pooled data from 6 studies (1980–2001) that diagnosed ADD or attention-deficit/hyperactivity disorder using formal criteria estimated a relative risk of 2.64 (95% CI 1.85, 3.78).[47] A more recent meta-analysis of pooled data from 5 studies (1998–2008) estimated combined effect sizes of −0.59 and −0.43 for ratings of ADD by parents and teachers, respectively.[81]

By contrast, meta-analyses of pooled data found small effect sizes for parent and teacher ratings of internalizing behaviors in children and adolescents born preterm compared with controls, and negligible effect sizes for externalizing behaviors.[81] These findings are corroborated by studies that reported lower rates in adolescents and adults born preterm than in full-term controls of risk-taking behaviors, including lower rates of illegal drug use, trouble with the law, and teen pregnancies, as well as higher rates of living with their parents.[51,97]

SUMMARY

Preterm birth is remarkable for its associated wide range of neurodevelopmental and functional outcomes. Although most children born preterm do not develop CP, rates of CP and minor neuromotor dysfunction are higher than in full-term controls. Children, adolescents, and young adults born preterm demonstrate a normal range of cognitive scores and mean scores within the normal range of intelligence, but their mean IQ scores are generally lower and their rate of ID and other cognitive impairments is higher than those of full-term controls. Their relative cognitive disadvantage remains statistically significant even when preterm children with CP, or visual or hearing impairment are excluded. At school age, children born preterm demonstrate higher rates of learning disability, grade retention, special education, ADD, and social-emotional problems than do peers born at term. Cognitive scores decrease and rates of CP, ID, neurodevelopmental disabilities, and school problems progressively increase with decreases in gestational age and BW categories.

Until more effective and efficient methods are devised for preventing preterm birth, prematurity will remain a significant public health problem in the United States. Nonetheless, the most remarkable aspect of all these findings is the resiliency of preterm infants. Current neonatal intensive care interventions for preterm infants are crude compared with the subtle, continuous adjustments of the mother's body for supporting the growth, development, and neuromaturation of the fetus. Yet the majority of preterm survivors are functional, contributing members of their communities. Many preterm children and adolescents with evidence of brain injury do relatively well in life.

Neuromaturation continues despite preterm exposure to the extrauterine environment. The preterm brain changes in response to injury, but neuromaturation continues. Alternative, functional neural circuits can be formed, although they are sometimes not as efficient as typical pathways. The development of the CNS is driven by genetic and epigenetic processes, in response to environmental input, movement, and responses. The most important challenge posed by preterm birth is to discover the best ways to protect the preterm infant and support his or her growth, organ development, and neuromaturation in the NICU and, after discharge, in the home and community.

REFERENCES

1. Behrman RE, Butler AS. Institute of Medicine (U.S.). Committee on understanding premature birth and assuring healthy outcomes. Preterm birth: causes, consequences, and prevention. Washington, DC: National Academies Press; 2007.
2. Mathews TJ, Minino AM, Osterman MJ, et al. Annual summary of vital statistics: 2008. Pediatrics 2011;127(1):146–57.
3. Mathews TJ, MacDorman MF. Infant mortality statistics from the 2006 period linked birth/infant death data set. Natl Vital Stat Rep 2010;58(17):1–31.
4. Hintz SR, Kendrick DE, Wilson-Costello DE, et al. Early-childhood neurodevelopmental outcomes are not improving for infants born at <25 weeks' gestational age. Pediatrics 2011;127(1):62–70.
5. Field DJ, Dorling JS, Manktelow BN, et al. Survival of extremely premature babies in a geographically defined population: prospective cohort study of 1994-9 compared with 2000-5. BMJ 2008;336(7655):1221–3.
6. Donohue PK, Boss RD, Shepard J, et al. Intervention at the border of viability: perspective over a decade. Arch Pediatr Adolesc Med 2009;163(10):902–6.
7. Doyle LW, Roberts G, Anderson PJ. Outcomes at age 2 years of infants <28 weeks' gestational age born in Victoria in 2005. J Pediatr 2010;156(1): 49.e1–53.e1.
8. Tomashek KM, Shapiro-Mendoza CK, Davidoff MJ, et al. Differences in mortality between late-preterm and term singleton infants in the United States, 1995–2002. J Pediatr 2007;151(5):450–6, 456 e451.
9. Khashu M, Narayanan M, Bhargava S, et al. Perinatal outcomes associated with preterm birth at 33 to 36 weeks' gestation: a population-based cohort study. Pediatrics 2009;123(1):109–13.
10. Stoll BJ, Hansen NI, Bell EF, et al. Neonatal outcomes of extremely preterm infants from the NICHD Neonatal Research Network. Pediatrics 2010;126(3):443–56.
11. Allen MC. Preterm outcomes research: a critical component of neonatal intensive care. Ment Retard Dev Disabil Res Rev 2002;8(4):221–33.
12. Allen MC. Assessment of gestational age and neuromaturation. Ment Retard Dev Disabil Res Rev 2005;11(1):21–33.
13. Engle WA. Age terminology during the perinatal period. Pediatrics 2004;114(5): 1362–4.
14. Allen M. Preterm development. In: Accardo PJ, editor. Capute & Accardo's neurodevelopmental disabilities in infancy and childhood, vol. 2. 3rd edition. Baltimore (MD): Paul H. Brookes Publications; 2008. p. 29–45.
15. Allen MC, Alexander GR. Gross motor milestones in preterm infants: correction for degree of prematurity. J Pediatr 1990;116(6):955–9.
16. Palisano RJ. Use of chronological and adjusted ages to compare motor development of healthy preterm and fullterm infants. Dev Med Child Neurol 1986;28(2): 180–7.
17. Hack M, DeMonterice D, Merkatz IR, et al. Rehospitalization of the very-low-birth-weight infant. A continuum of perinatal and environmental morbidity. Am J Dis Child 1981;135(3):263–6.
18. Williams J, Lee KJ, Anderson PJ. Prevalence of motor-skill impairment in preterm children who do not develop cerebral palsy: a systematic review. Dev Med Child Neurol 2010;52(3):232–7.
19. Johnson S, Fawke J, Hennessy E, et al. Neurodevelopmental disability through 11 years of age in children born before 26 weeks of gestation. Pediatrics 2009; 124(2):e249–57.

20. Himmelmann K, Hagberg G, Uvebrant P. The changing panorama of cerebral palsy in Sweden. X. Prevalence and origin in the birth-year period 1999–2002. Acta Paediatr 2010;99(9):1337–43.
21. Himmelmann K, Beckung E, Hagberg G, et al. Gross and fine motor function and accompanying impairments in cerebral palsy. Dev Med Child Neurol 2006;48(6): 417–23.
22. Ancel PY, Livinec F, Larroque B, et al. Cerebral palsy among very preterm children in relation to gestational age and neonatal ultrasound abnormalities: the EPI-PAGE cohort study. Pediatrics 2006;117(3):828–35.
23. Marret S, Ancel PY, Marpeau L, et al. Neonatal and 5-year outcomes after birth at 30-34 weeks of gestation. Obstet Gynecol 2007;110(1):72–80.
24. Sigurdardottir S, Thorkelsson T, Halldorsdottir M, et al. Trends in prevalence and characteristics of cerebral palsy among Icelandic children born 1990 to 2003. Dev Med Child Neurol 2009;51(5):356–63.
25. Bode MM, D'Eugenio DB, Forsyth N, et al. Outcome of extreme prematurity: a prospective comparison of 2 regional cohorts born 20 years apart. Pediatrics 2009;124(3):866–74.
26. Groenendaal F, Termote JU, van der Heide-Jalving M, et al. Complications affecting preterm neonates from 1991 to 2006: what have we gained? Acta Paediatr 2010;99(3):354–8.
27. Bodeau-Livinec F, Marlow N, Ancel PY, et al. Impact of intensive care practices on short-term and long-term outcomes for extremely preterm infants: comparison between the British Isles and France. Pediatrics 2008;122(5):e1014–21.
28. Woodward LJ, Moor S, Hood KM, et al. Very preterm children show impairments across multiple neurodevelopmental domains by age 4 years. Arch Dis Child Fetal Neonatal Ed 2009;94(5):F339–44.
29. Mikkola K, Ritari N, Tommiska V, et al. Neurodevelopmental outcome at 5 years of age of a national cohort of extremely low birth weight infants who were born in 1996-1997. Pediatrics 2005;116(6):1391–400.
30. Stahlmann N, Rapp M, Herting E, et al. Outcome of extremely premature infants at early school age: health-related quality of life and neurosensory, cognitive, and behavioral outcomes in a population-based sample in northern Germany. Neuropediatrics 2009;40(3):112–9.
31. Glinianaia SV, Rankin J, Colver A. Cerebral palsy rates by birth weight, gestation and severity in North of England, 1991–2000 singleton births. Arch Dis Child 2011;96(2):180–5.
32. de Kieviet JF, Piek JP, Aarnoudse-Moens CS, et al. Motor development in very preterm and very low-birth-weight children from birth to adolescence: a meta-analysis. JAMA 2009;302(20):2235–42.
33. Kuban KC, Allred EN, O'Shea TM, et al. Cranial ultrasound lesions in the NICU predict cerebral palsy at age 2 years in children born at extremely low gestational age. J Child Neurol 2009;24(1):63–72.
34. Maitre NL, Marshall DD, Price WA, et al. Neurodevelopmental outcome of infants with unilateral or bilateral periventricular hemorrhagic infarction. Pediatrics 2009; 124(6):e1153–60.
35. Nanba Y, Matsui K, Aida N, et al. Magnetic resonance imaging regional T1 abnormalities at term accurately predict motor outcome in preterm infants. Pediatrics 2007;120(1):e10–9.
36. Woodward LJ, Anderson PJ, Austin NC, et al. Neonatal MRI to predict neurodevelopmental outcomes in preterm infants. N Engl J Med 2006;355(7):685–94.

37. Staudt M, Pavlova M, Bohm S, et al. Pyramidal tract damage correlates with motor dysfunction in bilateral periventricular leukomalacia (PVL). Neuropediatrics 2003;34(4):182–8.

38. Abernethy LJ, Cooke RW, Foulder-Hughes L. Caudate and hippocampal volumes, intelligence, and motor impairment in 7-year-old children who were born preterm. Pediatr Res 2004;55(5):884–93.

39. Abernethy LJ, Klafkowski G, Foulder-Hughes L, et al. Magnetic resonance imaging and T2 relaxometry of cerebral white matter and hippocampus in children born preterm. Pediatr Res 2003;54(6):868–74.

40. Counsell SJ, Edwards AD, Chew AT, et al. Specific relations between neurodevelopmental abilities and white matter microstructure in children born preterm. Brain 2008;131(Pt 12):3201–8.

41. Hoon AH Jr, Stashinko EE, Nagae LM, et al. Sensory and motor deficits in children with cerebral palsy born preterm correlate with diffusion tensor imaging abnormalities in thalamocortical pathways. Dev Med Child Neurol 2009;51(9): 697–704.

42. Farooqi A, Hagglof B, Sedin G, et al. Chronic conditions, functional limitations, and special health care needs in 10- to 12-year-old children born at 23 to 25 weeks' gestation in the 1990s: a Swedish national prospective follow-up study. Pediatrics 2006;118(5):e1466–77.

43. Sommer C, Urlesberger B, Maurer-Fellbaum U, et al. Neurodevelopmental outcome at 2 years in 23 to 26 weeks old gestation infants. Klin Padiatr 2007; 219(1):23–9.

44. O'Connor AR, Wilson CM, Fielder AR. Ophthalmological problems associated with preterm birth. Eye 2007;21(10):1254–60.

45. Powls A, Botting N, Cooke RW, et al. Visual impairment in very low birthweight children. Arch Dis Child Fetal Neonatal Ed 1997;76(2):F82–7.

46. Smith BT, Tasman WS. Retinopathy of prematurity: late complications in the baby boomer generation (1946–1964). Trans Am Ophthalmol Soc 2005;103:225–34 [discussion: 234–6].

47. Bhutta AT, Cleves MA, Casey PH, et al. Cognitive and behavioral outcomes of school-aged children who were born preterm: a meta-analysis. JAMA 2002; 288(6):728–37.

48. Weisglas-Kuperus N, Hille ET, Duivenvoorden HJ, et al. Intelligence of very preterm or very low birthweight infants in young adulthood. Arch Dis Child Fetal Neonatal Ed 2009;94(3):F196–200.

49. Aylward GP. Cognitive and neuropsychological outcomes: More than IQ scores. Ment Retard Dev Disabil Res Rev 2002;8(4):234–40.

50. Johnson S. Cognitive and behavioural outcomes following very preterm birth. Semin Fetal Neonatal Med 2007;12(5):363–73.

51. Hack M, Flannery DJ, Schluchter M, et al. Outcomes in young adulthood for very-low-birth-weight infants. N Engl J Med 2002;346(3):149–57.

52. Allin M, Walshe M, Fern A, et al. Cognitive maturation in preterm and term born adolescents. J Neurol Neurosurg Psychiatry 2008;79(4):381–6.

53. Lefebvre F, Mazurier E, Tessier R. Cognitive and educational outcomes in early adulthood for infants weighing 1000 grams or less at birth. Acta Paediatr 2005; 94(6):733–40.

54. Ekeus C, Lindstrom K, Lindblad F, et al. Preterm birth, social disadvantage, and cognitive competence in Swedish 18- to 19-year-old men. Pediatrics 2010;125(1): e67–73.

55. Adams-Chapman I, Hansen NI, Stoll BJ, et al. Neurodevelopmental outcome of extremely low birth weight infants with posthemorrhagic hydrocephalus requiring shunt insertion. Pediatrics 2008;121(5):e1167–77.

56. Whitaker AH, Feldman JF, Lorenz JM, et al. Motor and cognitive outcomes in nondisabled low-birth-weight adolescents: early determinants. Arch Pediatr Adolesc Med 2006;160(10):1040–6.

57. Sherlock RL, Anderson PJ, Doyle LW. Neurodevelopmental sequelae of intraventricular haemorrhage at 8 years of age in a regional cohort of ELBW/very preterm infants. Early Hum Dev 2005;81(11):909–16.

58. Luu TM, Ment LR, Schneider KC, et al. Lasting effects of preterm birth and neonatal brain hemorrhage at 12 years of age. Pediatrics 2009;123(3):1037–44.

59. Patra K, Wilson-Costello D, Taylor HG, et al. Grades I-II intraventricular hemorrhage in extremely low birth weight infants: effects on neurodevelopment. J Pediatr 2006;149(2):169–73.

60. Dyet LE, Kennea N, Counsell SJ, et al. Natural history of brain lesions in extremely preterm infants studied with serial magnetic resonance imaging from birth and neurodevelopmental assessment. Pediatrics 2006;118(2):536–48.

61. Laptook A, Tyson J, Shankaran S, et al. Elevated temperature after hypoxic-ischemic encephalopathy: risk factor for adverse outcomes. Pediatrics 2008; 122(3):491–9.

62. Peterson BS, Vohr B, Staib LH, et al. Regional brain volume abnormalities and long-term cognitive outcome in preterm infants. JAMA 2000;284(15):1939–47.

63. Isaacs EB, Edmonds CJ, Chong WK, et al. Brain morphometry and IQ measurements in preterm children. Brain 2004;127(Pt 12):2595–607.

64. Yung A, Poon G, Qiu DQ, et al. White matter volume and anisotropy in preterm children: a pilot study of neurocognitive correlates. Pediatr Res 2007;61(6): 732–6.

65. Bohm B, Katz-Salamon M, Institute K, et al. Developmental risks and protective factors for influencing cognitive outcome at 5 1/2 years of age in very-low-birthweight children. Dev Med Child Neurol 2002;44(8):508–16.

66. Litt J, Taylor HG, Klein N, et al. Learning disabilities in children with very low birthweight: prevalence, neuropsychological correlates, and educational interventions. J Learn Disabil 2005;38(2):130–41.

67. Grunau RE, Whitfield MF, Davis C. Pattern of learning disabilities in children with extremely low birth weight and broadly average intelligence. Arch Pediatr Adolesc Med 2002;156(6):615–20.

68. Marlow N, Wolke D, Bracewell MA, et al. Neurologic and developmental disability at six years of age after extremely preterm birth. N Engl J Med 2005;352(1):9–19.

69. Anderson P, Doyle LW. Neurobehavioral outcomes of school-age children born extremely low birth weight or very preterm in the 1990s. JAMA 2003;289(24): 3264–72.

70. Foulder-Hughes LA, Cooke RW. Motor, cognitive, and behavioural disorders in children born very preterm. Dev Med Child Neurol 2003;45(2):97–103.

71. Saigal S, Hoult LA, Streiner DL, et al. School difficulties at adolescence in a regional cohort of children who were extremely low birth weight. Pediatrics 2000;105(2):325–31.

72. Rickards AL, Kelly EA, Doyle LW, et al. Cognition, academic progress, behavior and self-concept at 14 years of very low birth weight children. J Dev Behav Pediatr 2001;22(1):11–8.

73. Luu TM, Ment L, Allan W, et al. Executive and memory function in adolescents born very preterm. Pediatrics 2011;127(3):e639–46.

74. Taylor HG, Minich NM, Klein N, et al. Longitudinal outcomes of very low birth weight: neuropsychological findings. J Int Neuropsychol Soc 2004;10(2):149–63.
75. Marlow N, Hennessy EM, Bracewell MA, et al. Motor and executive function at 6 years of age after extremely preterm birth. Pediatrics 2007;120(4):793–804.
76. Isaacs EB, Edmonds CJ, Chong WK, et al. Cortical anomalies associated with visuospatial processing deficits. Ann Neurol 2003;53(6):768–73.
77. Pavlova M, Sokolov A, Krageloh-Mann I. Visual navigation in adolescents with early periventricular lesions: knowing where, but not getting there. Cereb Cortex 2007;17(2):363–9.
78. Peterson BS, Vohr B, Kane MJ, et al. A functional magnetic resonance imaging study of language processing and its cognitive correlates in prematurely born children. Pediatrics 2002;110(6):1153–62.
79. Gozzo Y, Vohr B, Lacadie C, et al. Alterations in neural connectivity in preterm children at school age. Neuroimage 2009;48(2):458–63.
80. Aarnoudse-Moens CS, Smidts DP, Oosterlaan J, et al. Executive function in very preterm children at early school age. J Abnorm Child Psychol 2009;37(7):981–93.
81. Aarnoudse-Moens CS, Weisglas-Kuperus N, van Goudoever JB, et al. Meta-analysis of neurobehavioral outcomes in very preterm and/or very low birth weight children. Pediatrics 2009;124(2):717–28.
82. Mulder H, Pitchford NJ, Hagger MS, et al. Development of executive function and attention in preterm children: a systematic review. Dev Neuropsychol 2009;34(4): 393–421.
83. Mulder H, Pitchford NJ, Marlow N. Processing speed and working memory underlie academic attainment in very preterm children. Arch Dis Child Fetal Neonatal Ed 2010;95(4):F267–72.
84. Strang-Karlsson S, Andersson S, Paile-Hyvarinen M, et al. Slower reaction times and impaired learning in young adults with birth weight <1500 g. Pediatrics 2010; 125(1):e74–82.
85. Anderson PJ, Doyle LW. Executive functioning in school-aged children who were born very preterm or with extremely low birth weight in the 1990s. Pediatrics 2004;114(1):50–7.
86. Nosarti C, Giouroukou E, Micali N, et al. Impaired executive functioning in young adults born very preterm. J Int Neuropsychol Soc 2007;13(4):571–81.
87. Skranes J, Evensen KI, Lohaugen GC, et al. Abnormal cerebral MRI findings and neuroimpairments in very low birth weight (VLBW) adolescents. Eur J Paediatr Neurol 2008;12(4):273–83.
88. Gimenez M, Junque C, Narberhaus A, et al. Correlations of thalamic reductions with verbal fluency impairment in those born prematurely. Neuroreport 2006; 17(5):463–6.
89. Narberhaus A, Segarra D, Caldu X, et al. Corpus callosum and prefrontal functions in adolescents with history of very preterm birth. Neuropsychologia 2008; 46(1):111–6.
90. Grunau RE, Whitfield MF, Fay TB. Psychosocial and academic characteristics of extremely low birth weight (< or =800 g) adolescents who are free of major impairment compared with term-born control subjects. Pediatrics 2004;114(6):e725–32.
91. Chyi LJ, Lee HC, Hintz SR, et al. School outcomes of late preterm infants: special needs and challenges for infants born at 32 to 36 weeks gestation. J Pediatr 2008;153(1):25–31.
92. Saigal S, den Ouden L, Wolke D, et al. School-age outcomes in children who were extremely low birth weight from four international population-based cohorts. Pediatrics 2003;112(4):943–50.

93. Morse SB, Zheng H, Tang Y, et al. Early school-age outcomes of late preterm infants. Pediatrics 2009;123(4):e622–9.
94. Mathiasen R, Hansen BM, Nybo Anderson AM, et al. Socio-economic achievements of individuals born very preterm at the age of 27 to 29 years: a nationwide cohort study. Dev Med Child Neurol 2009;51(11):901–8.
95. Lindstrom K, Winbladh B, Haglund B, et al. Preterm infants as young adults: a Swedish national cohort study. Pediatrics 2007;120(1):70–7.
96. Hille ET, Weisglas-Kuperus N, van Goudoever JB, et al. Functional outcomes and participation in young adulthood for very preterm and very low birth weight infants: the Dutch project on preterm and small for gestational age infants at 19 years of age. Pediatrics 2007;120(3):e587–95.
97. Cooke RW. Health, lifestyle, and quality of life for young adults born very preterm. Arch Dis Child 2004;89(3):201–6.
98. Moster D, Lie RT, Markestad T. Long-term medical and social consequences of preterm birth. N Engl J Med 2008;359(3):262–73.

Neuroprotective Approaches: Before and After Delivery

Lina F. Chalak, MD, MSCS[a],*, Dwight J. Rouse, MD[b]

KEYWORDS

- Cerebral palsy • Prematurity • Low birth weight
- Neuroprotection • Magnesium sulfate

Cerebral palsy is a leading cause of chronic childhood disability.[1] It is characterized by abnormal control of movement and posture, and resultant activity limitation. The genesis of cerebral palsy is nonprogressive damage or dysfunction of the developing fetal or infant brain.[2] Infants born preterm are especially vulnerable to cerebral palsy, the risk of which is inversely proportional to gestational age at birth. And because even at the extremes of viability, many if not most preterm infants now survive, the contribution of prematurity to the overall burden of cerebral palsy is substantial. For example, in a well-conducted population-based cohort study from Northern California, children born weighing less than 2500 g accounted for 47% of cerebral palsy cases, even though they accounted for only 5.3% of survivors. Those born weighing less than 1000 g at birth accounted for 8% of cerebral palsy cases but only 0.2% of survivors.[3]

RISK FACTORS FOR CEREBRAL PALSY AMONG PRETERM INFANTS

Certain factors have been associated with an increased risk of cerebral palsy among children who survive preterm birth. Perhaps the most well known is chorioamnionitis, both clinical and histologic. In a meta-analysis of 12 studies, 10 of which included only children who had been born preterm, Shatrov and colleagues[4] reported that clinical chorioamnionitis had an odds ratio (OR) of 2.42 (95% confidence interval [CI]

Dr Chalak is supported by Grant Number KL2RR024983, titled, "North and Central Texas Clinical and Translational Science Initiative" from the National Center for Research Resources (NCRR, NIH).

[a] Division of Neonatal-Perinatal Medicine, Department of Pediatrics, The University of Texas Southwestern Medical Center at Dallas, 5323 Harry Hines Boulevard, Dallas, TX 75390-9063, USA

[b] Division of Maternal-Fetal Medicine, Department of Obstetrics and Gynecology, Women & Infants Hospital of Rhode Island, The Warren G. Alpert School of Medicine of Brown University, 101 Dudley Street, Providence, RI 02905, USA

* Corresponding author.

E-mail address: lina.chalak@utsouthwestern.edu

Clin Perinatol 38 (2011) 455–470

doi:10.1016/j.clp.2011.06.012

0095-5108/11/$ – see front matter © 2011 Elsevier Inc. All rights reserved.

perinatology.theclinics.com

1.52–3.84) for cerebral palsy. In a meta-analysis of 8 studies that enrolled only children born preterm, histologic chorioamnionitis had an OR of 1.83 (95% CI 1.17–2.89).[4]

Using linked administrative databases, Gilbert and colleagues[5] compared the presence of recorded adverse intrapartum events and the risk of spastic quadriplegic or dyskinetic cerebral palsy among approximately 2500 children with cerebral palsy of these types and more than 87,000 controls. The investigators identified 6 diagnoses that they believed were likely to be associated with cerebral palsy: placental abruption, uterine rupture during labor, fetal distress, birth trauma, cord prolapse, and mild to severe birth asphyxia. The prevalence of any one of these diagnoses was more common among women who gave birth to children ultimately diagnosed with cerebral palsy than among those who gave birth to children without cerebral palsy, 37% versus 16%. As in the Shatrov meta-analysis, clinical chorioamnionitis was associated with a significantly increased risk of cerebral palsy (relative risk [RR] 1.5).

Multiple other studies have evaluated risk factors for cerebral palsy among preterm infants. Leveno[6] performed a secondary analysis of a randomized, double-blinded clinical trial of magnesium sulfate for the prevention of cerebral palsy. The objective was to evaluate antepartum, intrapartum, and neonatal factors related to the development of cerebral palsy among children born preterm. In all, he studied 39 risk factors. Women and their 1811 children (overall cerebral palsy rate = 5.5%) born between 24 and 32 weeks' gestation were included. In the final multivariable analysis, 7 factors were significantly associated with cerebral palsy (**Table 1**). It is worth noting that in this analysis, clinical chorioamnionitis was not associated with cerebral palsy (histologic chorioamnionitis was not evaluated).

POTENTIAL ANTENATAL NEUROPROTECTIVE APPROACHES

A review of the aforementioned risk factors might inform one's approach to the prevention of cerebral palsy among preterm infants. Unfortunately, only one of the associated factors, receipt of magnesium sulfate, has had this potential evaluated in a rigorous manner. Another factor not listed is the administration of maternal glucocorticoids for fetal lung maturation. Before these two, the authors review potential approaches targeted at other risk factors.

Treatment or Prevention of Chorioamnionitis

Both histologic and clinical chorioamnionitis are common among preterm deliveries. By definition, the diagnosis of histologic chorioamnionitis requires that the fetal

Table 1		
Risk factors for cerebral palsy in the BEAM[7] trial		
Factor (%)[a]	Adjusted Odds Ratio	95% Confidence Interval
Smoking (26)	1.86	1.11–3.10
Magnesium sulfate exposure (48)	0.58	0.35–0.95
Preterm labor (10)	1.98	1.06–3.71
Gestational age at delivery (by week)	0.76	0.68–0.85
Neonatal hypotension (18)	3.24	1.95–5.38
Intraventricular hemorrhage Grade III/IV (2.4)	5.96	2.50–14.24
PVL (1.9)	45.38	18.01–114.34

Abbreviation: PVL, periventricular leukomalacia.
[a] Percentage of cohort with condition or exposure.

membranes be examined microscopically. This procedure poses an obvious pragmatic impediment to targeting women for antenatal therapy, although various inflammatory markers that are more accessible, for example, amniotic fluid cytokines, might serve as surrogate markers. Clinical chorioamnionitis is often the consequence of expectantly managed preterm premature rupture of the membranes. Thus its prevention in many cases of threatened preterm birth would require a foreshortening of expectant management, which, by lowering the gestational age at delivery, very likely could be self-defeating from the standpoint of cerebral palsy prevention (see the effect of gestational age; **Table 1**). When clinical chorioamnionitis is diagnosed, standard management already includes the administration of broad-spectrum antibiotics and delivery to prevent immediate perinatal and/or maternal harms. Thus the potential to prevent and/or treat chorioamnionitis so as to lower the subsequent risk of cerebral palsy at present seems limited. In fact, data from the ORACLE II trial suggest that in the setting of preterm labor, administration of certain antibiotics to the mother may actually increase the risk of cerebral palsy.[8]

Prevention or Treatment of Placental Abruption, Uterine Rupture During Labor, and Cord Prolapse

These conditions are generally unpredictable and not preventable. When they do occur and are recognized, they are treated as emergencies and delivery is effected as quickly as possible so as to prevent the consequences of asphyxia, including hypoxic-ischemic encephalopathy (HIE), which in some cases is a precursor to cerebral palsy. Therefore, the potential to reduce the burden of cerebral palsy associated with these conditions is low, although some cases of uterine rupture during attempted vaginal birth after cesarean might be avoided by elective repeat cesarean delivery.

Avoidance of Birth Asphyxia

Although most cases of cerebral palsy are not related to an intrapartum event, some are and there are recognized essential criteria for allowing intrapartum oxygen deprivation to be considered as a possible cause of cerebral palsy among term infants.[9] The avoidance of birth asphyxia is a major focus of labor management for all deliveries. To that end, almost all women in the United States undergo continuous electronic fetal monitoring. Unfortunately, evidence that such monitoring reduces the risk of cerebral palsy is lacking. Indeed, in a multicentered trial of continuous electronic fetal monitoring versus periodic auscultation conducted among women who delivered prematurely, the risk of cerebral palsy was higher among children who had been monitored electronically than among those who had undergone periodic auscultation, 20% versus 8% (P<.03).[10]

Maternal Smoking

Maternal cigarette smoking during pregnancy increases the risk of low birth weight, stillbirth and, to a lesser degree, prematurity. The secondary analysis of Leveno[6] suggests that, independently, it almost doubles the risk of cerebral palsy. Some of this association may be due to residual confounding, but others have reported a similar, albeit less strong association. For instance, in a population-based study from Sweden, Thorngren-Jerneck and Herbst[11] reported that maternal smoking had an OR of 1.2 for cerebral palsy (95% CI 1.1–1.3). There appear to be good reasons beyond personal health to encourage and support pregnant women in efforts to stop smoking, and a reduction in the risk of cerebral palsy among their offspring might well be another one.

Corticosteroids for Fetal Maturation

Meta-analysis of multiple randomized clinical trials demonstrate that antenatal corticosteroids prior to preterm birth significantly reduce the risk of several adverse neonatal outcomes including death, respiratory distress syndrome, cerebroventricular hemorrhage, necrotizing enterocolitis, respiratory support, intensive care admissions, and systemic infections in the first 48 hours of life, with reductions ranging from 54% (necrotizing enterocolitis) to 20% (intensive care admissions). In a pooled analysis of 5 studies that included 904 children with follow-up from 2 to 6 years, corticosteroids were associated with a nonsignificant 40% reduction in the risk of cerebral palsy (RR 0.60, 95% CI 0.34–1.03).[12] A standard course of corticosteroids (reserved for women threatening to deliver before 34 weeks' gestation) is either 2 intramuscular doses of betamethasone, 12 mg, administered 24 hours apart, or 4 intramuscular doses of dexamethasone, 6 mg, administered 12 hours apart. This therapy clearly has short-term neonatal benefits, and the nearly significant reduction in the rate of cerebral palsy is suggestive of long-term neuroprotective benefit as well.

Magnesium Sulfate

In 1995 Nelson and Grether[13] reported a protective association between maternal receipt of magnesium sulfate ($MgSO_4$) and cerebral palsy among infants who delivered prematurely. In their case-control study, children with cerebral palsy had been exposed to $MgSO_4$ significantly less often than children without cerebral palsy (OR 0.14, 95 % CI 0.05–0.51). This association persisted after control for multiple confounders.

Soon after the Nelson and Grether study, 3 separate multicentered, placebo-controlled trials of antenatal $MgSO_4$ for fetal neuroprotection were performed. In these trials the inclusion and exclusion criteria as well as the dosing of $MgSO_4$ were not exactly similar (**Table 2**). The first of the 3 trials to be reported was the Australian trial of Crowther and colleagues.[14] The investigators enrolled 1062 women in whom delivery was anticipated before 30 weeks' gestation and found that the risk of moderate or severe cerebral palsy was significantly lower among children in the $MgSO_4$ group, 3.4% versus 6.6% (RR 0.51, 95% CI 0.29–0.91). Moreover, stillbirth or death before age 2 occurred less frequently in the children born to mothers randomized to $MgSO_4$, 13.8% versus 17.1% (RR 0.83, 95% CI 0.64–1.09).

Table 2
Characteristics and outcomes of the 3 largest trials of $MgSO_4$[a] for the prevention of cerebral palsy

Trial	Mothers (N)	Gestational Age at Study Entry	$MgSO_4$ Dose	Cerebral Palsy[b]	Death or Cerebral Palsy
Crowther et al[14]	1062	<30 wk	4 g load; 1 g/h	RR 0.51; 95% CI 0.29–0.61	RR 0.83 95% CI 0.66–1.03
Rouse et al[7]	2241	<32 wk	6 g load; 2 g/h	RR 0.55 95% CI 0.32–0.95	RR 0.97 95% CI 0.77–1.23
Marret et al[15]	573	<33 wk	4 g load only	OR 0.69 95% CI 0.41–1.19	OR 0.80 95% CI 0.58–1.10

Abbreviations: CI, confidence interval; OR, odds ratio; RR, relative risk.
[a] Magnesium sulfate.
[b] Moderate or severe (Crowther, Rouse); any (Marret).

The second trial to be reported was the BEAM trial, in which 2241 women at imminent risk of delivery between 24 and 31 weeks' gestation were enrolled in the United States.[7] As in the Australian trial, children in the $MgSO_4$ group had a significantly lowered risk of moderate or severe cerebral palsy, 1.9% versus 3.5% (RR 0.55, 95% CI 0.32–0.95), an absolute risk reduction of 1.6%. Among the children of women randomized prior to 28 weeks, the relative risk reduction was comparable (RR 0.45, 95% CI 0.23–0.87) but the absolute reduction in risk was larger—3.4%—because the overall rates of moderate or severe cerebral palsy were higher, 2.7% versus 6.1%. $MgSO_4$ significantly reduced the combined rate of all grades of cerebral palsy ($P = .004$, **Table 3**) but had no significant effect on the risk of fetal or infant death.

The third trial to be reported was the French trial of Marret and colleagues.[15] In this trial 573 mothers were randomly allocated to a 4-g intravenous bolus of $MgSO_4$ or to a placebo. Children in the $MgSO_4$ group had a lower risk of cerebral palsy, 7.0% versus 10.2% (RR 0.69, 95% CI 0.41–1.2) and a lower risk of death, 9.7% versus 11.3% (RR 0.85, 95% CI 0.55–1.3).

The results of these 3 trials and 2 others form the basis for a Cochrane Systematic Review that includes 6145 children.[16] In this review, $MgSO_4$ was found to significantly reduce the risk of cerebral palsy (RR 0.68, 95% CI 0.54–0.87) but to have no effect on fetal or infant mortality (RR 1.04, 95% CI 0.92–1.17). Four of the 5 trials (4446 children) were conducted for the express purpose of evaluating the fetal neuroprotective effectiveness of $MgSO_4$. In analyses confined to these 4 trials, $MgSO_4$ reduced both the risk of cerebral palsy and the risk of the combined outcome of cerebral palsy or fetal/infant death (RR 0.85, 95% CI 0.74–0.98). The meta-analysis of Conde-Aguedo and Romero[17] reaches similar conclusions (**Fig. 1**; **Table 4**).[18,19]

Based on the data from the BEAM trial, to prevent one case of moderate or severe cerebral palsy requires treating 63 women with threatened delivery prior to 32 weeks, and 29 women with threatened delivery prior to 28 weeks.[7] For comparison, approximately 100 women with preeclampsia need to be treated with $MgSO_4$ to prevent eclampsia.[20] $MgSO_4$ for neuroprotection is highly cost-effective. Conde-Aguedo and Romero estimated the incremental cost of preventing a case of cerebral palsy with $MgSO_4$ to be $10,291.[17] By contrast, the average lifelong cost of cerebral palsy has been estimated to be almost $1 million.[21]

Used appropriately, $MgSO_4$ is very safe: there were no life-threatening events in more than 3000 maternal exposures in the Cochrane Review. During use, maternal reflexes should be closely monitored (neuromuscular depression occurs at Mg^{2+} concentrations of 10 mEq/L and above) as should urine output (as Mg^{2+} is renally excreted). A high level of vigilance is necessary when $MgSO_4$ is used in women with renal dysfunction. If hypermagnesemia is suspected, serum Mg^{2+} concentration should be measured and discontinuation of the $MgSO_4$ infusion considered. Respiratory depression (and cardiopulmonary arrest, which is very rare) is treated with 1 g of intravenous calcium gluconate, discontinuation of $MgSO_4$, and ventilatory support as necessary.[22]

Table 3		
Cerebral palsy rates in the BEAM[7] trial		
Cerebral Palsy	**Magnesium Sulfate (%)**	**Placebo (%)**
Mild	2.2	3.7
Moderate	1.5	2.0
Severe	0.5	1.6

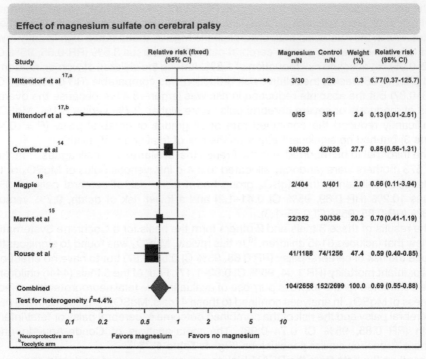

Fig. 1. Effect of magnesium sulfate on cerebral palsy. (*Modified from* Conde-Aguedo A, Romero R. Antenatal magnesium sulfate for the prevention of cerebral palsy in preterm infants less than 34 weeks' gestation: a systematic review and meta-analysis. Am J Obstet Gynecol 2009;200:603; with permission.)

POSTNATAL NEUROPROTECTION

Birth asphyxia is a global burden; worldwide, 4 million newborns are affected every year, of which 1 million die and an additional 1 million have significant disability. In the United States alone, between 1 and 4 per 1000 newborns delivered at term have asphyxia resulting from a fetal insult.[23] Despite improvements in obstetric and neonatal care, perinatal cerebral hypoxic-ischemic injury continues to cause cerebral palsy, mental retardation, and epilepsy.[24]

Encephalopathy of prematurity is a complex mixture of HIE and secondary maturational and trophic disturbances, as more than one-third of brain growth takes place between 32 and 40 weeks of gestation.[25] Moreover, it is difficult to diagnose early HIE clinically in the late preterm infant because signs may be lacking or mistaken for developmental immaturity.[26] This part of the review summarizes the key challenges for implementation of effective postnatal neuroprotective therapies, and discusses neuroprotective (treatment and prevention) options available after delivery.

Challenges for Implementation of Effective Neuroprotective Therapies

Physiology of the hypoxic-ischemic insult leads to a limited therapeutic window

This insult is caused by impaired cerebral blood flow (CBF) as a consequence of a substantial interruption of maternal and/or fetal placental blood flow and gas exchange. At the cellular level, the reduction in CBF and oxygen delivery initiates

Table 4
Effect of magnesium sulfate on cerebral palsy and pediatric mortality

Outcome	No. of Trials	No. of Events/Total Number		Relative Risk (95% CI)
		Magnesium	No Magnesium	
Cerebral palsy	6	104/2658	152/2699	0.69 (0.55–0.88)
Moderate/severe cerebral palsy	3	45/2169	72/2218	0.64 (0.44–0.92)
Mild cerebral palsy	3	54/2169	74/2218	0.74 (0.52–1.04)
Total pediatric mortality	6	401/2658	400/2699	1.01 (0.89–1.14)
Fetal mortality	5	17/2254	22/2298	0.78 (0.42–1.46)
Under 2 y of corrected age mortality	5	217/2254	220/2298	1.00 (0.84–1.19)
Death or cerebral palsy	6	505/2658	551/2699	0.92 (0.83–1.02)

Abbreviation: CI, confidence interval.
Modified from Conde-Aguedo A, Romero R. Antenatal magnesium sulfate for the prevention of cerebral palsy in preterm infants less than 34 weeks' gestation: a systematic review and meta-analysis. Am J Obstet Gynecol 2009;200:603; with permission.

a cascade of deleterious biochemical events, resulting in a switch to anaerobic metabolism.[27,28] It is often forgotten that severe fetal asphyxia is also associated with substantial alterations in other organs as well, due to the redistribution of cardiac output.[27] The switch to anaerobic metabolism leads to secondary energy failure and neuronal death within hours to days after resuscitation.[28] The interval between the primary insult and the development of permanent injury results in a limited window (less than 6 hours) for therapeutic interventions to improve brain outcome.

Time and duration of the fetal insult are not clearly defined
The relative contribution of antepartum, intrapartum, and postpartum insults in the pathogenesis of HIE is difficult to quantitate, as antepartum factors might also predispose to acute intrapartum events. Intrapartum asphyxia is estimated to account for 80% of HIE, and because of the short therapeutic window, is a prerequisite for effective implementation of neuroprotective interventions.[29]

Other organs are more severely affected and contribute to further injury
The fetal circulatory response to hypoxemia and asphyxia is a rapid centralization of blood flow in favor of the vital organs, brain, heart, and adrenals, at the expense of almost all other peripheral organs. Only at the nadir of severe asphyxia do the adaptive mechanisms fail and does brain damage occur.[27] The brain and heart are "spared" in early mild hypoxemia whereas the other organs are not. Thus, in HIE they are very likely to be more severely affected and for longer periods than the brain and heart, due to preferential redistribution of cardiac output. Experimental models have demonstrated quantitatively different organ response to asphyxia induced via repeated brief versus prolonged arrest of uterine blood flow.[28]

The etiology of brain injury in the preterm newborns is multifaceted
Multiple biological risks and causative factors can contribute to an abnormal neurodevelopmental outcome; some occur before or at birth, and others are related to comorbidities during maturation of the developing brain.[30] Potential mechanisms of injury in the preterm newborn in addition to hypoxia-ischemia include severe intracranial hemorrhage, perinatal infection and chorioamnionitis,[31] hypoglycemia,[32] postnatal

steroid administration,[33,34] environmental exposures, and genetic influences. Intraventricular hemorrhage (IVH) and periventricular leukomalacia (PVL) are the two primary signs of acute brain injury in the premature infant, contributing significantly to abnormal neurodevelopmental outcome.[35] Infants who have suffered major complications of prematurity, such as chronic lung disease at discharge, are at greater risk of abnormal neurodevelopmental outcomes.[36] This fact illustrates the need for preventative therapies for high-risk newborns, along with therapeutic interventions following a hypoxic-ischemic insult.

Postnatal Interventions: Past, Present, and Future

Hypothermia is the only neuroprotective therapy available in term newborns with HIE, but how does this translate to the preterm newborn?

Until 2006 the treatment of birth asphyxia was only supportive, with no specific neuroprotective therapy. Moderate hypothermia (33°–34°C) is the only neuroprotective therapy that has been shown in recent large trials to reduce hypoxic-ischemic brain injury when initiated within 6 hours after the insult.[37–39] Hypothermia reduces cerebral metabolism, stabilizes the blood-brain barrier, and prevents seizures. In addition, hypothermia inhibits glutamate and nitric oxide (NO) release, reduces apoptosis, and suppresses microglia activation.[40] Meta-analysis of the large randomized hypothermia trials have reported a 24% reduction in death or disability, with a significantly reduced RR of 0.76 (95% CI 0.65–0.89) and a number needed to treat of 6.[41] To date, 13 randomized controlled trials have been published on the experience of hypothermia therapy in 1440 term neonates with moderate or severe encephalopathy after perinatal asphyxia.[42] Therapeutic hypothermia was confirmed to be associated with a reduced risk of death or disability at 18 months and to also reduce individual outcomes of mortality, severe cerebral palsy, and cognitive and psychomotor delay.[40] At present, hypothermia is the only intervention shown to improve neurologic outcome in full-term newborn infants after HIE.

Barriers to Implementation of Therapeutic Hypothermia in the Preterm Newborn

Can induced therapeutic hypothermia be applied in preterm newborns for neuroprotection?

Direct translation of hypothermia to preterm infants is not assumed because of differences in the pattern of injury and their greater potential susceptibility to the adverse effects of hypothermia. Encephalopathy of prematurity is a complex mixture of HIE and secondary maturational and trophic disturbances.[43] The classic feature of brain injury in preterm infants is white matter injury, predominantly PVL. Although cystic PVL occurs infrequently, diffuse white matter injury, with selective loss of immature oligodendrocytes, remains a nearly universal problem.[44,45] Imaging studies have recently shown that PVL is associated not only with reduced white matter volumes and ventricular enlargement but also reduced volume and complexity of cerebral cortical gray matter. This finding of reduced brain growth has been associated with poor neurodevelopmental outcomes in preterm neonates.[46] This finding will further complicate the response to hypothermia or any other neuroprotective therapy in preterm infants.

Safety issues preclude immediate application of hypothermia in preterm newborns

Historical data suggest that mild hypothermia is associated with increased mortality in preterm newborns.[47,48] Silverman and colleagues[47] reported in 1958 an increased mortality in newborns under1000 g who were kept in incubators at 28.7°C. Their axillary temperature average was 31°C in the first 5 days of life. There are no gestational age–specific randomized trials addressing the effect of mild hypothermia (33°–34°C) on mortality. Theoretical concerns of safety related to therapeutic mild hypothermia include coagulopathy, thrombogenesis, cardiac arrhythmia, superficial cold injury, metabolic acidosis, and increased requirements for inotrope support.[49] None of these adverse events were confirmed by large randomized hypothermia trials.[50] In meta-analysis of term newborns undergoing therapeutic hypothermia, the side effects were limited to physiologic bradycardia, mild thrombocytopenia, and scalp edema with head cooling.[41] It appears that mild to moderate therapeutic hypothermia is well tolerated and has a good safety record in term newborns with encephalopathy. The known systemic side effects of hypothermia still represent theoretical safety concerns in preterm newborns in whom hypothermia might promote hypotension, increased oxygen consumption, worsening pulmonary hypertension, jaundice, or increased risk for infection. In all likelihood, assessment of hypothermia in later preterm infants will reveal fewer problems than in those born at 32 weeks' gestation or less, because the frequency of confounding problems related to prematurity will be substantially lower. Thus late preterm newborns (33–35 weeks) will have to be targeted first in upcoming large randomized controlled trials to establish safety and efficacy.

The screening process has not been well defined in preterm newborns
Despite the steadily increasing number of late preterm births in the United States, where 12% of all live births are less than 37 weeks gestational age,[51] it is challenging to adequately power studies of late preterm infants with HIE prospectively, as HIE occurs in 1 to 2 per 1000 of all births. Moreover, it is difficult to diagnose early HIE clinically in the late preterm infant because signs may be lacking or mistaken for developmental immaturity. Normal preterm infants typically have systematic developmental differences in primitive reflexes, tone, and posture.[52] Pertinent literature describing HIE incidence in preterm infants is limited to a 10 years' retrospective report at Parkland Memorial Hospital[53] that identified 62 neonates born between 31 and 36 weeks gestational age with an umbilical arterial pH of less than 7.00. Seven of these newborn infants were diagnosed as having moderate or severe HIE (1.3/1000) per Sarnat criteria, but only 2 of those newborns were of 33 to 35 weeks' gestation. The authors have more recently reviewed the late preterm infants (33–35 weeks) to assess the frequency and incidence of HIE when using a screening assessment for metabolic acidosis and encephalopathy that are similar to published guidelines In term newborns. Of the 2.5% late preterm newborns who met screening criteria for the presence of physiologic fetal acidosis, 27% were identified with moderate to severe HIE (estimated incidence 5/1000).[54] This study is providing basic information that is needed to design randomized trials in this patient population.

In summary, hypothermia has not been tested for safety or efficacy as a neuroprotective therapy for preterm newborns, and should first be studied in large, multicenter randomized clinical trials of older preterm infants (33–35 weeks) who have metabolic acidosis and clinical encephalopathy. These infants present the closest clinical parallel to term infants who have acute encephalopathy, and thus are the most likely to benefit while being at the least risk for hypothermia-associated complications.

OTHER INTERVENTIONS THAT CAN OFFER ADDITIVE NEUROPROTECTION

Postnatal administration of medications to reduce severe IVH has historically included the use of phenobarbital,[55–57] vitamin E,[58] ethamyslate,[59] and indomethacin.[60] This

IVH prevention armamentarium has not borne out over time, with the exception of indomethacin, which is discussed first. In addition, the authors review caffeine, NO, and erythropoietin (Epo), each of which were subsequently found to also have neuroprotective effects.

Indomethacin

Indomethacin acts via nonspecific inhibition of cyclooxygenase, leading to decreased prostaglandin synthesis. Indomethacin is believed to prevent IVH through effects on blood flow and on basement membrane maturation by improving cerebral autoregulation.[60–62] Indomethacin has been shown to promote maturation of the germinal matrix in beagle pups and inhibit the alterations in blood-brain barrier permeability.[63,64] Three studies have demonstrated a significant reduction in the incidence of severe IVH in infants who received indomethacin but failed to show differences in long-term follow-up, with no reduction in the risk of cerebral palsy.[65] Subgroup analysis on the basis of gender revealed a decreased rate of IVH in male infants.[66]

Indomethacin appears to hold the most promise in the prevention of severe hemorrhage, but does not translate into long-term neurodevelopmental benefit. It is possible that it should be reserved for newborns at greatest risk for severe IVH, but further studies are needed.

Nitric Oxide

NO is an endogenous intercellular signaling molecule produced by NO synthase that regulates vascular tone in the pulmonary and systemic circulation. Schreiber and colleagues[67] reported a single-center, blinded randomized controlled trial where preterm infants of less than 34 weeks' gestation were randomly assigned to receive NO (5–10 ppm) or placebo while intubated in the first week of life. Main findings in this trial of preterm infants were that NO patients had a significantly reduced RR (0.76) of death or chronic lung disease. The overall incidence of IVH and PVL did not differ between NO and placebo-treated infants, but the study reported an unexpected marked 47% risk reduction in grades III or IV IVH and PVL in NO-treated infants. A follow-up study at 2 years corrected for age[68] confirmed that the surviving NO-treated patients had approximately half the risk of abnormal neurodevelopmental outcome compared with placebo. This finding remained significant after adjusting for known confounders such as birth weight, sex, socioeconomic status, ventilation, and exposure to corticosteroids.

Although such clinical evidence suggests that NO could provide effective neuroprotection, studies using animal models of hypoxic-ischemic injury indicate that endogenous NO, when combined with an increase in reactive oxygen species production, can lead to formation of peroxynitrite and subsequent neuronal injury and death.[69,70] Provision of NO is a promising therapy that could result in improved neuroprotection, but needs to be further studied.

Caffeine

Caffeine is commonly prescribed to prevent or treat apnea in preterm infants, and has been recently shown in a large trial by Schmidt and colleagues,[71] when started at a median of 3 days after birth until 36 weeks adjusted gestational age, to reduce the rates of cerebral palsy and neurodevelopmental impairment in these infants. Postulated neuroprotective effects include a direct neuroprotective effect, as well as an effect secondary to reduction of apnea and the need for assisted ventilation and, subsequently, chronic lung disease. The protection offered with caffeine remains significant even after adjustment of confounding variables, further suggesting a direct neuroprotective effect. A meta-analysis of 21 studies found likely neuroprotective benefit from early caffeine administration.[72] Further, a new ongoing trial (NCT00809055) is refining dosage recommendations and mechanisms of neuroprotection.

Erythropoietin

Epo, the primary regulator of red blood cell production, has been shown to be broadly protective against hypoxic-ischemic and inflammatory injuries. The mechanisms by which Epo exerts its neuroprotective and neurotropic effects include the inhibition of glutamate release, modulation of intracellular calcium metabolism, induction of anti-apoptotic factors, reduction of inflammation, inhibition of NO-mediated injury, and direct antioxidant effects.[73] Recent experimental studies, as well as trials including adult patients, highly favor Epo as a neuroprotective agent.[74,75] As an added bonus for its use in ameliorating neonatal brain injury, Epo has been widely used in preterm infants to prevent or treat anemia of prematurity. It is considered safe and well tolerated in preterm infants.[76,77] Epo dosages range from 100 to 400 U/kg administered every other day for 6 weeks or until 36 weeks corrected gestational age. The long-term neurologic outcome of preterm infants who received Epo for prevention of blood transfusion for anemia of prematurity has been reported in only few small studies, mostly with no significant reduction in abnormal outcomes.[78,79] Two studies have reported a correlation between Mental Developmental Index scores and cumulative Epo dosage.[80,81] An additional post hoc analysis reported higher developmental index scores at 18 to 22 months' corrected age selectively for infants with Epo serum concentrations of 500 mU/m.[82] Zhu and colleagues[83] reported the first trial of Epo neuroprotection in term newborns with moderate to severe HIE, where Epo was administered at either 300 or 500 U/kg every other day for 2 weeks. Epo administration in those newborns with HIE at term resulted in improved neurologic examinations, as well as decreased death, disability, and incidence of cerebral palsy at 18 months.

Evidence from animal experiments reveals that Epo must be given in high doses at the beginning or within a short critical time period after the onset of brain injury in order to achieve a significant effect. Optimal dosing remains to be addressed before Epo can be recommended for clinical use as a neuroprotective therapy in preterm newborns.

SUMMARY OF MOST PROMISING POSTNATAL NEUROPROTECTIVE THERAPIES

While hypothermia has emerged as a front runner in neuroprotective therapy in the term newborn with HIE, ongoing large multicenter trials are attempting to optimize this effect. Such studies of term newborns with HIE include studies of initiation of hypothermia beyond 6 hours (Laptook, NCT00614744), deeper (32°C vs 33.5°C), and longer duration (72 vs 120 hours) of hypothermia (Shankaran, NCT01192776), as well as optimization of the rewarming phase (Chalak, substudy within NCT01192776). Large randomized multicenter hypothermia trials involving the late preterm newborn are being considered for the future, and will address the safety of hypothermia therapy in this high-risk population. Epo trials are under way with the aim of confirming its neuroprotective effect in term newborns with HIE (NCT00719407).

No new single postnatal neuroprotective therapy has emerged for the preterm newborn. By contrast, a multitude of safe, efficacious therapies such as caffeine, NO, and indomethacin, already used in neonatal regimens, have subsequently been found to have additive neuroprotective effects. Prenatal administration of corticosteroids and magnesium appears to be beneficial according to the most recent literature reviewed, and postnatal Epo administration promises to be neuroprotective therapy candidate in the preterm, for which large randomized trials are currently under way in Switzerland (NCT00413946), China (NCT00910234), and New Mexico (NCT01207778).

REFERENCES

1. Kuban KC, Leviton A. Cerebral palsy. N Engl J Med 1994;330:188–95.
2. Bax M, Goldstein M, Rosenbaum P, et al, Executive Committee for the Definition of Cerebral Palsy. Proposed definition and classification of cerebral palsy, April 2005. Dev Med Child Neurol 2005;47:571–6.
3. Cummins SK, Nelson KB, Grether JK, et al. Cerebral palsy in four northern California counties, births 1983 through 1985. J Pediatr 1993;123:230–7.
4. Shatrov M, Birch S, Lam L, et al. Chorioamnionitis and cerebral palsy: a meta-analysis. Obstet Gynecol 2010;116:387–92.
5. Gilbert W, Jacoby B, Xing G, et al. Adverse obstetric events are associated with significant risk of cerebral palsy. Am J Obstet Gynecol 2010;203:328,e1–5.
6. Leveno K. Antecedents to cerebral palsy in preterm infants. Am J Obstet Gynecol 2009;201:S181.
7. Rouse DJ, Hirtz DG, Thom E, et al. A randomized, controlled trial of magnesium sulfate for the prevention of cerebral palsy. N Engl J Med 2008;359:895–905.
8. Kenyon S, Pike K, Jones D, et al. Childhood outcomes after prescription of antibiotics to pregnant women with spontaneous preterm labour: a 7-year follow-up of the ORACLE II trial. Lancet 2008;372:1319–27.
9. The American College of Obstetricians and Gynecologists Task Force on Neonatal Encephalopathy and Cerebral Palsy. Neonatal encephalopathy and cerebral palsy: defining the pathogenesis and pathophysiology. Washington, DC: ACOG; 2003. p. xviii.
10. Shy K, Luthy D, Forrest C, et al. Effects of electronic fetal-heart-rate monitoring, as compared with periodic auscultation, on the neurologic development of premature infants. N Engl J Med 1990;322:588–93.
11. Thorngren-Jerneck K, Herbst A. Perinatal factors associated with cerebral palsy in children born in Sweden. Obstet Gynecol 2006;108(6):1499–505.
12. Roberts D, Dalziel S. Antenatal corticosteroids for accelerating fetal lung maturation for women at risk of preterm birth. Cochrane Database Syst Rev 2006;3: CD004454.
13. Nelson KB, Grether JK. Can magnesium sulfate reduce the risk of cerebral palsy in very low birthweight infants? Pediatrics 1995;95:263–9.
14. Crowther CA, Hiller JE, Doyle LW, et al. Effect of magnesium sulfate given for neuroprotection before preterm birth. A randomized controlled trial. JAMA 2003;290:2669–76.
15. Marret S, Maroeau L, Follet-Bouhamed C, et al. [Effect of magnesium sulphate on mortality and neurologic morbidity of the very preterm newborn with two-year neurologic outcome: results of the prospective PREAMAG trial]. Gynecol Obstet Fertil 2008;36:278–88 [in French].
16. Doyle LW, Crowther CA, Middleton P, et al. Magnesium sulphate for women at risk of preterm birth for neuroprotection of the fetus. Cochrane Database Syst Rev 2009;1:CD004661.
17. Conde-Aguedo A, Romero R. Antenatal magnesium sulfate for the prevention of cerebral palsy in preterm infants less than 34 weeks' gestation: a systematic review and meta-analysis. Am J Obstet Gynecol 2009;200:595–609.
18. Mittendorf R, Covert R, Boman J, et al. Is tocolytic magnesium sulphate associated with increased total paediatric mortality? Lancet 1997;350:1517–8.

19. Magpie Trial follow-up study collaborative group. The Magpie Trial: a randomized trial comparing magnesium sulphate with placebo for pre-eclampsia. Outcome for children at 18 months. Br J Obstet Gynaecol 2007;114:289–99.
20. Lucas MJ, Leveno KJ, Cunningham FG. A comparison of magnesium sulfate with phenytoin for the prevention of eclampsia. N Engl J Med 1995;333:201–5.
21. Honeycutt A, Dunlap L, Chen H, et al. Economic costs associated with mental retardation, cerebral palsy, hearing loss, and vision impairment: United States, 2003. MMWR Morb Mortal Wkly Rep 2004;53:57–9.
22. Cunningham FG, Leveno K, Bloom S, et al. Williams obstetrics. 23rd edition. New York: McGraw-Hill Medical Publishing; 2009. p. 738.
23. Bryce J, Boschi-Pinto C, Shibuya K, et al. WHO estimates of the causes of death in children. Lancet 2005;365(9465):1147–52.
24. Levene ML, Kornberg J, Williams TH. The incidence and severity of post-asphyxial encephalopathy in full-term infants. Early Hum Dev 1985;11(1):21–6.
25. Volpe JJ. Brain injury in premature infants: a complex amalgam of destructive and developmental disturbances. Lancet Neurol 2009;8(1):110–24.
26. Shalak L, Perlman JM. Hypoxic-ischemic brain injury in the term infant-current concepts. Early Hum Dev 2004;80(2):125–41.
27. Jensen A, Garnier Y, Berger R. Dynamics of fetal circulatory responses to hypoxia and asphyxia. Eur J Obstet Gynecol Reprod Biol 1999;84(2):155–72.
28. Lorek A, Takei Y, Cady EB, et al. Delayed ("secondary") cerebral energy failure after acute hypoxia-ischemia in the newborn piglet: continuous 48-hour studies by phosphorus magnetic resonance spectroscopy. Pediatr Res 1994;36(6):699–706.
29. Volpe JJ. Neurology of the newborn. Major Probl Clin Pediatr 1981;22:1–648.
30. Neubauer AP, Voss W, Kattner E. Outcome of extremely low birth weight survivors at school age: the influence of perinatal parameters on neurodevelopment. Eur J Pediatr 2008;167(1):87–95.
31. Wu YW, Colford JM Jr. Chorioamnionitis as a risk factor for cerebral palsy: a meta-analysis. JAMA 2000;284(11):1417–24.
32. Salhab WA, Wyckoff MH, Laptook AR, et al. Initial hypoglycemia and neonatal brain injury in term infants with severe fetal acidemia. Pediatrics 2004;114(2):361–6.
33. O'Shea TM, Kothadia JM, Klinepeter KL, et al. Randomized placebo-controlled trial of a 42-day tapering course of dexamethasone to reduce the duration of ventilator dependency in very low birth weight infants: outcome of study participants at 1-year adjusted age. Pediatrics 1999;104(1 Pt 1):15–21.
34. Shinwell ES, Karplus M, Reich D, et al. Early postnatal dexamethasone treatment and increased incidence of cerebral palsy. Arch Dis Child Fetal Neonatal Ed 2000;83(3):F177–81.
35. Shalak L, Perlman JM. Hemorrhagic-ischemic cerebral injury in the preterm infant: current concepts. Clin Perinatol 2002;29(4):745–63.
36. Jeng SF, Hsu CH, Tsao PN, et al. Bronchopulmonary dysplasia predicts adverse developmental and clinical outcomes in very-low-birthweight infants. Dev Med Child Neurol 2008;50(1):51–7.
37. Shankaran S, Laptook AR, Ehrenkranz RA, et al. Whole-body hypothermia for neonates with hypoxic-ischemic encephalopathy. N Engl J Med 2005;353(15):1574–84.
38. Gluckman PD, Wyatt JS, Azzopardi D, et al. Selective head cooling with mild systemic hypothermia after neonatal encephalopathy: multicentre randomised trial. Lancet 2005;365(9460):663–70.

39. Azzopardi DV, Strohm B, Edwards AD, et al. Moderate hypothermia to treat peri-natal asphyxial encephalopathy. N Engl J Med 2009;361(14):1349–58.
40. Laptook AR. Use of therapeutic hypothermia for term infants with hypoxic-ischemic encephalopathy. Pediatr Clin North Am 2009;56(3):601–16.
41. Spitzmiller RE, Phillips T, Meinzen-Derr J, et al. Amplitude-integrated EEG is useful in predicting neurodevelopmental outcome in full-term infants with hypoxic-ischemic encephalopathy: a meta-analysis. J Child Neurol 2007;22(9): 1069–78.
42. Shah PS. Hypothermia: a systematic review and meta-analysis of clinical trials. Semin Fetal Neonatal Med 2010;15(5):238–46.
43. Kinney HC. The encephalopathy of prematurity: one pediatric neuropathologist's perspective. Semin Pediatr Neurol 2009;16(4):179–90.
44. Inder TE, Anderson NJ, Spencer C, et al. White matter injury in the premature infant: a comparison between serial cranial sonographic and MR findings at term. AJNR Am J Neuroradiol 2003;24(5):805–9.
45. Inder TE, Huppi PS, Warfield S, et al. Periventricular white matter injury in the premature infant is followed by reduced cerebral cortical gray matter volume at term. Ann Neurol 1999;46(5):755–60.
46. Bhutta AT, Anand KJ. Abnormal cognition and behavior in preterm neonates linked to smaller brain volumes. Trends Neurosci 2001;24(3):129–30 [discussion: 131–2].
47. Silverman WA, Fertig JW, Berger AP. The influence of the thermal environment upon the survival of newly born premature infants. Pediatrics 1958;22(5):876–86.
48. Day RL, Caliguiri L, Kamenski C, et al. Body temperature and survival of prema-ture infants. Pediatrics 1964;34:171–81.
49. Gunn AJ, Wyatt JS, Whitelaw A, et al. Therapeutic hypothermia changes the prognostic value of clinical evaluation of neonatal encephalopathy. J Pediatr 2008;152(1):55–8, 58,e51.
50. Shankaran S, Pappas A, Laptook AR, et al. Outcomes of safety and effectiveness in a multicenter randomized, controlled trial of whole-body hypothermia for neonatal hypoxic-ischemic encephalopathy. Pediatrics 2008;122(4):e791–8.
51. Raju TN, Higgins RD, Stark AR, et al. Optimizing care and outcome for late-preterm (near-term) infants: a summary of the workshop sponsored by the National Institute of Child Health and Human Development. Pediatrics 2006;118(3):1207–14.
52. Volpe JJ. Neurologic outcome of prematurity. Arch Neurol 1998;55(3):297–300.
53. Salhab WA, Perlman JM. Severe fetal acidemia and subsequent neonatal encephalopathy in the larger premature infant. Pediatr Neurol 2005;32(1):25–9.
54. Chalak LF, Rollins N, Morris MC, et al. Screening, neuroimaging findings and outcomes in 33–35 weeks preterm newborns with HIE. APS-SPR; 2010.
55. Bedard MP, Shankaran S, Slovis TL, et al. Effect of prophylactic phenobarbital on intraventricular hemorrhage in high-risk infants. Pediatrics 1984;73(4):435–9.
56. Donn SM, Roloff DW, Goldstein GW. Prevention of intraventricular haemorrhage in preterm infants by phenobarbitone. A controlled trial. Lancet 1981;2(8240): 215–7.
57. Kuban KC, Leviton A, Krishnamoorthy KS, et al. Neonatal intracranial hemorrhage and phenobarbital. Pediatrics 1986;77(4):443–50.
58. Sinha S, Davies J, Toner N, et al. Vitamin E supplementation reduces frequency of periventricular haemorrhage in very preterm babies. Lancet 1987;1(8531): 466–71.
59. Morgan ME, Benson JW, Cooke RW. Ethamsylate reduces the incidence of peri-ventricular haemorrhage in very low birth-weight babies. Lancet 1981;2(8251): 830–1.

60. Ment LR, Oh W, Ehrenkranz RA, et al. Low-dose indomethacin and prevention of intraventricular hemorrhage: a multicenter randomized trial. Pediatrics 1994; 93(4):543–50.
61. Pourcyrous M, Busija DW, Shibata M, et al. Cerebrovascular responses to therapeutic dose of indomethacin in newborn pigs. Pediatr Res 1999;45(4 Pt 1):582–7.
62. van Bel F, Klautz RJ, Steendijk P, et al. The influence of indomethacin on the autoregulatory ability of the cerebral vascular bed in the newborn lamb. Pediatr Res 1993;34(2):178–81.
63. Ment LR, Oh W, Ehrenkranz RA, et al. Low-dose indomethacin therapy and extension of intraventricular hemorrhage: a multicenter randomized trial. J Pediatr 1994;124(6):951–5.
64. Leffler CW, Busija DW, Fletcher AM, et al. Effects of indomethacin upon cerebral hemodynamics of newborn pigs. Pediatr Res 1985;19(11):1160–4.
65. Linder N, Haskin O, Levit O, et al. Risk factors for intraventricular hemorrhage in very low birth weight premature infants: a retrospective case-control study. Pediatrics 2003;111(5 Pt 1):e590–5.
66. Ment LR, Vohr BR, Makuch RW, et al. Prevention of intraventricular hemorrhage by indomethacin in male preterm infants. J Pediatr 2004;145(6):832–4.
67. Schreiber MD, Gin-Mestan K, Marks JD, et al. Inhaled nitric oxide in premature infants with the respiratory distress syndrome. N Engl J Med 2003;349(22):2099–107.
68. Mestan KK, Marks JD, Hecox K, et al. Neurodevelopmental outcomes of premature infants treated with inhaled nitric oxide. N Engl J Med 2005;353(1):23–32.
69. Marks JD, Schreiber MD. Inhaled nitric oxide and neuroprotection in preterm infants. Clin Perinatol 2008;35(4):793–807, viii.
70. Gunasekar PG, Kanthasamy AG, Borowitz JL, et al. NMDA receptor activation produces concurrent generation of nitric oxide and reactive oxygen species: implication for cell death. J Neurochem 1995;65(5):2016–21.
71. Schmidt B, Roberts RS, Davis P, et al. Long-term effects of caffeine therapy for apnea of prematurity. N Engl J Med 2007;357(19):1893–902.
72. Winckworth LC, Powell E. Question 1. Does caffeine treatment for apnoea of prematurity improve neurodevelopmental outcome in later life? Arch Dis Child 2010;95(9):757–9.
73. Dame C, Juul SE, Christensen RD. The biology of erythropoietin in the central nervous system and its neurotrophic and neuroprotective potential. Biol Neonate 2001;79(3–4):228–35.
74. McPherson RJ, Juul SE. Erythropoietin for infants with hypoxic-ischemic encephalopathy. Curr Opin Pediatr 2010;22(2):139–45.
75. Ehrenreich H, Hasselblatt M, Dembowski C, et al. Erythropoietin therapy for acute stroke is both safe and beneficial. Mol Med 2002;8(8):495–505.
76. Maier RF, Obladen M, Muller-Hansen I, et al. Early treatment with erythropoietin beta ameliorates anemia and reduces transfusion requirements in infants with birth weights below 1000 g. J Pediatr 2002;141(1):8–15.
77. Ohlsson A, Aher SM. Early erythropoietin for preventing red blood cell transfusion in preterm and/or low birth weight infants. Cochrane Database Syst Rev 2006;3: CD004863.
78. Newton NR, Leonard CH, Piecuch RE, et al. Neurodevelopmental outcome of prematurely born children treated with recombinant human erythropoietin in infancy. J Perinatol 1999;19(6 Pt 1):403–6.
79. Ohls RK, Ehrenkranz RA, Das A, et al. Neurodevelopmental outcome and growth at 18 to 22 months' corrected age in extremely low birth weight infants treated with early erythropoietin and iron. Pediatrics 2004;114(5):1287–91.

80. Brown MS, Eichorst D, Lala-Black B, et al. Higher cumulative doses of erythropoi-
    etin and developmental outcomes in preterm infants. Pediatrics 2009;124(4):
    e681–7.
81. He JS, Huang ZL, Yang H, et al. [Early use of recombinant human erythropoietin
    promotes neurobehavioral development in preterm infants]. Zhongguo Dang Dai
    Er Ke Za Zhi 2008;10(5):586–8 [in Chinese].
82. Bierer R, Peceny MC, Hartenberger CH, et al. Erythropoietin concentrations and
    neurodevelopmental outcome in preterm infants. Pediatrics 2006;118(3):
    e635–40.
83. Zhu C, Kang W, Xu F, et al. Erythropoietin improved neurologic outcomes in
    newborns with hypoxic-ischemic encephalopathy. Pediatrics 2009;124(2):
    e218–26.

Care at the Edge of Viability: Medical and Ethical Issues

Marlyse F. Haward, MD[a],*, Nancy W. Kirshenbaum, MD[b],
Deborah E. Campbell, MD[a]

KEYWORDS

- Periviability - Ethics - Decision-making - Extreme prematurity

MEDICAL ISSUES
General Considerations

When critically examining the ethical issues for infants born extremely preterm, at 22 to 25 weeks' gestation, a review of neonatal outcomes and its limitations is necessary to help families and the perinatal community in making shared informed decisions. The complexity of this process must take into consideration the chances for survival when such an early birth occurs, the range of complications experienced by these infants once born, and the impact of both acute and long-term health and developmental care needs for the infant and families. The woman or couple must interpret this information within their moral framework, deciding which course of action—comfort care or resuscitation with a trial of intensive care—should be pursued in the delivery room.

Informed decision-making requires knowledge about fetal development at this critical period, including the degree of physiologic development necessary to sustain life outside the womb, even with currently available therapies. Not only are infants born in this periviable period susceptible to injury sustained from preterm birth but also their neurodevelopmental processes are changed so that the normal migration and connectivity patterns in the brain are altered permanently, leading to errors in brain development. No technological advancements have been able to address this insult to development. Thus, although survival has improved for these extremely preterm babies, the neurologic and developmental sequelae they experience have not. In addition, the potential for survival at 22 to 25 weeks is not an all-or-none phenomenon. Biologic variability in organ maturation and function among individual fetuses contributes

The authors have nothing to disclose.
[a] Division of Neonatology, Albert Einstein College of Medicine, Children's Hospital at Montefiore, 1601 Tenbroeck Avenue, 2nd Floor, Bronx, NY 10461, USA
[b] Department of Obstetrics & Gynecology, Albert Einstein College of Medicine, Montefiore Medical Center, 1601 Tenbroeck Avenue, 1st Floor, Bronx, NY 10461, USA
* Corresponding author.
E-mail address: mhaward@montefiore.org

to difficulty in accurately predicting the likelihood of a particular outcome before the infant's birth. Discussion must therefore encompass not only what is possible but also what is probable in terms of treatment options and outcomes.[1] Maternal health and pregnancy complications further affect survival rates and long-term outcomes. Education and support are essential for the perinatal team members to assure they offer appropriate consistent information and assistance to families.

Injury versus alterations in development: prematurity versus immaturity

Developmentally, at 22 weeks' gestation, although all major organs are present, their structure and function are at different phases and extremely immature. This circumstance poses significant challenges for physicians trying to promote survival with minimal morbidity. Unique to infants born at 22 to 25 weeks' gestation and different from older preterm infants is the structural and developmental immaturity of the lungs and brain. Damage to these organs and secondarily to the gastrointestinal tract has the greatest impact on the chance for survival and the degree of functional impairment. In particular, normal neuronal migration, starting at 18 weeks, is arrested at birth and does not continue to follow the same pattern as in children who remain in utero or in later-born preterm infants whose neurons have completed migration. Although review of the developmental contribution of each organ system is beyond the scope of this article, interventions proven efficacious for older preterm infants may be physiologically and developmentally ineffective in the extremely immature baby.

Methodological themes important to review

Statistics The manner in which outcome statistics are reported affects how outcome data are interpreted. Survival statistics are significantly higher if only infants admitted to the intensive care unit are considered (10/100), compared with all live births (10/150) or with all live births and still births (10/200).[2] Likewise, rates of disability reported for all live births (eg, 10/100 = 10%) versus rates reported on only those who survive (eg, 10/40 = 25%) will be different if a large number of infants die before discharge.[3] The specific denominators used to describe these rates vary based on institutional and national policies, making comparability between cohorts difficult.[4]

Birth weight versus gestational age Until recently, most cohort analyses have focused on birth weight categories. These cohorts include infants who are more developmentally mature but are small for gestational age. Cohorts whose upper limits include older infants will seem to have better survival statistics than cohorts whose upper limits are younger.[5] Gestational age definitions are themselves subject to uncertainty based on dating methods.[6] The National Institutes of Health Center for Child Health and Human Development (NICHD) Neonatal Research Network[7] notes that a difference of 100 g is equivalent in survival to an additional 1 week in utero, and an additional day in utero increases survival by 4%.[8] Because of these difficulties, the outcomes literature has started to report cohorts with gestational ages.

Differences in management styles Survival statistics can also reflect delivery room management styles and can vary by center and within regions and countries. Proactive strategies have resulted in increased live births and survival rates compared with less-aggressive management styles.[9–11] Some international comparisons of varied management approaches have shown increased morbidities in the total population,[9] whereas others have reported similar rates of morbidities.[10,11] It has been argued that management strategies can result in self-fulfilling prophecies, whereby less-aggressive management at lower gestational ages results in decreased survival.[6]

Cohorts: center, multicenter, regional, international Regional cohorts representing tertiary referral centers with large sample sizes may be subject to referral biases, which can be resolved by using geographic (population-based) cohorts. Center-specific cohorts collect detailed data but may have limited sociodemographic diversity making generalization difficult. Epoch comparisons allow for evaluation of trends over time reflecting changing management strategies and survival indices.

MEDICAL OUTCOMES
Survival to Hospital Discharge

Table 1 summarizes survival rates by gestational age for live born infants reported in the United States,[12,13] Europe,[14–18] Canada,[19] and Japan.[20,21] These data illustrate the worldwide variation in survival rates based on nation-specific approaches to care and when data are presented for the entire population, live births, or neonatal intensive care unit (NICU) admissions. A review of the NICHD database reveals survival rates of 6% for infants at 22 weeks, 26% at 23 weeks, 55% at 24 weeks, and 72% at 25 weeks.[12] These rates are comparable to 2009 data from the Vermont Oxford Neonatal Network (VON), a multicenter multinational database; reported survival rates were 5% at 22 weeks, 33% at 23 weeks, and 61% at 24 weeks.[13] Of the infants in the NICHD cohort who survived, 100% at 22 weeks' gestation experienced morbidity at discharge, 92% at 23 weeks, and 91% at 24 weeks. Survival at 22 weeks' gestation was significantly more likely to be influenced by delivery room resuscitation practices than at 25 weeks, suggesting potentially higher survival rates if all infants been resuscitated.

In the EPICure study, a population-based cohort of infants born between 20 and 25 weeks' gestation in the United Kingdom and Ireland during 1995, 1%, 11%, 26%, and 44% of infants born at 22, 23, 24, and 25 weeks' gestation, respectively, were discharged alive from the NICU.[14] Some studies provide survival data as all births and all live births[15] or admissions to the NICU.[16] The Swedish EXPRESS group, who reported on live births, showed that survival rates were higher at 22 and 23 weeks than the NICHD or VON cohorts: 12% at 22 weeks, 54% at 23 weeks, 71% at 24 weeks, and 82% at 25 weeks. Survival rates at 1 year were 9.8%; 53%, 67%, and 82%, respectively.[15] In the Norwegian Extreme Prematurity Study, survival rates among NICU admissions were 39% at 23 weeks, 60% at 24 weeks, and 80% at 25 weeks. No infants at 22 weeks were admitted to the NICU, and the risk of not being resuscitated increased with decreasing gestational age.[16]

Neurodevelopmental Outcomes After Extremely Preterm Birth

Numerous outcome studies have been reported in recent years from single-center, multicenter, and national cohorts of extremely preterm children. Significant variation exists in outcomes, partly related to the chronologic age at evaluation, criteria used to classify disability and functional capacity, and attrition among the group whose outcome is described. The two largest cohorts of children born since the mid-1990s for whom sequential outcome data by week of gestation are cited are the NICHD Neonatal Network and EPICure Study Group. The earliest outcomes that correlate with later severe disability are reported at 18 to 22 months' and at 30 months' corrected age by the NICHD[22] and EPICure Group, respectively.[14] Subsequent time points when outcomes have been reported are 6 to 8 years of age[23,24] and 10 to 12 years of age.[25] Assessments at 8 years of age most accurately predict academic achievement and performance outcomes into young adulthood.

Table 1
Survival rates to hospital discharge among infants born 22 to 25 weeks' gestation

Cohort	Year	Denominator	22 Wk	23 Wk	24 Wk	25 Wk
NICHD (United States)[12]	2003–2007	Live births	6%	26%	55%	72%
VON (Multinational)[13]	2009	Live births	5%	33%	61%	—
Canadian Neonatal Network (Chan et al, 2001)[19]	1996–1997	Population-based	1%	17%	44%	68%
EPIBel (Vanhaesebrouck et al, 2004)[18]	1999–2000	Population-based	0%	6%	29%	56%
EPICure (United Kingdom, Ireland)[14]	1995	Population-based (LB + SB)	1%	11%	26%	44%
EXPRESS (Sweden)[15]	2004–2007	Live births	12%	54%	71%	82%
		Population-based	7%	34%	60%	73%
Norwegian Infant Study[16]	1999–2000	Admissions to NICU	0	39%	60%	80%
		Population-based	0	16%	44%	66%
Switzerland (Fischer et al, 2009)[17]	2000–2004	Population-based	0%	5%	30%	50%
Japan: Single Center[20]	1991–2006	Live births	25%	47%	50%	—
Japan: Multicenter[21]	2003		36%	75%	75%	—

Abbreviations: LB, live birth; NICU, Neonatal Intensive Care Unit; SB, Stillbirth.

The NICHD has reported that the likelihood of a favorable outcome with neonatal intensive care can be better estimated by evaluating four factors in addition to gestational age: female or male sex, exposure or nonexposure to antenatal corticosteroids, single versus multiple birth, and birth weight.[7] The infant's sex not only impacts the chance for survival but also has implications for longer-term cognitive and functional outcomes.[26] **Table 2** provides an overview of the rates of death and severe neurodevelopmental impairment among infants enrolled in the NICHD Network. Death or severe to profound disability is common among the few survivors born at 22 weeks' gestation. Similarly, intact outcomes for infants at 23 and 24 weeks' gestation are extremely poor. By 25 weeks' gestation, however, greater equipoise is seen, as rates of death and severe disability approach 50%.[7]

Hintz and colleagues[27] recently reported that early childhood neurodevelopmental outcomes are not improving for infants born before 25 weeks' gestation. Despite advances in perinatal care practices, infants born between 2002 and 2004 did not experience fewer adverse outcomes (moderate-severe cerebral palsy [11% vs 14.9%], cognitive impairment [IQ<70; 44.9% vs 51%], or developmental delays [50.1% vs 58.7%]) at 18 to 22 months' corrected age compared with an earlier cohort of infants born between 1999 and 2001.

The EPICure Study Group has reported longitudinal outcome data through 11 years of age for their population of 4004 infants born in 1995. Of this group, 811 infants with gestational ages less than 26 weeks were admitted to the NICU; 314 babies survived to hospital discharge. Among survivors, 92% (283/302), 78% (241/308), and 71% (219/307) were evaluated at 30 months' corrected age, 6 years, and 11 years of age, respectively. Neurocognitive outcomes and composite disability rates are summarized in **Table 3**.[24,26] Overall, only 16% of survivors between 22 and 25 weeks' gestation are disability-free; 39% have mild impairments that affect functioning, with 45% exhibiting moderate to severe impairments. Extremely preterm children have a mean IQ significantly below that of their classmates (83.7 [SD 18.0] vs 104.1 [SD 11.1]), modified only slightly through controlling for socioeconomic status and

Table 2
Rates of death and severe neurodevelopmental impairment among infants enrolled in the NICHD Network

Gestational Age (Completed Wk)	Death Before NICU Discharge	Outcomes at 18–22 Months' Corrected Age		
		Death	Death/Profound Neurodevelopmental Impairment	Death/Moderate to Severe Neurodevelopmental Impairment
Outcomes for all infants in the sample				
22 wk	95%	95%	98%	99%
23 wk	74%	74%	84%	91%
24 wk	44%	44%	57%	72%
25 wk	24%	25%	38%	54%
Outcomes Only for Mechanically Ventilated Infants in the Sample				
22 wk	79%	80%	90%	95%
23 wk	63%	63%	76%	87%
24 wk	40%	41%	55%	70%
25 wk	23%	24%	37%	54%

Data from Tyson JE, Parikh NA, Langer J, et al. Intensive care for extreme prematurity: moving beyond gestational age. N Engl J Med 2008;358:1672–81.

Table 3
Neurocognitive function and degree of disability at 6 years,[24] and 11 years[26]

Outcome Age 6 Y	≤23 Wk	24 Wk	25 Wk	Outcome Age 11 Y	≤23 Wk	24 Wk	25 Wk
Cognition (%)				**Cognition (%)**			
No disability	25	21	33	No disability	35	26	34
Severe disability	25	27	17	Mild	26	27	30
				Moderate	22	26	25
				Severe	17	21	10
Neuromotor (%)				**Neuromotor (%)**			
No disability	70	75	79	No disability	78	78	86
Cerebral palsy	16	19	10	Cerebral palsy, mild	9	9	7
				Cerebral palsy, moderate	4	4	2
				Cerebral palsy, severe	9	9	5
Overall disability (%)				**Overall disability (%)**			
No disability	12	14	24	No disability	13	16	17
Severe disability	25	29	28	Mild	39	30	44
No disability	1	3	8	Moderate	26	33	28
(original birth cohort)				Severe	22	21	11

excluding children untestable because of severe impairments (20 vs 15.5 points difference).

The infants sex and gestational age have independent effects on outcomes. Serious disability was more common among extremely preterm boys (53%) than preterm girls (38%), with boys scoring eight points lower than girls. Serious disability was identified in 53% of children born at 23 to 24 weeks' gestation compared with 39% of children born at 25 weeks. Mean cognitive scores at 23, 24, and 25 weeks' gestation were 82.9 (SD 21.2), 79.6 (20.8), and 86.1 (15.3), respectively. Among children with significant disability, 75% had impairment in one domain (cognition, vision, hearing, neuromotor function), 17% in two domains, and 8% in three.[26]

Studies in a single center in Japan, where all infants receive intensive care beginning at 22 weeks' gestation, showed that 67% (2 of 3 survivors) had significant neurologic disability and 100% had cerebral palsy. At 23 and 24 weeks' gestation the risks of disability were 40% and 45%, respectively, and risks for cerebral palsy were 62% and 28%, respectively.[20]

Health and Behavioral Outcomes

Poor health outcomes affect preterm infants more than term controls[28,29] and show gestational age effects.[30] Behavioral differences, including autism spectrum disorder, and inattention type attention deficit hyperactivity disorder (ADHD)[31] are more prevalent among preterm infants.[30] Adult psychiatric disorders, schizophrenia, and externalizing and internalizing behaviors are up to 10-fold more likely to occur in low-birth-weight children.[30] Preterm children have been reported to either show fewer risk-taking behaviors[28,32] or be similar to the general population.[30] These studies, however, reflect preterm adolescents/young adults who were more mature at birth.

Social Relationships and Quality of Life Perceptions

Despite these differences, many studies show higher-than-anticipated overall quality of life perceptions by the preterm individuals and their families.[32] Patterns of adjustment give surprisingly favorable perceptions of quality of life for many preterm adolescents and young adults,[29,31] despite the lower likelihood of finding a life partner,[30] increased perceived difficulties in romantic relationships and finding a job, lesser scholastic achievement, and poorer athletic abilities.[33] Other reports suggest no differences in overall independence and social relationships.[34] Self-reports of quality of life by preterm adolescents are high despite parental reports of more frequent issues with depression and ADHD.[31] A meta-analysis focused on quality of life studies highlighted the differences in self-reports and parental reports. In general, self-reports suggest no differences between the teen/young adulthood perception of quality of life and term controls despite objective measures and parental reports suggesting the contrary.[35]

ETHICS
Overview

The four cardinal principles of beneficence, nonmaleficence, autonomy, and justice that guide medical ethics frequently conflict when questions related to neonatal intensive care and delivery room management arise for extremely preterm infants. These principles are briefly defined in **Table 4** followed by discussion about the tensions inherent in neonatal decision-making. Professional guidelines are reviewed and a culturally and ethically sensitive approach to decision-making offered.

Table 4 Ethical Principles	
Beneficence	Duty of the physician to take action to prevent harm or actively promote welfare of the patient[70]
Nonmaleficence	Duty of the physician to "above all (or first) do no harm."[70] Passive action[70]
Autonomy Respect for Autonomy[a]	"Self"- auto and "rule"-nomos[59] "…at minimum, to acknowledge that person's right to hold views, to make choices and to take actions based on personal values and beliefs."[59] Norm guiding medical decision-making for competent patients[41]
Distributive Justice	Balance between the patients' rights to medical care and the fair allocation of resources and social burdens within society[59]

[a] For neonates, respect for autonomy applies to surrogate decision-making, accepted to be the parent's responsibility, acting on behalf of the best interests of the child.[61]

Principles

Table 4 defines the principles of beneficence, nonmaleficence, autonomy, and justice.

Framework for Ethical Decision-Making

Sound evidence-based ethical decisions cannot be made without evaluating what is known and predictable and what is unknown and unpredictable.[36] The struggle in decision making for these marginally viable infants begins with the data. When outcomes are clearly beneficial[37] or "predictably good enough,"[38] there is little ethical conflict and treatment is mandatory.[38,39] When treatment is deemed futile[37] and society judges the cost to be unacceptably high relative to benefit,[39] then it is mandatory not to provide treatment. In fact, as argued by Paris and Reardon,[40] it should be considered ethical and moral to not offer options for futile treatment because this undermines patient autonomy, misinforming patients that options exist when they do not. When outcomes are "uncertain" or "ambiguous,"[37,38] however, society might reasonably, although not universally, consider the cost to be acceptable in relation to the value.[39] Treatment choices should be available and explained to the decision makers.

The health care team should thoroughly assess the mitigating factors that may influence prognosis. A fetus' initial prognosis may change based on complicating antenatal and/or postnatal factors. Thus, open and transparent multidisciplinary communication between health professionals and the family is crucial to sustain trust and foster collaborative decision-making. Given the uncertainty and unpredictability of outcomes and significant associated health burdens for the infant and family, the perinatal community supports a process of shared decision-making between the physician and the family. Parents of extremely immature infants are permitted to interpret information within the context of their own moral values.[41,42] The exact gestational ages at which these boundaries are set have been shown to vary among physicians, disciplines, health care institutions, and countries.[43,44] The tensions inherent in neonatal decision-making must be explored to understand the variability in professional guidelines.

TENSIONS IN ETHICAL NEONATAL DECISION-MAKING FOR EXTREMELY PRETERM INFANTS
Futility: Is it a Legitimate Concept to Justify Care Boundaries for Extremely Immature Infants?

The inherent limitations must be understood when defining futility. Quantitative definitions propose labeling futile interventions as those consistently resulting in treatment failures when provided consecutively to 100 patients.[45] Operationalizing this definition in the context of the extremely immature neonate is problematic given limitations in the outcomes evidence and ethical concerns in obtaining this data.[36] Defining futility qualitatively attempts to isolate the term *futile* from judgments related to the value of the intended outcome, which are values inevitably heterogeneous in any society.[46] Futility can also be defined as qualitative effects to the "whole person" rather than brief effects of treatment.[45,47,48] However, this effect/benefit dyad is inseparable from the values assigned to the effectiveness of a particular outcome.[46]

Futility arguments based on distributive justice rest on cost analyses, assessment of benefits and burdens, and the ability to predict outcomes.[46,47] A review of hospitalization and posthospitalization costs in industrialized countries has shown increased health care cost trends with decreasing gestational age and birth weight, increasing survival and morbidities at lower gestational ages, and costs far exceeding what would be anticipated based on the proportion of infants born.[49–51] In addition, hidden costs such as sibling effects and the impact on family functioning are rarely considered.[36,49] The question becomes whether these resources would be better allocated toward preventive measures to decrease rates of preterm birth.[52] Unfortunately, factors predictive of resource expenditures before birth remain elusive and therefore cannot be used in a decision analysis.[42,53–57]

Lastly, attempts at resolving the futility debate balance concepts of best interests, patient autonomy and physician duties. Kopelman[58] argues that the best interests standard depends on assessments of benefits and burdens; maximizing short- and long-term interests while allowing subjective latitude as long as an objective minimum standard of care is met. This standard weighs the rights and duties of the patient against rights and duties to others. She argues that the "Best Interests' Standard permits within socially sanctioned limits, and established rights and duties, individualized decision-making including attention to such decisions as when to seek to maintain biologic life and when to seek comfort care." Discussions of physician duties often cite the Hippocratic Oath, which states "I will use treatment to help the sick according to my ability and judgment, but I will never use it to injure or wrong them."[59] Implicit are principles of beneficence and nonmaleficence. When the patients' best interests are not clear and are potentially harmed is when conflict with physician duties arises and attempts to define futility begin. However, no consensus has been obtained with this approach, reiterating the multidimensional "complex network of relational obligations, which can be negotiated in one way under certain circumstances and in another way when the situation changes."[47]

These arguments, however, are not meant to imply that all demands for treatment should be honored. Physicians have an obligation to protect patients from treatment that involves risk for inexcusable harm without ultimately altering imminent, inevitable death.[6] Fine and colleagues[60] note that no clear guidance is available from professional organizations on conflict resolution when parents want to continue treatment that physicians feel does not further the infant's best interests.

The authors suggest that using "futility" as a reason for limiting care is misleading and too dependent on subjective interpretations. In constructing the boundaries of the "gray zone," it would be preferable to describe limits based on care that minimally promotes a socially and culturally defined goal, congruent with a family's moral framework, and ethically acceptable based on empirical outcomes evidence and evidence-based best interests principles. The burden of proof would then no longer lie in showing that a treatment fails but rather that a treatment meets an acceptable level of success with respect to the defined goal.

Surrogate Decision-Making: The Concept and Role of the Parent

For patients who lack decisional capacity, the medical community advocates for a surrogate decision-maker. In adult populations, this representative makes decisions believed to be consistent with the patient's wishes, executing "substituted judgment." For infants, whose wishes are unknown, decision-making uses the best interests standard, and the representatives who can best ascertain these interests are generally accepted to be the infant's parents.[61] They are expected to possess adequate knowledge and information to make informed decisions, be committed to the child's interests while emotionally stable, and be able to make reasoned judgments.[59] This role is rarely disputed unless physicians feel the parents do not meet these qualifications.

Determining a child's best interests is complex. It requires an assessment of how a "reasonable person" (or the infant as an older individual) would weigh the benefits and burdens of disabilities and overall perceptions about quality of life.[62] Furthermore, perceptions of disability are often presumed worse by those without disability.[63] Whether the best interests of the child should be considered in isolation of the family's interests is also disputed,[64] because burdens on families after the birth of an extremely preterm infant are significant.[65]

Shared Decision-Making: The "Responsibility"

Many professional organizations support a process of shared decision-making between the physician and the parents[66–69] under conditions of uncertainty in which significant burdens to the infant and family could ensue. What exactly is shared decision-making: a process, a decisional responsibility, or both? The authors argue that it should be a process with decisional responsibility based on parental preferences. Without fulfilling certain requirements in this process, the resulting decisional outcomes can be biased. Shared decision-making does not preclude autonomous decision-making. Rather, by fulfilling the tenets of informed consent, the processes of shared decision-making support autonomous decision making.

Informed consent requires adherence to five principles: disclosure, comprehension, voluntariness, competence, and decision or consent.[70] Disclosure requires that complete information about the treatment and its risks, and the risks and benefits of forgoing treatment, is communicated.[70,71] The inherent challenge is that the extent of the disclosure can be based either on professional standards,[70] reasonable person standards (information that a minimum number of people would deem important in making these decisions),[72] or a subjective standard in which the physician decides what information is the most salient to share.[70] Comprehension signals the decision-maker's capacity to assimilate and articulate this information. Voluntariness reflects the decision maker's right to be free of any coercive influences on their decision. Competence requires an ability to integrate the information and assimilate it in terms that are both accurate and relevant to the circumstances, weighing benefits and burdens, to come to a consistent choice. Finally the last step, the consent or decision signifies autonomous decision-making.

Shared decision making also requires a reciprocal exchange of information. Physicians should communicate medical information objectively to the parent in exchange for information about the parent's values and moral ideals.[41] Informed consent and shared decision making have been suggested to differ in the final tenet: consent or decision. In shared decision making, the physician's role has been proposed to include active participation, sharing in the decisional responsibility, and providing recommendations. In the informed consent model, patients or surrogate decision makers make the decision independently without physician recommendations.[73,74]

In principle, processes supporting informed consent and autonomous decision-making are the norm. In practice, several leading ethicists have suggested that this last step, the end-of-life decision-making responsibility, can be too overwhelming for some parents,[75,76] especially as it relates to withdrawal of care for neonates. Unquestionably, asking surrogates to physically sign a do not resuscitate order increases stress and produces feelings akin to "signing a death warrant."[77] The anguish, psychological distress, and suffering that accompany these end-of-life decisions are important to recognize because despite the ethical equivalence of withdrawal and noninitiation of care, the psychological consequences have the potential to be widely divergent.[75] This fact suggests that the "wait and see approach," which itself is disputed as an effective prognostic tool,[42,54–57] may have limited applicability in this difficult decision.

Despite hesitations concerning the burdens of parental responsibility, studies of parental perceptions about end-of-life decision-making after withdrawal of care from sick neonates showed that most parents felt it was their responsibility, as part of their parental duty, to make these decisions on behalf of their infant.[78–80] These beliefs remain consistent over time; parental guilt was not related to withdrawal of care but rather to their less-active participation in the decision-making process.[79]

Families' exhibit varied decision-making preferences. Zupancic and colleagues,[81] identified that physicians are poor at determining which decision-making style families favor. Respecting a family's right to determine their desired level of participation in decision-making is both legal and ethical. If a family chooses not to participate in decision-making, this should be respected as an autonomous decision; under these circumstances forcing a decision disrespects their choices.[82] Qualitative research has shown that when parents are confronted with a decision-making style that differs from their expectations, they are less confident about their decisions.[83] Even when the decision-making approach is less autonomous, physicians have a responsibility to explore and formulate management decisions consistent with the parent's moral framework. Parents must be engaged in a process of consent and assent: consent to give the physicians decisional discretion and assent for the actual management decision.

Assent Versus Consent: The Role of Physician Recommendations

The difference between assent and consent is subtle. Assent traditionally means concurrence of opinion, whereas consent usually denotes permission. Assent requires physician recommendation, whereas it can be argued to be discretionary in a consent process. Physician recommendations have been criticized for introducing bias based on physician values, perpetuating a perceived power hierarchy between the physician and the patient.[84,85] Clinically, both assent and consent models have been described in end-of-life decision-making in adult and neonatal settings.[74,83] In neonatal settings, two paradigms are common: one in which a physician neutrally presents objective information, allowing parents to decide independently to consent to a particular course of action, and another in which physicians propose a course of action to which parents assent. The fact that two paradigms exist is not surprising given the lack of consensus among professional organizations.[67] The American Academy of Pediatrics (AAP) Committee on Bioethics advocates for a negotiated model, in which parental moral values guide decision-making, whereas the AAP Committee on Fetus and Newborn suggests an expertise model, in which physicians are more directive in assessing the best interests of the infant.[68,69,86] In adult end-of-life decision-making, four practices have been described: physicians taking an informative role, a facilitative role, a collaborative role, or a directive role.[74] Physicians seldom deviated from their consultative styles, rarely giving recommendations even when requested by surrogates.[74,83]

For parents who favor active participation in decision-making without physician recommendations, consent models may be appropriate, whereas for those who desire a more passive role, assent models with physician recommendations may be preferable. Assent models can incorporate physician recommendations either by asking for agreement or concurrence with a proposed plan of action or requiring dissent to a proposed course of action, also known as *default* models. The difference between these approaches rests on whether the parent must make an active decision. Use of defaults (disagreement with the proposed course of treatment) may be an important communication strategy under certain circumstances, lessening the burden of decision-making feared by some parents. Feudtner and colleagues[87] suggest that when a child's death is imminent and the goal is to determine whether to halt or continue therapy, using default options would not be unreasonable because they would permit parents to achieve a desired goal without needing to actively decide to withdraw care.[87] However, processes involving default models for a recommended course of care can exert powerful effects on decisional behaviors, and therefore must be used with caution.

Quality of Life Versus Sanctity of Life

Subjective judgments about quality of life and sanctity of life are central to decision-making. Parents must rapidly assimilate medical information under conditions of uncertainty, incorporating quality of life and sanctity of life perceptions, to judge the overall value of a particular decision. They may be at a disadvantage if long-term issues were not addressed prenatally,[88] because their attention is directed toward the immediate effects of interventions without consideration of long-term consequences.[88,89] Unintentionally failing to address the longer-term outcomes and their meaning to families may lead to misperceptions about future expectations.

What is quality of life and who is best suited to make these assessments? Quality of life might be considered a minimum standard for life beyond biologic existence. That minimum standard is not easy to define, is highly subjective, and varies based on who is making the assessment.[34] According to the social sciences, a minimal standard would require sufficient functioning to engage in life tasks that bring enjoyment and satisfaction.[90] Others suggest a minimum standard requires "capacity for symbolic interaction and communication" or "potential for cognitive development and interaction."[91,92]

Sanctity of life also has inconsistent definitions. Vitalists' mark conception as the initiation of life, whereas others, such as the Nuffield Council on Bioethics, "...regard the moment of birth, which is straight forward to identify, and usually represents a significant threshold in potential viability, as the significant moral and legal point of transition for judgments about preserving life." The Nuffield Council makes no statement on the moral status of the embryo or fetus.[66] Even with this variability, these concepts can be operationalized through identifying how they motivate decision-making. Physicians can then assist parents in maximizing those goals.[93] Difficulty arises when these values are not clearly identified or when they are present in degrees.

Maternal Versus Fetal Rights

Unique to the obstetrician's role is the dual responsibility of caring for two patients, the mother and fetus, simultaneously. Historically, a focus of maternal–fetal conflicts has involved maternal refusal of treatments deemed clearly beneficial for the fetus, such as refusal of a cesarean section for a term fetus at risk. On balance is a woman's right to autonomy versus the best interests of the fetus. Professional guidelines recommend that although everything possible must be attempted to protect the best interests of the fetus, these interests are insufficient to override the pregnant woman's right to autonomy. The American College of Obstetricians and Gynecologists has stated that "respect for the right of individual patients to make their own choices about their health care is fundamental."[94] Risk/benefit analyses can help justify strong recommendations, and even warrant assent approaches under these circumstances, but cannot take away a woman's right to decide what happens to her body.

The impending birth of an extremely preterm fetus has an added dimension related to personhood: at what point does a fetus possess rights and liberties? Related to this argument, and poignantly controversial, are questions surrounding the spectrum and overlap of the pregnant woman's termination rights against viability boundaries for the fetus. The perinatal team is acutely aware of the legal and political landscape, making this apparent inconsistency especially treacherous to navigate.

Can a Physician Refuse to Resuscitate?

Mercurio[6] explores three potential reasons why physicians can refuse resuscitation based on the principles of futility, distributive justice, and best interests. Futility has been rejected for reasons cited previously. Distributive justice, he also argues, is difficult for an individual physician to justify until society has upheld the idea of withholding intensive care based on resource allocation. The third argument justifies refusal based on the best interests of the infant. This stance is supported by the Hippocratic Oath and professional medical organizations. On forgoing life-sustaining medical treatment, the AAP Committee on Bioethics endorses overriding parental decisions when "those views clearly conflict with the interests of the child."[68] Best interests standards have been the primary guide for treatment decisions in never-competent patients, whose wishes and desires are unknown[95] and surrogates are charged with guarding those interests. However, a surrogate's decisions can be questioned when unilateral demands for, or refusal of, treatments conflicts with the patient's best interests.[96]

Can a Physician Refuse to Perform a Cesarean Section for an Extremely Preterm Fetus?

Competing principles of beneficence, nonmaleficence, and patient autonomy complicate matters for the perinatal/obstetric team caring for the woman and fetus. This conflict can be approached in two ways: first, weighing the risks and benefits for both patients, and then evaluating whether the intention and the likely result based on medical evidence are equivalent and acceptable. Ultimately, physicians reserve the right to use their own medical judgment and refuse to perform a procedure deemed harmful and of no benefit to a patient. The risk for harm can be immediate or long-term. Certainly any risk likely to result in imminent death should not be considered mandatory or ethical and would violate the principle of nonmaleficence. Even when harm is not an immediate consequence of an intervention, if no realistic probability of the desired outcome exists based on sound medical evidence and multidisciplinary assessments, then it is reasonable for a physician to override a patient's demand for treatment that is without clear benefit.

Unique Circumstances: Medical Decision-Making During the Prenatal Consultation

The threatened delivery of an extremely preterm fetus poses complicated medical and ethical challenges for physicians and families. The information available for deliberation is incomplete, may not reflect current management for this unique population of infants, and must be communicated under less-than-ideal circumstances of emotional distress and time constraints.[97,98] Personal beliefs, values, knowledge about outcomes, and emotional exhaustion caused by conflicts over treatment decisions by members of the woman's health care team may influence how information is presented to families and the type of support offered.[99]

During the consultation, physicians must explore the parent's values and expectations about decision-making, respecting their autonomy as surrogate decision-makers. Physicians should follow best interests standards and begin a process of shared decision-making, with responsibility for decisions dictated by parental preferences. Parents must rapidly assimilate new and evolving information and determine how their moral framework will guide their deliberation. When appropriate, recommendations can be given and models of assent followed. All members of the perinatal team must participate in the consultation process, bridging gaps for parents as they transition from antenatal to postnatal care issues. The multidisciplinary deliberations must be transparent for parents to understand potential uncertainties compounding the evolving clinical prognoses and to avoid feelings of mistrust. Boundaries of care should be constructed based on best available evidence and decisional discretion permitted for gestational ages when clinical and ethical equipoise exists.

Practically speaking, most of the empirical work on decision-making for extremely preterm infants during the prenatal consultation has focused on physician behaviors and parental recall, knowledge, and satisfaction with the process of prenatal consultation.[100,101] Only a few studies have focused specifically on the parental decision-making process.[80,83] Physician behavior, however, is a poor proxy for parental preferences. Survey assessments delineating physician practices have shown inconsistencies in resuscitation of infants born between 23 and 24 weeks, which cannot be attributed solely to variations in parental preferences, because nearly half of the physicians do not alter their behavior based on parental preferences.[43,44,64,81,88,102–104]

Perceptions of a good outcome can vary among disciplines. Despite this discrepancy, however, recommendations for delivery room management are frequently more similar among disciplines than not.[104] Initial obstetric assessments of prognosis, however, can dictate whether neonatal consultations are obtained.[105] Neonatal and obstetric assessments of prognosis can act independently or can interplay, impacting behaviors across disciplines.

Several studies have queried parents retrospectively about which factors have been most helpful to them when withdrawing life support from their children/infants. These studies are prone to retrospective biases based on the infant's outcome and parental adjustment. Some studies report on thematically related but intrinsically different decisions. Nonetheless, they inform the medical community about issues parents find important: clear information; visual deterioration; repetitive conversations; pain and suffering; the infant's bleak prognosis[78,79]; reliance on spirituality, hope,[80] and religion[106,107]; and parents' own interpretations of the infant's condition.[80,83] The parents' frame of reference is different from the physicians': parents view decisions initially from the perspective of the impending loss of the pregnancy and their chance at parenthood. Parents express the need for support and the opportunity to explore the meaning of uncertainty to augment the factual information provided. In contrast, physicians approach decisions from a medical perspective already focused on the to-be-born infant.[83,108] Only when the decision-making style fits their expectations do parents become confident in their decisions. Few physicians believe that discussing nonmedical facts with parents is part of their role, resulting in little exploration of parental values. This lack of communication compromises their ability to help parents interpret risks and benefits according to the family's moral framework.[109] Clearly, under conditions of emotional distress, what is communicated shows poor concordance with what is heard or remembered.[80,81,103,110] If parents cannot recall that they had a choice, how can the process be informed? External factors may influence their perception of options.[107] Physicians may be reluctant to offer choices based on their beliefs.[64] Parents who present to a tertiary care center may expect that the only option is resuscitation and may not be informed of the contrary.[98]

Research optimizing risk communication has been limited. The general public's awareness of issues related to extreme prematurity is limited,[89] and is impacted by the way in which information is presented.[107] A series of investigators and parents have advocated for increased education of the general public, especially those who are pregnant,[89] and for consideration of initiatives to create advance directives for pregnancies threatened with preterm delivery.[111] If the goal is to optimize parental decision-making and permit parents to make decisions consistent with their own moral framework, then continued research is needed into the process, factors that impede or promote an informed decision, and strategies to maximize consistent and stable decisions for parents. As stated by Paris and Reardon,[112] "treatment decisions for extremely premature newborns whose course is uncertain or ambiguous remains with those who bear responsibility for the infant — the parents."

Professional Guidelines

Principles of justice preclude physicians individually determining the limits of viability. Rather, professional medical organization guidelines provide standards based on which individualized factors can be considered in an attempt to provide decision-makers with some prognostic guidance.[7] International guidelines are remarkably similar, supporting parental discretion at 23 and 24 weeks. Several countries suggest resuscitation and intensive care is experimental at less than 23 weeks' gestation, supporting provision of compassionate care.[113] A few countries consider providing resuscitation or intensive care on parental insistence at 22 weeks' gestation (United Kingdom, Germany, Canada, United States). At greater than 25 weeks' gestation, most countries support intensive care, with the Netherlands considering care mandatory at 26 weeks and essentially mandatory at 25 weeks.[113] Parental expectations of participation in medical decisions about infants born extremely preterm vary by country.[43,114] Recommendations for parental involvement, the degree to which physicians direct care, and views on trials of therapy also vary. Within the United States, several state initiatives have attempted to construct guidelines; however, professional organizations struggle to provide guidance without making treatment mandatory, because this has the potential to increase liability risks when taken out of context. Some organizations designate boundaries based on short-term burdens of pain and suffering (Switzerland); others on long-term consequences. Many countries do not stratify based on gestational age; those that do not base recommendations on assessments made and information gained after birth or based on trials of intensive care (Germany, Singapore).[113]

Obstetric recommendations range from aggressive management that includes intrapartum fetal monitoring, tocolysis, glucocorticoids, and cesarean delivery to nonintervention. Intermediate approaches that attempt to avoid an operative delivery may be used, but add further complexity to the decision process because the fetus may experience additional compromise. The challenge for the obstetrician is identifying the fetus for which nonintervention is the appropriate option given a poor prognosis versus the fetus who would fare well if the intrapartum care was managed intensively.[115] Cesarean section for fetal indications is generally not recommended at less than 25 weeks' gestation, and antenatal steroids, although recommended[116] from 24 weeks' gestation, are inconsistently administered. In their comparison of international guidelines, Pignotti and Donzelli[113] noted that none of the reviewed practice parameters addressed antenatal corticosteroid administration at less than 24 weeks' gestation, with the United States recommending use after 24 weeks and the Netherlands after 25 weeks.

Whenever possible, the use of local data should be incorporated in prenatal consultations, adhering to social and cultural norms. Constructing intrainstitutional guidelines is an important way to support parental decision-making. Inconsistent messages received from different providers have been shown to increase parental distress.[117] To address this issue, a multidisciplinary effort to improve the quality of prenatal consultations and decisional satisfaction was successfully undertaken in Oregon. It provided caregivers an opportunity to incorporate their expertise with local and national outcomes and create clear and effective communication interventions to improve consistency and quality among providers.[117] These standardized evidence-based guidelines encompass obstetric and neonatal care options specific to the periviable period, offering counseling recommendations for pregnancies less than 27 weeks, including gestations less than 23 weeks.[115]

SUMMARY

Decision-making for extremely immature preterm infants at the margins of viability is ethically, professionally, and emotionally complicated. Expectant parents are suddenly thrust onto an emotional roller coaster, needing to urgently decide the fate of their unborn child while their thought processes are confounded by feelings of guilt, grief, and disbelief. They must not only incorporate the uncertainty of the medical prognostic information but also balance this new information against their values and moral framework, questioning the meaning of life and altering their world order. For some parents this may be their first experience with this decisional process, whereas for others it is a road too familiar.

This ethical dilemma has reached new dimensions as technology collides with the margins of human physiologic capacity. Interventions previously shown to improve outcomes may be of trivial benefit to these extremely immature infants. The professional community has not given definitive recommendations, appropriately leaving decisional discretion to the physician and the woman/couple to jointly decide care options at gestational ages at which the burdens of survival are significant and risks of burdensome long-term outcomes are not inconsequential. The heterogeneity of societal values and parental preferences should guide the physician–parent encounter, and the processes of shared decision-making should be encouraged.

The authors encourage that a standard for prenatal consultation be developed that would incorporate an assessment of parental decision-making preferences and styles, a communication process involving a reciprocal exchange of information, and effective strategies for decisional deliberation, guided by and consistent with parental moral framework. They recommend that all professional caregivers who provide perinatal consultations or end-of-life counseling for extremely preterm infants be sensitive to these issues and be taught flexibility in counseling techniques adhering to consistent guidelines. Emphasis must shift away from physician beliefs and behaviors about the boundaries of viability. Research must be focused on parental decisional processes to understand how they construct a minimally acceptable outcome and make life and death decisions under conditions of prognostic uncertainty.

ACKNOWLEDGMENTS

The authors wish to thank Shlomo Shinnar, MD, PhD, for his thoughtful perspectives in the review of this manuscript.

REFERENCES

1. Blackmon L. Biologic limits of viability: implications for clinical decision making. Neoreviews 2003;4(6):e140–6.
2. Evans DJ, Levene MI. Evidence of selection bias in preterm survival studies: a systematic review. Arch Dis Child Fetal Neonatal Ed 2001;84:F79–84.
3. Hack M, Wilson-Costello D. Trends in the rates of CP associated with neonatal intensive care of preterm children. Clin Obstet Gynecol 2008;51(4):763–74.
4. Draper ES. Evaluating and comparing neonatal outcomes. Arch Dis Child Fetal Neonatal Ed 2010;95:F158–9.
5. Lorenz JM, Wooliever DE, Jetton JR, et al. A quantitative review of mortality and developmental disability in extremely premature newborns. Arch Pediatr Adolesc Med 1998;152:425–35.
6. Mercurio MR. Physicians' refusal to resuscitate at borderline gestational age. J Perinatol 2005;25:685–9.
7. Tyson JE, Parikh NA, Langer J, et al. Intensive care for extreme prematurity-moving beyond gestational age. N Engl J Med 2008;358:1672–81.
8. Fanaroff AA, Stoll BJ, Wright LL, et al. Trends in neonatal morbidity and mortality for very low birthweight infants. Am J Obstet Gynecol 2007;196:147, e1–8.
9. Lorenz JM, Paneth N, Jetton JR, et al. Comparison of management strategies for extreme prematurity in New Jersey and the Netherlands: outcomes and resource expenditure. Pediatrics 2001;108:1269–74.
10. Håkansson S, Farooqi A, Holmgren PA, et al. Proactive management promotes outcome in extremely preterm infants: a population based comparison of two perinatal management strategies. Pediatrics 2004;114:58–64.
11. Saigal S, den Ouden L, Wolke D, et al. School-age outcomes in children who were extremely low birth weight from four International population-based cohorts. Pediatrics 2003;112:943–50.
12. Stoll BJ, Hansen NI, Bell EF, et al. Neonatal outcomes of extremely preterm infants from the NICHD Neonatal Research Network. Pediatrics 2010;126: 443–56.
13. Hobar JD, Carpenter J, Kenny M, et al. Very Low Birth Weight (VLBW) database summary for infants 501–1500 grams. Available at: https://nightingale.vtoxford.org/summaries.aspx. Accessed January 4, 2011.
14. Wood NS, Marlow N, Costeloe K, et al. Neurologic and developmental disability after extremely preterm birth. N Engl J Med 2000;343:378–84.
15. Express Group. One year survival of extremely preterm infants after active perinatal care in Sweden. JAMA 2009;301(21):2225–33.
16. Markestad T, Kaaresen P, Rønnestad A, et al. Early death, morbidity, and need of treatment among extremely premature infants. Pediatrics 2005;115:1289–98.
17. Fischer N, Steurer MA, Adams M, et al. Survival rates of extremely preterm infants: (gestational age <26 weeks) in Switzerland: impact of the Swiss guidelines for the care of infants born at the limit of viability. Arch Dis Child Fetal Neonatal Ed 2009;94:F407–13.
18. Vanhaesebrouck P, Allegaert K, Bottu J, et al. The EPIBEL Study: outcomes to discharge from hospital for extremely preterm infants in Belgium. Pediatrics 2004;114:663–75.

19. Chan K, Ohlsson A, Synnes A, et al. Survival, morbidity, and resource use of infants of 25 weeks' gestational age or less. Am J Obstet Gynecol 2001;185:220–6.

20. Iijima S, Arai H, Ozawa Y, et al. Clinical patterns in extremely preterm (22 to 24 weeks of gestation) infants in relation to survival time and prognosis. Am J Perinatol 2009;26:399–406.

21. Kusauda S, Fujimura M, Sakuma I, et al. Morbidity and mortality of infants with very low birth weight in Japan: center variation. Pediatrics 2006;118:e1130–8.

22. Hintz SR, Kendrick DE, Vohr BR, et al. Changes in neurodevelopmental outcomes at 18 to 22 months' corrected age among infants of less than 25 weeks' gestational age born in 1993–1999. Pediatrics 2005;115:1645–51.

23. Marlow N, Hennessy EM, Bracewell MA, et al. Motor and executive function at 6 years of age after extremely preterm birth. Pediatrics 2007;120:793–804.

24. Marlow N, Wolke D, Bracewell MA, et al. Neurologic and developmental disability at six years of age after extremely preterm birth. N Engl J Med 2005;352(1):9–19.

25. Johnson S, Hennessy E, Smith R, et al. Academic attainment and special educational needs in extremely preterm children at 11 years of age: the EPICure study. Arch Dis Child Fetal Neonatal Ed 2009;94:F283–9.

26. Johnson S, Fawke J, Hennessey E, et al. Neurodevelopmental disability through 11 years of age in children born before 26 weeks' gestation. Pediatrics 2009; 124:e249–57.

27. Hintz SR, Kendrick DE, Wilson-Costello DE, et al. Early-childhood neurodevelopmental outcomes are not improving for infants born at 25 weeks' gestational age. Pediatrics 2011;127:62–70.

28. Hack M, Flannery DJ, Schluchter M, et al. Outcomes in young adulthood for very low birth weight infants. N Engl J Med 2002;346:149–57.

29. Saigal S, Stoskopf B, Boyle M, et al. Comparison of current health, functional limitations and health care use of young adults who were born with extremely low birth weight and normal birth weight. Pediatrics 2007;119:e562–73.

30. Moster D, Lie RT, Markestad T. Long term medical and social consequence of preterm birth. N Engl J Med 2008;359:262–73.

31. Saigal S, Pinelli J, Hoult L, et al. Psychopathology and social competencies of adolescents who were extremely low birth weight. Pediatrics 2003;111:969–75.

32. Hille E, Weisglas-Kuperus N, van Goudoever JB, et al. Functional outcomes and participation in young adulthood for very preterm and very low birthweight infants: the Dutch Project on preterm and small for gestational age infants at 19 years of age. Pediatrics 2007;120:e587–95.

33. Grunau RE, Whitfield MF, Fay TB. Psychosocial and academic characteristics of extremely low birth weight (<800gm) adolescents who are free of major impairment compared with term-born control subjects. Pediatrics 2004;114:e725–32.

34. Saigal S, Stoskopf B, Pinelli J, et al. Self perceived health related quality of life of former extremely low birth weight infants at young adulthood. Pediatrics 2006; 118:1140–8.

35. Zwicker JG, Harris SR. Quality of life of formerly preterm and very low birth weight infants from preschool age to adulthood: a systematic review. Pediatrics 2008;121:e366–76.

36. Tyson JE, Stoll BJ. Evidence-based ethics and the care and outcome of extremely premature infants. Clin Perinatol 2003;30:363–87.

37. Abram MB. Deciding to forego life-sustaining treatment: a report on ethical, medical, and legal issues in treatment decisions. Washington, DC: President's

Commission for the Study of Ethical Problems in Medicine and Biomedical and Behavioral Research; 1983. p. 218–9.

38. Lantos JD, Meadow WL. Neonatal bioethics: the moral challenges of medical innovation. Baltimore (MD): Johns Hopkins University Press; 2006.

39. Tyson JE. Evidenced-based ethics and the care of premature infants. Future Child 1995;5(1):197–213.

40. Paris JJ, Reardon FE. Physician refusal of requests for futile or ineffective interventions. Camb Q Healthc Ethics 1992;1:127–34.

41. Charles C, Whelan T, Gafni A, et al. What do we mean by partnership in making decisions about treatment. BMJ 1999;319(7212):780.

42. Leuthner SR, Lorenz JM. Can rule-based ethics help in the NICU? Available at: http://virtualmentor.ama-assn.org/site/archives.html. Accessed June 28, 2011.

43. De Leeuw R, Cuttini M, Nadai M, et al. Treatment choices for extremely preterm infants: an international perspective. J Pediatr 2000;137:608–15.

44. Partridge JC, Freeman H, Weiss E, et al. Delivery room resuscitation decisions for extremely low birth weight infants in California. J Perinatol 2001;21:27–33.

45. Schneiderman LJ, Jecker NS, Jonsen AR. Medical futility: its meaning and ethical implications. Ann Intern Med 1990;112(12):949–54.

46. Truog RD, Brett AS, Frader J. The problem with futility. N Engl J Med 1992;326: 1560–4.

47. Helft PR, Siegler M, Lantos J. The rise and fall of the futility movement. N Engl J Med 2000;343:293–6.

48. Veatch RM, Spicer CM. Medically futile care: the role of the physician in setting limits. Am J Law Med 1992;18:15–36.

49. Petrou S, Eddama O, Mangham L. A structured review of the recent literature on the economic consequences of preterm birth. Arch Dis Child Fetal Neonatal Ed 2011;96:F225–32. DOI: 10.1136/adc.2009.161117.

50. Cuevas KD, Silver DR, Brooten D, et al. The cost of prematurity: hospital charges at birth and frequency of rehospitalizations and acute care visits over the first year of life. Am J Nurs 2005;105:56–64.

51. Gilbert WM, Nesbitt TS, Danielsen B. The cost of prematurity: quantification by gestational age and birth weight. Obstet Gynecol 2003;102:488–92.

52. Zupancic JA. Dangerous economics: resource allocation in the NICU. Can Med Assoc J 1992;146(6):1073–6.

53. Ardagh M. Futility has no utility in resuscitation medicine. J Med Ethics 2000;26: 396–9.

54. Meadow W, Lagatta J, Andrews B, et al. Just in time: ethical implications of serial predictions of death and morbidity for ventilated premature infants. Pediatrics 2008;121:732–40.

55. Meadow W, Frain L, Ren Y, et al. Serial assessment of mortality in the neonatal intensive care unit by algorithm and intuition: certainty, uncertainty and informed consent. Pediatrics 2002;109(5):878–87.

56. Singh J, Fanaroff J, Andrews B, et al. Resuscitation in the gray zone of viability: determining physician preferences and predicting infant outcomes. Pediatrics 2007;120:519–26.

57. Donovan EF, Tyson JE, Ehrenkranz RA. Inaccuracy of Ballard scores before 28 weeks' gestation. National Institute of Child and Human Development Neonatal Research Network. J Pediatr 1999;135(2):147–52.

58. Kopelman L. The best interests standard for incompetent or incapacitated persons of all ages. J Law Med Ethics 2007;35(1):187–96.

59. Beauchamp TL, Childress JF. Principles of biomedical ethics. 5th edition. New York: Oxford University Press; 2001.
60. Fine RL, Whitfield JM, Carr BL, et al. Medical futility in the neonatal intensive care unit: hope for a resolution. Pediatrics 2005;116:1219–22.
61. American Academy of Pediatrics Committee on Fetus and Newborn. The initiation or withdrawal of treatment for high-risk newborns. Pediatrics 1995;96:362–4.
62. Campbell AG, McHaffie HE. Prolonging life and allowing death: infants. J Med Ethics 1995;21(6):339.
63. Saigal S, Stoskopf BL, Feeny D, et al. Differences in preferences for neonatal outcomes among health care professionals, parents and adolescents. JAMA 1999;281(21):1991–7.
64. Peerzada JM, Richardson DK, Burns JP. Delivery room decision-making at the threshold of viability. J Pediatr 2004;145(4):492–8.
65. Forman V. This lovely life. New York: Houghton Mifflin Harcourt Publishing Company; 2009.
66. Critical Care Decisions in Fetal and Neonatal Medicine. Ethical issues: Nuffield Counsel on Bioethics. Available at: www.nuffieldbioethics.org. Accessed April 6, 2010.
67. Leuthner SR. Decisions regarding resuscitation of the extremely premature infant and models of best interest. J Perinatol 2001;21:193–8.
68. AAP Committee on Bioethics. Guidelines on forgoing life-sustaining medical treatment. Pediatrics 1994;93:532–6.
69. AAP Committee on Bioethics. Ethics and the care of critically ill infants and children. Pediatrics 1996;98:149–52.
70. Faden RR, Beauchamp TL. A history and theory of informed consent. New York: Oxford University Press; 1986.
71. Kon AA. Healthcare providers must offer palliative treatment to parents of neonates with hypoplastic left heart syndrome. Arch Pediatr Adolesc Med 2008;162(9):844–9.
72. Feudtner C. Ethics in the midst of a therapeutic evolution. Arch Pediatr Adolesc Med 2008;162(9):854–7.
73. Emanuel EJ, Emanuel LL. Four models of the physician-patient relationship. JAMA 1992;267:2221–6.
74. White DB, Malvar G, Karr J, et al. Expanding the paradigm of the physician's role in surrogate decision-making: an empirically derived framework. Crit Care Med 2010;38:743–50.
75. Paris JJ, Graham N, Schreiber MD, et al. Has the emphasis on autonomy gone too far? Insights from Dostoevsky on parental decision making in the NICU. Special section: the power of choice: autonomy, informed consent and the right to refuse. Camb Q Healthc Ethics 2006;15:147–51.
76. Montello M, Lantos J. The Karamazov complex: Dostoevsky and DNR orders. Perspect Biol Med 2002;45:190–9.
77. Sulmacy DP, Sood JR, Texlera K, et al. A prospective trial of a new policy eliminating signed consent for do not resuscitate orders. J Gen Intern Med 2006;21:1261–8.
78. McHaffie HE, Laing IA, Parker M, et al. Deciding for imperiled newborns: medical authority or parental autonomy? J Med Ethics 2001;27:104–9.
79. McHaffie HE, Lyon AJ, Hume R. Deciding on treatment limitation for neonates: the parents' perspective. Eur J Pediatr 2001;160:339–44.

80. Boss RD, Hutton N, Sulpar LJ, et al. Values parents apply to decision-making regarding delivery room resuscitation for high risk newborns. Pediatrics 2008; 122:583–9.
81. Zupancic JA, Kirpalani H, Barrett J, et al. Characterizing doctor-parent communication in counseling for impending preterm delivery. Arch Dis Child Fetal Neonatal Ed 2002;87:F113–7.
82. Meisel A, Kuczewski M. Legal and ethical myths about informed consent. Arch Intern Med 1996;156:2521–6.
83. Payot A, Gendron S, Lefebvre F, et al. Deciding to resuscitate extremely premature babies: how do parents and neonatologists engage in the decision? Soc Sci Med 2007;64:1487–500.
84. Truog RD. Doctor if this were your child what would you do? Commentary. Pediatrics 1999;103(1):153–5.
85. White DB, Evans LR, Bautista CA, et al. Are physicians' recommendations to limit life support beneficial or burdensome? Am J Respir Crit Care Med 2009; 180:320–5.
86. AAP, Committee on Fetus and Newborn and ACOG, Committee on Obstetric Practice. Perinatal care at the threshold of viability. Pediatrics 1995;96: 974–6.
87. Feudtner C, Munson D, Morrison W. Framing permission for halting or continuing life-extending therapies. Virtual Mentor 2008;10(8):506–10.
88. Schroeder J. Ethical issues for parents of extremely premature infants. J Paediatr Child Health 2008;44:302–4.
89. Martinez AM, Partridge JC, Yu V, et al. Physician counseling practices and decision making for extremely preterm infants in the Pacific Rim. J Paediatr Child Health 2005;41:209–14.
90. McCullough LB. Neonatal ethics at the limits of viability. Pediatrics 2005;116: 1019–21.
91. Rhoden NK. Treatment dilemmas for imperiled newborns: why QOL counts. S C Law Rev 1985;58(6):1283–347.
92. Robertson JA. Extreme prematurity and parental rights after baby doe. Hastings Cent Rep 2004;34:32–9.
93. Chiswick M. Parents and end of life decisions in neonatal practice. Arch Dis Child Fetal Neonatal Ed 2001;85:1–3.
94. American College of Obstetricians and Gynecologists. Ethical decision making in obstetrics and gynecology. Available at: http://www.acog.org/from_home/ publications/ethics/co390.pdf. Accessed June 17, 2011.
95. Caplan A, Cohen CB. Imperiled newborns. Hastings Cent Rep 1987;17(6):1–52.
96. Paris JJ, Schreiber MD. Parental discretion in refusal of treatment for newborns: a real but limited right. Clin Perinatol 1996;23:573–81.
97. Harrison H. Counseling parents of extremely premature babies. Lancet 1997; 349(9047):289.
98. Janvier A, Barrington KJ. The ethics of neonatal resuscitation at the margins of viability: informed consent and outcomes. J Pediatr 2005;147:579–85.
99. Yoon JD, Rasinski KA, Curlin FA. Conflict and emotional exhaustion in obstetricians and gynecologists: a national survey. J Moral Educ 2010;36:731–5.
100. Paul DA, Epps S, Leef KH, et al. Prenatal consultation with a neonatologist prior to preterm delivery. J Perinatol 2001;21:431–7.
101. Blanco F, Suresh G, Howard D, et al. Ensuring accurate knowledge of prematurity outcomes for prenatal counseling. Pediatrics 2005;115:e478–87.

102. Doron MW, Veness-Meehan KA, Margolis LH, et al. Delivery room resuscitation decisions for extremely premature infants. Pediatrics 1998;102(3):574–82.

103. Keenan H, Doron M, Seyda B. Comparison of mothers' and counselors' perceptions of pre-delivery counseling for extremely premature infants. Pediatrics 2005;116(1):104–11.

104. Lavin JP, Kantak A, Ohlinger JM, et al. Attitudes of obstetric and pediatric health care providers toward resuscitation of infants who are born at the margins of viability. Pediatrics 2006;118:S169–76.

105. Martinez AM, Weiss E, Partridge JC, et al. Management of extremely low birth weight infants: perceptions of viability and parental counseling practices. Obstet Gynecol 1998;92:520–4.

106. Hammerman C, Kornbluth E, Lavie O, et al. Decision making in the critically ill neonate: cultural background v individual life experiences. J Med Ethics 1997; 23:164–9.

107. Haward MF, Murphy RO, Lorenz JM. Message framing and perinatal decisions. Pediatrics 2008;122:109–18.

108. Britt DW, Evans WJ, Mehta SS, et al. Framing the decision: determinants of how women considering multifetal pregnancy reduction as a pregnancy-management strategy frame their moral dilemma. Fetal Diagn Ther 2004; 19(3):232–40.

109. Bastek TK, Richardson DK, Zupancic JA, et al. Prenatal consultation practices at the border of viability; a regional survey. Pediatrics 2005;116:406–13.

110. Koh TH, Jarvis C. Promoting effective communication in neonatal intensive care units by audiotaping doctor-patient conversations. Int J Clin Pract 1998;52:27–9.

111. Catlin A. Thinking outside the box: prenatal care and the call for a prenatal advanced directive. J Perinat Neonatal Nurs 2005;19:169–76.

112. Paris J, Reardon F. Bad cases make bad law: HCA vs. Miller is not a guide for resuscitation of extremely premature newborns. J Perinatol 2001;21(8):541–4.

113. Pignotti MS, Donzelli G. Perinatal care at the threshold of viability: an international comparison of practical guidelines for the treatment of extremely preterm births. Pediatrics 2008;121:e193–8.

114. Orfali K. Parental role in medical decision-making: fact or fiction? A comparative study of ethical dilemmas in French and American neonatal intensive care units. Soc Sci Med 2004;58(10):2009–22.

115. Tomlinson MW, Kaempf JW, Ferguson LA, et al. Caring for the pregnant woman presenting at periviable gestation: acknowledging the ambiguity and uncertainty. Am J Obstet Gynecol 2010;202:529.e1–6.

116. Effect of corticosteroids for fetal maturation on perinatal outcomes. NIH Consens Statement 1994;12(2):1–24.

117. Kaempf JW, Tomlinson M, Arduzza C, et al. Medical staff guidelines for periviability pregnancy counseling and medical treatment of extremely premature infants. Pediatrics 2006;117:22–9.

Morbidity and Mortality in Late Preterm and Early Term Newborns: A Continuum

William A. Engle, MD

KEYWORDS

- Late preterm • Early term • Late term • Morbidity • Mortality
- Outcomes • Unplanned delivery • Elective delivery

Late preterm and early term newborns are at higher risk for morbidities and mortality during and after the birth hospitalization than infants born at exactly 39 weeks' (39 0/7) gestation to 40 weeks plus 6 days' (40 6/7) gestation. Similarly, newborns delivered before 34 0/7 weeks' gestation or after 41 6/7 weeks' gestation are at higher risk than term infants for complications and death. This article defines late preterm, early term, and late term; summarizes outcomes for these infants; outlines management priorities for the neonate and mother/fetus dyad; reviews causes for births before 39 weeks' gestation; and should stimulate research and development of new, effective, and safe care strategies.

Categorizing groups of newborns is valuable to focus attention on common causes of negative outcomes and to develop care strategies to address these causes. However, categorization is arbitrary and blurs the fact that outcomes generally correlate with gestational age.[1–9] Biologic variability further complicates the comparison of outcomes within gestational age categories. A secondary purpose of this article is to highlight several important clinical outcomes that are strongly associated with gestational age. Furthermore, it poses the question of whether 34 weeks' gestation is an optimal surrogate for fetal maturity and target for delivery when urgent delivery is not indicated for the safety and health of a woman or her fetus.

DEFINITIONS

Late preterm and early term newborns include infants that are categorized as infants born at 34 0/7 to 36 6/7 weeks' gestation and 37 0/7 to 38 6/7 weeks' gestation,

Disclosures: The author has nothing to disclose.
Section of Neonatal-Perinatal Medicine, Indiana University School of Medicine, Riley Research Room 208, 699 Riley Drive, Indianapolis, IN 46202, USA
E-mail address: wengle@iupui.edu

Clin Perinatol 38 (2011) 493–516
doi:10.1016/j.clp.2011.06.009
0095-5108/11/$ – see front matter © 2011 Elsevier Inc. All rights reserved.

respectively (**Fig. 1**). Late preterm was defined by participants at a 2005 workshop of the Eunice Kennedy Shriver National Institutes of Child Health and Human Development of the National Institutes of Health to address an emerging body of evidence that such infants had higher rates of morbidity and mortality than was generally understood.[10] Early term was more recently coined to focus attention on the risks for morbidity and mortality in such infants compared with other term infants born later in the term category (late term, 39 0/7–41 6/7 weeks' gestation). The primary goals of defining late preterm and early term are to more accurately describe outcomes and focus care strategies, better understand the causes of births at these gestational categories, and stimulate research and development of care strategies to minimize the number of these births, if possible.

MAGNITUDE OF LATE PRETERM AND EARLY TERM BIRTHS

The percentage of live births in the United States that were born late preterm increased between 1990 and 2006 from 7.3% to 9.14%, a 25% increase.[11] This increase accounted for 84% of the increase in the rate of prematurity during that same 16-year period. During 2007 and 2008, the percentage of live births that were late preterm decreased by 3% to 8.77% of all live births (about 15,000 fewer late preterm births). Although this trend is encouraging, the percentage of live births born late preterm remains substantially greater than in 1990 (7.3%) and, assuming about 4 million births in the United States each year, equates to 351,000 late preterm births. That fewer infants are being born during the late preterm period reflects positively on the initial educational efforts of many advocacy groups such as the American Congress of Obstetricians and Gynecologists; American Academy of Pediatrics; National Institutes of Health; Centers for Disease Control; Association of Women's Health, Obstetric and Neonatal Nurses; and March of Dimes.

Early term births account for about 23% and 20% of all live births in the United States and France, respectively.[9,12] If 4 million live births occur annually in the United States, early term births will account for about 920,000 births.[13] The early term population of mothers and infants has received some attention by investigators who have described higher risks of morbidity, especially respiratory, compared with infants born at 39 0/7 to 41 6/7 weeks' gestation.[9,14–16] To address concerns about the respiratory morbidity in early term infants, the American Congress of Obstetricians and

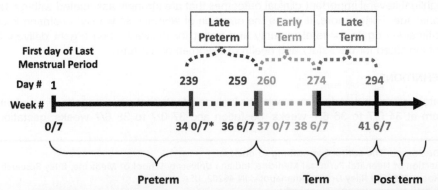

Fig. 1. Definitions of late preterm, early term, and late term. Asterisk (*) indicates completed weeks' gestation and equals the number of 7-day intervals from the first day of LMP. (*Adapted from* Engle WA, Kominiarek M. Late preterm infants, early term infants, and timing of elective deliveries. Clin Perinatol 2008;35:326; with permission.)

Gynecologists updated their 1996 recommendation that elective cesarean or induction of labor (eg, elective delivery) before 39 weeks' gestation be performed only after fetal maturity is proved and the appropriate clinical circumstances are present.[17,18] The impact of such recommendations, hospital policy changes, and educational efforts on clinical practice are being evaluated, with initial evidence indicating a significant reduction in elective deliveries (28% vs 3%) and several maternal and neonatal morbidities, without an increase in stillbirths (**Table 1**).[1,2,9,19–22]

CONSEQUENCES OF LATE PRETERM AND EARLY TERM BIRTHS
Acute Medical Morbidities and Mortality

Late preterm and early term infants are physiologically and metabolically less mature than late term infants. Risks of respiratory distress and death and/or a severe neurologic disorder are inversely associated with gestational age (**Figs. 2** and **3**).[3,6,8,9,23,24] In a population-based study of 150,426 live-born infants, severe respiratory failure (ie, treatment with mechanical ventilation and/or nasal continuous positive airway pressure) decreased from 20% at 34 weeks' gestation to 0.3% at 39 to 41 weeks' gestation, with a reduction in relative risk of severe respiratory failure between 34 and 38 weeks by a factor of 2 to 3 for each additional week of gestation.[9] The risk of death and/or a severe neurologic disorder defined by ischemic encephalopathy, grade 3 or 4 intraventricular hemorrhage, cystic periventricular leukomalacia, and/or seizures decreased from 1.7% at 34 weeks' gestation to 0.15% to 0.16% at 38 to 41 weeks' gestation (see **Fig. 3**). Need for resuscitation in the delivery room, especially ventilation with a manual resuscitator, also has been shown to be significantly more frequent as gestational age decreases from 41 6/7 weeks to 34 0/7 weeks.[25] Significant factors influencing need for manual resuscitation included gestational age, twin gestation, maternal hypertension, nonclear amniotic fluid, nonvertex presentation, cesarean delivery, birth weight less than 2500 g, and male sex.

Table 1
Change in elective deliveries after implementation of a policy to avoid elective deliveries before 39 weeks of gestation

Outcome	Period 1: 37,686 Deliveries (%)	Period 2: 122,718 Deliveries (%)
Elective deliveries before 39 weeks' gestation (elective inductions or labor and cesareans)	28	3*
Indicated inductions of labor	18.0	16.4
Maternal morbidity		
Cesarean for fetal distress	11	6*
Postpartum anemia	1.6	0.5*
Stillbirths	0.09	0.03*
Preeclampsia	0.6	0.8*
Neonatal morbidity		
Meconium aspiration	1.1	0.6*
Apgar score at 1 min <5	3.0	2.4*
Respiratory distress syndrome	0.5	0.6
Neonatal mechanical ventilation	0.4	0.4

*P<0.05.
Data from Oshiro BT, Henry E, Wilson J, et al. Decreasing elective deliveries before 39 weeks of gestation in an integrated health care system. Obstet Gynecol 2009;113:804–11.

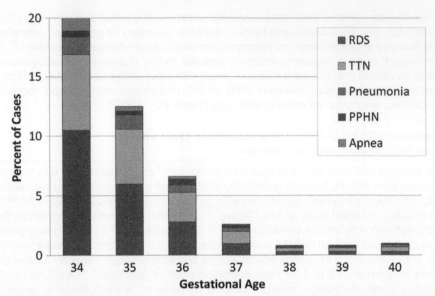

Fig. 2. Respiratory morbidity according to gestational age. n = 233,844. PPHN, persistent pulmonary hypertension of the newborn; RDS, Respiratory Distress Syndrome; TTN, transient tachypnea of the newborn. (*Data from* Hibbard JU, Wilkins I, Sun L, et al. Consortium on Safe Labor, Respiratory morbidity in late preterm births. JAMA 2010;304:423.)

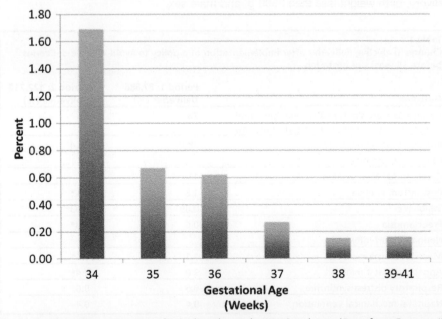

Fig. 3. Death and/or severe neurologic disorder and gestational age. (*Data from* Gouyon JB, Vintejoux A, Sagot P, et al. Neonatal outcome associated with singleton birth at 34–41 weeks of gestation. Int J Epidemiol 2010;39:772.)

In a retrospective analysis of 26,170 late preterm and 377,638 term infants, late preterm infants experienced morbidity during the birth hospitalization 7 times more frequently than term infants (22% vs 3.0%, respectively).[26] In this large population-based study, morbidity was defined as a hospital stay greater than 5 nights and a life-threatening condition; a hospital stay less than or equal to 5 nights and transfer to a higher level of care medical facility; or death before initial hospitalization discharge. Gestational age was significantly correlated with morbidity risk with the lowest risk at 39 and 40 weeks' gestation (**Fig. 4**).

In a cohort of 264 infants of women with healthy pregnancies other than spontaneous onset of preterm labor at 24 0/7 to 33 6/7 weeks' gestation, adverse medical morbidity of late preterm infants during the birth hospitalization was compared with that of moderately preterm (32 0/7–33 6/7 weeks' gestation) and term (≥37 0/7 weeks' gestation) infants.[23] Betamethasone was given to 98% of the women. Medical morbidity was defined as a composite outcome that included intraventricular hemorrhage, witnessed seizures, treatment of apnea/bradycardia, home monitoring, treatment with mechanical ventilation or continuous positive airway pressure, necrotizing enterocolitis, gastroesophageal reflux, hypoglycemia, longer than 4 days to achieve full per os or nasogastric feedings, antibiotics for sepsis, treatment with phototherapy, blood transfusion, and temperature instability. The incidence of adverse neonatal medical morbidity during the birth hospitalization decreased by 23% with each week of advancing gestational age at delivery between 32 and 39 completed weeks after controlling for race, chorioamnionitis, sex, and time between betamethasone administration and delivery (relative risk, 0.77; 95% confidence interval, 0.71–0.84) (**Fig. 5**).

Similar outcomes for 2478 late preterm infants of women with low-risk, spontaneous singleton deliveries and 7434 term infants were reported in a retrospective analysis of births from a single institution.[8] Respiratory (mechanical ventilation, respiratory

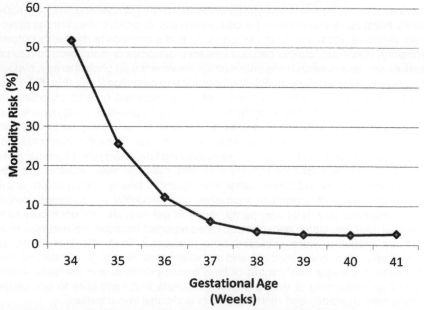

Fig. 4. Neonatal morbidity versus gestational age. (*Data from* Shapiro-Mendoza CK, Tomashek KM, Kotelchuck M, et al. Effect of late-preterm birth and maternal medical conditions on newborn morbidity risk. Pediatrics 2008;121:e227.)

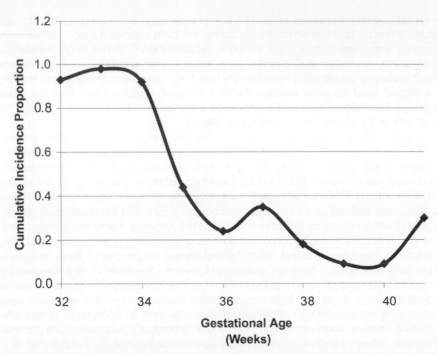

Fig. 5. Composite adverse neonatal outcome. (*Data from* Bastek JA, Sammel MD, Paré E, et al. Adverse neonatal outcomes: examining the risks between preterm, late preterm, and term infants. Am J Obstet Gynecol 2008;199:367,e6.)

distress syndrome, transient tachypnea of the newborn, persistent pulmonary hypertension), infectious (culture-proved sepsis, meningitis, or pneumonia), central nervous system (seizures, intraventricular hemorrhage), and a composite morbidity outcome (respiratory, infectious, central nervous system morbidities or admission to neonatal intensive care, death, necrotizing enterocolitis, treatment with phototherapy, hypoglycemia, or hypothermia) were inversely proportional to gestational age (**Fig. 6**).[8] Potential negative effects on infant outcomes of other maternal or fetal disorders that contribute to late preterm and early term births (such as preeclampsia, hypertension, preterm premature rupture of membranes, diabetes, intrauterine growth restriction, oligohydramnios, fetal acidosis, cervical incompetence, abruptio placentae, fetal demise, cesarean delivery because of nonreassuring fetal heart rate, placental abruption, placenta previa, suspected chorioamnionitis, maternal fever, induction of labor, cesarean deliveries for indications other than dystocia, breech presentation, or prior cesarean delivery, and congenital anomalies) and frequently encountered confounders (eg, maternal age, fetal sex, parity, mode of delivery) did not contribute to the gestational age–associated neonatal outcomes reported because mother/fetus dyads with these problems were excluded from analyses.[8] Thus, the immaturity, and presumptively incomplete medical and developmental recovery, of late and early term infants is a major determinant of long-term morbidities and mortality. A more complete understanding of the pathobiologic events that contribute to late preterm and early term morbidity and mortality awaits additional investigation.

Late preterm infants have been determined to be at higher risk than early and late term infants for complications that are similar to those encountered by moderately preterm infants during and after the birth hospitalization.[8,9,23,26–30] Hypothermia

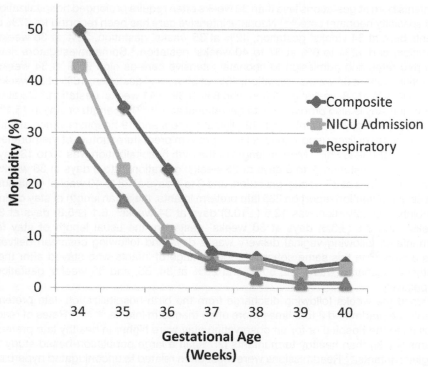

Fig. 6. Rate of neonatal morbidity versus gestational age. NICU, neonatal intensive care unit. (*Data from* Melamed N, Klinger G, Tenenbaum-Gavish K, et al. Short-term neonatal outcome in low-risk, spontaneous, singleton, late preterm deliveries. Obstet Gynecol 2009; 114:258.)

(10% vs 0%), hypoglycemia (16% vs 5%), respiratory distress (29% vs 4%), jaundice (54% vs 38%), feeding problems (32% vs 7%), and admission to intensive care occur more frequently during the birth hospitalization.[27] Late preterm infants also are treated with intravenous fluids (27% vs 5%), evaluated for sepsis (37% vs 13%), and receive mechanical ventilation (3.4% vs 0.9%) more frequently than term infants.

Early term infants are at higher risk for morbidities, especially respiratory disorders, death, and/or severe neurologic disorders, and neonatal intensive care unit admissions, than late term infants.[3,8,9,23,31] In an analysis of 2,527,766 women with live, singleton, cephalic, term pregnancies during 2003, 8.3% were delivered at 37 weeks' gestation, 19.4% at 38 weeks' gestation, 30.2% at 39 weeks' gestation, 32.1% at 40 weeks' gestation, and 10% at 41 weeks' gestation.[31] Births at 37 weeks' gestation (0.45% vs 0.14%; adjusted odds ratio, 3.12; 95% confidence interval, 2.90–3.38) and 38 weeks' gestation (0.19% vs 0.14%; adjusted odds ratio, 1.30; 95% confidence interval, 1.19–1.43) were at significantly higher risk of hyaline membrane disease. The need for mechanical ventilation in neonates born at 37 weeks' gestation (0.57% vs 0.28%; adjusted odds ratio, 2.20; 95% confidence interval 1.88–2.18) and 38 weeks' gestation (0.32% vs 0.28%; adjusted odds ratio, 1.15; 95% confidence interval 1.08–1.23) were also found to be significantly greater in frequency than that in neonates born at 39 weeks' gestation.[5,7,9,15,31,32] In absolute numbers, infants born at 37 and 38 weeks' gestation account for about 1850 cases of hyaline membrane disease and 2770 cases of neonatal mechanical ventilation each year in the United States.

Infants born at gestations less than 39 weeks often require prolonged hospitalization and specialty neonatal care.[3,31] Neonatal intensive care has been reported for 67% of infants born at 34 weeks' gestation, 42% at 35 weeks' gestation, 22% at 36 weeks' gestation, and 12% to 6% at 37 to 40 weeks' gestation.[3] Some investigators have reported rates and admission to neonatal intensive care as high 96% at 34 weeks' gestation, 80% at 35 weeks' gestation, 43% at 36 weeks' gestation, 18% at 37 weeks' gestation, 9% at 38 weeks' gestation, and 6% at 39 to 41 weeks' gestation.[9] Duration of hospital stay is also proportional to gestational age.[27,33–38] Length of stay in 15,136 late preterm singleton infants from 12 clinical centers and 19 hospitals varied slightly with cause for delivery (spontaneous labor, preterm premature rupture of membranes, indicated, or unknown).[33] Median length of the birth hospitalization was 10 to 13 days at 34 weeks' gestation, 7 to 8 days at 35 weeks' gestation, 5 to 6 days at 36 weeks' gestation, 5 days at 37 weeks' gestation, and 3 to 4 days at 38 to 40 weeks' gestation. In a single-institution report on 235 late preterm infants, the mean length of stay during the birth hospitalization was 12.6 (±10.6) days at 34 weeks', 6.1 (±5.8) days at 35 weeks', and 3.8 (±3.6) days at 36 weeks' gestation; the usual length of stay for term infants following vaginal delivery was 2 days and following cesarean delivery was 3 days.[35] In this same cohort, the percentage of infants who stayed after their mothers' discharge was 75%, 50%, and 25% at 34, 35, and 36 weeks' gestation, respectively.

During the weeks following discharge from the birth hospitalization, late preterm infants are readmitted 2 to 3 times more often than term infants.[36,39,40] Rates of readmission to the hospital or for an observation stay were higher in healthy late preterm infants (4.3%) than healthy term infants (2.7%) in a large population-based study of singleton infants.[41] Readmissions were most often related to unconjugated hyperbilirubinemia, feeding problems, and suspected infection. Oral feeding problems may only become apparent after the mother's breast milk supply increases and the infant's oromotor skills are challenged. In a retrospective review of 282 late preterm infants, reasons for readmission or emergency outpatient visits were respiratory distress, apnea (apparent life-threatening event), fever, jaundice, vomiting, and crying.[39] Risk factors for readmission include a primigravida mother, breastfeeding, maternal complications during labor and delivery, public insurance, and east Asian heritage. Never being admitted to a neonatal intensive care unit during the birth hospitalization also increased risk for readmission to the hospital.[40] Such factors are useful to identify mother-infant dyads that most benefit from close monitoring, emphasis on breast-feeding education, and screening for hyperbilirubinemia and feeding difficulties before discharge. Readmission rates for early term and late term infants have yet to be described.

Many late preterm infants are clinically well and do not experience significant short-term medical complications. Because of limited available data, risk factors for medical complications in early term infants must be extrapolated from those associated with late preterm delivery. Several risk factors for morbidity in late preterm infants have been identified by investigators (**Box 1**).[4,8,23,24,26,34] In a prospectively evaluated cohort of 548 consecutively born late preterm neonates without major congenital anomalies, chromosomal disorders, or congenital infections (percentage of infants 14% at 34 weeks' gestation, 34% at 35 weeks' gestation, and 52% at 36 weeks' gestation), 30% of cases suffered morbidity during the birth hospitalization.[4] Of cases with morbidity, 44% had more than 1 morbid condition. In addition to gestational age, a dominant factor, risk factors for morbidity included small for gestational age (odds ratio 4.18), multiple gestation (odds ratio 3.68), lack of antenatal corticosteroid administration (odds ratio 4.03), emergency cesarean delivery (odds ratio 1.43), and antepartum hemorrhage

---

Box 1
Risk factors for morbidity during the birth hospitalization in late preterm infants

- Younger gestational age
- Small for gestational age
- Multiple gestation
- Lack of antenatal corticosteroid administration
- Emergency cesarean delivery
- Elective cesarean delivery
- Complicated vaginal delivery
- Antepartum hemorrhage
- Hypertensive disorders of pregnancy
- Maternal diabetes
- Maternal pulmonary, cardiac, or renal disease
- Apgar score less than 7 at 5 minutes
- Male
- Racial or ethnic minority
- Lower levels of maternal education
- Primiparae or grand multiparae
- Maternal smoking
- Public insurance

(odds ratio 3.07).[4] In a case-control study comparing short-term neonatal outcomes in 2478 late preterm versus 7434 term infants delivered after spontaneous low-risk deliveries (ie, absent multiple gestation, preterm premature rupture of membranes, maternal medical illnesses, or fetal complications), the rate of morbidities decreased as gestational age increased from 34 to between 39 and 40 weeks (see **Fig. 6**).[8] Risk factors for a composite morbidity involving respiratory, infectious, or nervous system complications; neonatal death; necrotizing enterocolitis; need for phototherapy; hypoglycemia; or hypothermia included younger gestational age and male sex. Risk factors for respiratory complications (ie, respiratory distress syndrome, transient tachypnea of the newborn, pulmonary hypertension, or need for ventilator support) included younger gestational age, male sex, multiparity, cesarean delivery, complicated vaginal delivery and Apgar score less than 7 at 5 minutes.[8,24] Elective and emergent cesarean delivery are both associated with higher rates of morbidities in late preterm and term infants, with lowest rates at gestational ages of 38 to 40 weeks.[42] In late preterm infants delivered by elective cesarean and compared with those delivered vaginally, adverse outcomes included birth depression (41.1% vs 24.0%; relative risk, 1.7; *P*<.001), special care admission (46.0% vs 25.0%; relative risk, 1.84; *P* = .001), and respiratory morbidity (18.9% vs 8.8%; relative risk, 2.15; *P*<.001).[42]

In a retrospective analysis of 26,170 late preterm and 377,638 term infants, late preterm infants experienced morbidity during the birth hospitalization 7 times more frequently than term infants (22% vs 3.0%, respectively).[26] In this large population-based study, morbidity was defined as a hospital stay greater than 5 nights and a life-threatening condition; a hospital stay less and or equal to 5 nights and transfer to a higher level of care medical facility; or death before initial hospitalization discharge. Gestational age was significantly correlated with morbidity risk, with the lowest risk at 39 and 40 weeks' gestation (see **Fig. 4**).[26] Late preterm infants were more likely than term infants to have the following characteristics: male sex, racial or ethnic minority, lower levels of maternal education, primiparae or grand multiparae, maternal smoking, and public insurance. Sociodemographic risk factors for morbidity among late preterm infants included being classified as non-Hispanic white or Hispanic race. Several maternal conditions were found to have a greater than additive effect with late preterm gestation (ie, an interaction) on risk for morbidity. For example, the expected additive joint effect (adjusted risk ratio) of late preterm gestation and maternal antepartum hemorrhage was 7.1; the actual adjusted risk ratio was 12.3 (95% confidence interval, 11.5–13.1). Other maternal conditions that increased morbidity risk with a greater than additive effect included hypertensive disorders of pregnancy (adjusted risk ratio, 10.9; 95% confidence interval, 10.4–11.5); diabetes mellitus (adjusted relative risk, 9.2; 95% confidence interval, 8.6–9.9); and maternal lung, (adjusted relative risk, 9.3; 95% confidence interval, 8.6–10.1), cardiac (adjusted relative risk, 8.7; 95% confidence interval, 7.5–10.0), or kidney disease (adjusted relative risk, 10.5; 95% confidence interval, 8.9–12.4).

Mortality has long been known to be associated with gestational age, with the lowest mortality in infants born at 39 to 40 weeks (**Tables 2** and **3**).[5,8,21,34,43,44] In a landmark report, Kramer and colleagues[43] performed a population-based cohort study of births in the United States and Canada between 1985 and 1995. After correcting for congenital anomalies, the most frequent cause for mortality in late preterm infants, the risk of early neonatal death (4.5-fold to 5.6-fold), late neonatal death (2.0-fold to 2.9-fold), postneonatal death (2.0-fold to 2.6-fold), and infant mortality (2.5-fold to 3.2-fold) were significantly greater than for term infants.[43,45] Furthermore, Kramer and colleagues[43] found that late preterm infants contributed significantly more to overall neonatal and infant mortality than infants born at 32 to 33 weeks' gestation because of the higher prevalence of late preterm births. Although neonatal and infant mortalities have declined, the risks of death in late preterm and early term infants compared with late term infants continues to be significantly greater.[5,34,45] Tomashek and colleagues[45] found infant mortality to be threefold higher in late preterm infants between 1995 and 2002; causes for late preterm infant deaths were predominantly

Table 2
Neonatal mortality and gestational age in a 2001 cohort from the United States

Weeks of Gestation	Neonatal Mortality per 1000 Live Births	
	Rate	RR (95% CI)
34	7.1	9.5 (8.4–10.8)
35	4.8	6.4 (5.6–7.2)
36	2.8	3.7 (3.3–4.2)
37	1.7	2.3 (2.1–2.6)
38	1.0	1.4 (1.3–1.5)
39	0.8	1.00 (reference)
40	0.8	1.0 (0.9–1.1)
41	0.8	1.1 (0.9–1.2)

Early term, 37 to 38 weeks' gestation; late preterm, 34 to 36 weeks' gestation.
Abbreviations: CI, confidence interval; RR, relative risk.
Data from Reddy UM, Ko CW, Raju TNK, et al. Delivery indications at late-preterm gestations and infant mortality rates in the United States. Pediatrics 2009;124:236.

Table 3 Neonatal mortality and gestational age in a 2001 cohort from the United States		
	Infant Mortality per 1000 Live Births	
Weeks of Gestation	**Rate**	**RR (95% CI)**
34	11.8	5.4 (4.9–5.9)
35	8.6	3.9 (3.6–4.3)
36	5.7	2.6 (2.4–2.8)
37	4.1	1.9 (1.8–2.0)
38	2.7	1.2 (1.2–1.3)
39	2.2	1.00 (reference)
40	2.1	0.9 (0.9–1.0)
41	2.2	1.1 (1.0–1.1)

Early term, 37–38 weeks' gestation; late preterm, 34–36 weeks' gestation.
Data from Reddy UM, Ko CW, Raju TNK, et al. Delivery indications at late-preterm gestations and infant mortality rates in the United States. Pediatrics 2009;124:236.

congenital malformations, sudden infant death syndrome, accidents, diseases of the circulatory system, intrauterine hypoxia, and birth asphyxia; these 6 diagnoses accounted for 66% of deaths. Early neonatal mortality (<7 days from birth) was sixfold greater, late neonatal mortality (7–27 days from birth) threefold greater, and postneonatal mortality (28–364 days from birth) twofold greater than in term infants.[45] Weight for gestational age, especially when cases with congenital anomalies are excluded, significantly affects mortality at all gestational ages.[46] Although infants who are large for gestational age increase risk for infant mortality through 38 weeks' gestation, being small for gestational age has a greater impact. For example, after excluding infants with congenital anomalies, late preterm male and female infants who are small for gestational age have a 14-fold and sixfold risk, respectively, of dying within the first year after birth than term female infants.

Long-term Morbidities

Long-term outcomes affected by late preterm and, to some extent, early term births involve school performance, behavioral problems, social and medical disabilities, and mortality (**Tables 4–7**).[7,47–57] Although the absolute risk of poor long-term

Table 4 School-age outcomes and healthy late preterm infants				
Outcome	**Age (y)**	**% Near Term N = 22,552**	**% Full Term N = 164,628**	**RR (95% CI) Adjusted**
Developmental delay/disability	0–3	4.24	2.96	1.36 (1.29–1.43)
PreK at 3[a]	3	4.46	3.89	1.13 (1.08–1.19)
PreK at 4[a]	4	7.40	6.60	1.10 (1.05–1.14)
Not ready to start school	4	5.09	4.40	1.04 (1.00–1.09)
Exceptional student education	5	13.30	11.88	1.10 (1.07–1.13)
Retention in kindergarten	5	7.96	6.17	1.11 (1.07–1.15)
Suspension in kindergarten	5	1.80	1.22	1.19 (1.10–1.29)

[a] Referral to Florida part B program, prekindergarten program for children with disabilities.
Data from Morse SB, Zheng H, Tang Y, et al. Early school-age outcomes of late preterm infants. Pediatrics 2009;123:e626.

Table 5
Gestational age and risk of hyperkinetic disorder (attention-deficit hyperactivity disorder [ADHD])

Gestational Age (wk)	Controls n = 20,100	ADHD n = 834	Adjusted RR (95% CI)
<34	298	34	2.7 (1.8–4.1)
34–36	544	37	1.7 (1.2–2.5)
37–39	6629	298	1.1 (0.9–1.3)
40–42	12,365	456	Reference
43–44	264	9	1.0 (0.5–2.0)

Data from Linnet KM, Wisborg K, Agerbo E. Gestational age, birth weight, and the risk of hyperkinetic disorder. Arch Dis Child 2006;9:656.

outcomes in infants born late preterm and early term are small, the risks are significantly greater than if born at 39 to 40 weeks' gestation.[49] Intelligence quotients were assessed in a matched pairs analysis of 168 late preterm and 168 term infants.[51] The risk of having full-scale and performance intelligence quotient scores of less than 85 was twice as likely in the late preterm group (21% vs 12%). In addition, internalizing and attention problems were more than twofold to threefold more frequent than in term infants. School performance in late preterm infants, especially reading skills and need for special education, lags behind that of term infants when assessed between kindergarten and grade 5.[56] In a small cohort of 53 healthy late preterm infants (34–36 weeks' gestation) at 14 to 15 years of age raised in families with higher incomes and educational status than in the general population in the United States, no difference was found in cognition, achievement, and socioemotional and behavioral

Table 6
Medical outcomes in Norwegian people aged 20 to 36 years by gestational age

	Gestational Age (%)					RR 95% CI 34–36 vs ≥37
	23–27 N = 362	28–30 N = 1,686	31–33 N = 6,591	34–36 N = 32,187	≥37 N = 853,309	
Cerebral palsy	9.1	6.0	1.9	0.3	0.1	2.7 (2.2–3.3)
Mental retardation	4.4	1.8	1.0	0.7	0.4	1.6 (1.4–1.8)
Schizophrenia	0.6	0.1	0.2	0.2	0.1	1.3 (1.0–1.7)
Disorders of psychological development, behavior, and emotion	2.5	0.7	0.3	0.3	0.2	1.5 (1.2–1.8)
Other major disabilities	4.1	2.2	0.5	0.3	0.2	1.5 (1.2–1.8)
Any disability affecting working capacity	10.6	8.2	4.2	2.4	1.7	1.4 (1.3–1.5)

Abbreviation: N, number.
Data from Moster D, Lie RT, Markestad T. Long-term medical and social consequences of preterm birth. N Engl J Med 2008;359:262–73.

Table 7
Social outcomes in Swedish people aged 23 to 29 years by gestational age

	Gestational Age (%)					
	24–28 N = 317	29–32 N = 2,630	33–36 N = 19,166	37–38 N = 68,541	39–41 N = 431,656	P Value
Postsecondary education	26	34	36	38	40	.001
Employed in 2002	68	70	73	73	74	.001
Social welfare in 2002	5.0	3.0	2.8	2.2	1.8	.001
Lives with parents	18	18	17	17	15	.001
Disability (sickness pension, disability allowance, disability assistance)	13.2	5.6	2.7[a]	1.9[a]	1.5	.001

Abbreviation: N, number.
[a] Attributable risk for disability: 74% of all disability is associated with birth at 33 to 38 weeks' gestation because of large N (vs high incidence in more preterm infants). n = 522,310, 23 to 29 years old.
Data from Lindstrom K, Winbladh B, Haglund B, et al. Preterm infants as young adults: a Swedish national cohort study. Pediatrics 2007;120:74.

development compared with term infants.[57] Additional information is needed to confirm whether these observations can be generalized.

Several early school and developmental outcomes in 161,804 children in Florida who were born between 34 and 41 weeks' gestation with a length of hospital stay less than 4 days (ie, healthy) were analyzed.[49] Outcomes improved with advancing gestational age. However, late preterm infants were at significantly greater risk of having adverse outcomes compared with term infants (see **Table 4**). For example, developmental delay or disability was present in 4.2% of late preterm infants compared with 3.0% of term infants (adjusted relative risk, 1.36; 95% confidence interval 1.29–1.43). The incidence of cerebral palsy and developmental delay/cognitive dysfunction is also higher at lower gestational ages (**Fig. 7**).[7] Late preterm infants were greater than threefold more likely to have a diagnosis of cerebral palsy than term infants (hazard ratio, 3.39; 95% confidence interval, 2.54–4.52) and at slightly but significantly higher risk for developmental delay/cognitive dysfunction (hazard ratio, 1.25; 95% confidence interval, 1.10–1.54). One-third of late preterm infants have academic difficulties when evaluated at 7 years of age. In an evaluation of 1,682,441 singleton Norwegian children born between 37 and 44 weeks' gestation, early term infants were also more likely than infants born at 40 weeks' gestation to have a diagnosis of cerebral palsy.[50] The prevalence of cerebral palsy in infants born at 37 weeks' gestation was 1.91 per 1000 children (relative risk, 1.9; 95% confidence interval, 1.6–2.4) and at 38 weeks' gestation was 1.25 per 1000 children (relative risk, 1.3; 95% confidence interval, 1.1–1.6).

Behavior problems, especially attention-deficit hyperactivity disorder, are also more common in late preterm infants than in term infants (adjusted relative risk, 1.7; 95% confidence interval, 1.2–2.5) (see **Table 5**).[52,54] During early adulthood, late preterm and early term infants carry a higher risk for hospitalization for psychiatric illnesses than late term infants.[47] The rate of psychiatric hospitalizations in a cohort of 573,869 Swedish adolescents and young adults was found to be dependent on gestational age with highest risk at the lowest gestational ages. After adjustment for age, sex, housing, social welfare, socioeconomic status, parental psychiatric disorder,

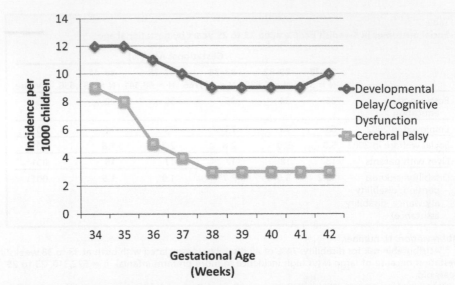

Fig. 7. Developmental delay/cognitive dysfunction, cerebral palsy, and gestational age. (*Data from* Petrini JR, Dias T, McCormick MC, et al. Increased risk of adverse neurologic development for late preterm infants. J Pediatr 2009;154:174.)

low Apgar score, and intrauterine growth restriction, the incidence of psychiatric illness in late preterm infants (3%; odds ratio, 1.16; 95% confidence interval, 1.07–1.26) and early term infants (2.6%; odds ratio, 1.06; 95% confidence interval, 1.01–1.12) was significantly greater than in late term infants (2.4%). From a public health perspective, late preterm and early term infants are targets for interventions and services because 85% of cases of psychiatric disorders in people born before 39 weeks' gestation are attributable to those born at 34 to 38 weeks' gestation.

Medical and social morbidities increase with decreasing gestational age (see **Table 6**).[55] In a cohort of 903,402 Norwegian infants born alive without congenital anomalies and followed through early adulthood, infants born late preterm had significantly higher risks for cerebral palsy; cognitive dysfunction; schizophrenia; disorders of psychological development, behavior, and emotion; other major disabilities such as blindness, poor vision, hearing loss, and epilepsy; and any medical disability that severely affected working capacity. Of 522,310 Swedish young adults, both late preterm and early term infants were less successful than infants born at 39 weeks' gestation or greater in postsecondary education, employment, and living apart from parents and were at higher risk for receiving social welfare benefits and disabilities (see **Table 7**).[48]

MANAGEMENT OF LATE PRETERM AND EARLY TERM INFANTS

The focus of care of late preterm and early term infants is individualized depending on the specific medical and social issues that may occur. Counseling of women by pediatric and obstetric caregivers about the possible outcomes for late preterm and term infants is important when delivery of such infants is indicated so that families are informed of possible morbidities, admission to neonatal intensive care, prolonged birth hospitalizations, and readmission for hospital care. If delivery of late preterm or early term infants is requested, it is important for caregivers to share the gestational age–specific risks of induction of labor and cesarean delivery and the risks of morbidity and mortality. Anticipation of the common medical, developmental, behavioral, educational, and social problems experienced by these groups of infants alerts caregivers and families to monitor for such problems during the birth hospitalization and throughout childhood. During the birth hospitalization, monitoring and treating for frequent problems such as respiratory distress, apnea, jaundice, hypoglycemia, hypothermia, possible infection, and poor oral feeding is indicated (**Table 8**). During the weeks following discharge, especially if discharged within 3 to 4 days from birth, jaundice, poor feeding, and suspected sepsis may prompt readmission to the hospital or emergency outpatient evaluation. Education of mothers and families before discharge to home from the birth hospitalization about problems that may lead to hospital readmission is recommended. Such education is particularly important for infants born late preterm who are born to first-time and/or breastfeeding mothers, and mothers with complications of labor and delivery, public financing, or Asian/ Pacific Islander descent. Early intervention and developmental services for late preterm and early term infants may be indicated, especially for those who have problems with cognition, learning, behavior, psychiatric, or medical morbidities.

CAUSES OF LATE PRETERM AND EARLY TERM BIRTHS

Preterm births have increased for many reasons including demographic changes of women who become pregnant (such as delayed childbearing), infertility treatments, increased maternal age, increased multiple gestations, and maternal comorbid conditions including obesity.[58] Several risk factors have been identified for late preterm and, by extrapolation, early term births.[58–60] Late preterm birth has been associated with chorioamnionitis (relative risk, 3.1; 95% confidence interval, 2.6–3.7), hypertension (relative risk, 2.5; 95% confidence interval, 2.3–2.7), and preterm premature rupture of membranes (relative risk, 1.7; 95% confidence interval, 1.6–1.7).[34,59] Previous preterm delivery (odds ratio, 7.2; 95% confidence interval, 1.6–33.2), short (<12 months) interpregnancy interval (odds ratio, 4.1; 95% confidence interval, 2.2–7.5), and early pregnancy bleeding (odds ratio, 7.6; 95% confidence interval, 1.3–3.8) have also been found to increase risk for late preterm delivery.[59]

It is estimated that 20% to 32% of late preterm births are indicated because of an adverse maternal (eg, preeclampsia, 46%; placental abruption, 14%; fetal compromise, 18%; and other indications such as obesity, 20%) or fetal condition (eg, oligohydramnios, intrauterine growth restriction), 25% to 32% for preterm premature rupture of membranes, 30% to 55% for spontaneous preterm labor, and 6.1% unknown.[33,58,61–64] In a study of birth indications by gestational age at a university-based delivery service, spontaneous labor occurred in 79% of 149 late preterm infants, 59% of 100 early term infants, and 48% of 50 late term infants (**Table 9**).[65] Indications for births that were found more often in late preterm and at an intermediate frequency in early term infants compared with late term infants included spontaneous rupture of membranes (50% in late preterm infants, 27% in early term infants, and 18% in late term infants, respectively); spontaneous labor or spontaneous rupture of membranes (93%, 69%, and 54%, respectively); and spontaneous rupture of membranes and labor (36%, 17%, and 12%, respectively). Pregestational diabetes was equally common at 34 to 38 weeks' gestation and less common in late term infants. Hypertensive disorders and nonreassuring fetal heart rate were more common causes of births of early and late term infants than late preterm infants. It is unknown whether these data can be generalized to other populations.

An understanding of the contribution of unintended or elective deliveries on the number of late preterm and early term infants is emerging. In a group of 514 singleton

Table 8
Management of late preterm and early term infants: guidelines from a single institution

Admission criteria	• Infants born at 35 wk completed gestation and greater with a birth weight of ≥1800 g are eligible for admission to the Newborn Nursery • Infants born at less than 35 wk completed gestation or <1800 g will be admitted to the Special Care Nursery • Infants born at 35 wk or greater who have required positive pressure ventilation in the delivery room will be observed for at least 6 h in the Special Care Nursery before transfer to the Newborn Nursery
Normal transition	• All infants have a period of physiologic transition after delivery. Although some late preterm and early term infants are at a higher risk of delayed transition than infants born at term gestation, some may successfully transition with initial attention to temperature regulation by their mothers and health care providers
Temperature regulation	• Late preterm infants have a higher risk of hypothermia in the first days after birth because of decreased white and brown fat stores and increased surface area • Temperature maintenance is improved with use of a hat • Temperature should be taken and recorded every hour for the first 6 h after birth, then every 6 h until discharge • If the temperature is found to be less than 36.0°C, the infant should be swaddled and a hat should be placed on the head. If at 30 min the temperature remains less than 36.0°C, the infant should be placed under a radiant warmer for rewarming. A second failure of maintaining temperature greater than 36.0°C will necessitate transfer to the Special Care Nursery
Feeding	• Late preterm infants are at a greater risk of poor feeding and subsequent dehydration during the first days after birth. This is because of their neurologic immaturity. Therefore, they require close observation and documentation of their feeding skills • Intake and output should be recorded for all newborns. Weights should be recorded daily. Obtain Special Care Nursery consult for weight loss of >3% daily or total of 7% of birth weight • At least 1 feeding every 12 h for the first 2 d after birth should be observed by a trained caregiver to document feeding ability. If the infant is breastfeeding, a lactation specialist should observe the feeding for position, latch, and milk transfer • If the infant is not capable of adequate feeding, consultation with the Special Care Nursery staff is warranted before beginning a supplementation strategy
Glycemic control	• Late preterm infants born to mothers who are on medication for diabetes (type I, type II, or gestational) will follow the policy for infants of diabetic mothers • Late preterm infants are at higher risk of hypoglycemia because of immature glycogenolysis, immature gluconeogenesis, and hormonal dysregulation • Blood glucose levels should be checked at 1 hour after birth and every 4 h until greater than 50 mg/dL twice, consecutively • If blood glucose levels are <50 mg/dL, refer to hypoglycemia protocol

(continued on next page)

Table 8 (continued)	
Jaundice	• Late preterm infants are at higher risk of jaundice requiring intervention because of hepatic immaturity and potential feeding difficulties • Transcutaneous bilirubin measurements should be obtained and documented daily. Refer to American Academy of Pediatrics Guidelines on Treatment of Hyperbilirubinemia for threshold for intervention
Respiratory distress or Apnea	• Late preterm infants have a higher incidence of respiratory distress after delivery for several reasons, including delayed clearance of fetal lung fluid, relative surfactant deficiency, and immature hormone levels • Normal transition includes variable respiratory rates, ranging from 25 to 100 breaths per minute during the first hours after delivery. Generally, the respiratory rate decreases to 40–60 breaths per minute by 2 h after delivery • Central cyanosis is always pathologic and consultation with the Special Care Nursery staff should be immediately obtained • Documented apnea episodes of >20 s requires transfer to the Special Care Nursery for monitoring
Discharge criteria	• Late preterm infants are at a higher risk of morbidities, rehospitalization, and mortality. Therefore, precautions and education beyond that provided to parents of term infants are required • Accurate gestational age has been determined • Infant is >48 h chronologic age • Postdischarge medical care has been arranged, with a follow-up visit scheduled for 24 to 48 h after discharge. A home visit by a home-health nurse in the first 72 h after discharge is also encouraged. If the infant is discharged after about 7 d of age or longer and has met all discharge criteria and resolved all medical issues, a follow-up visit within 7 d of discharge may be recommended • The infant has had stable vital signs for the 24 h before discharge, including an axillary temperature of 36.5 to 37.4°C in an open crib with appropriate clothing, respiratory rate less than 60 breaths per minute, and heart rate 100–160 beats per minute • Twenty-four hours of successful feeding, either by breast or bottle. Documentation of feeding success for 4 feedings by health care provider is complete • Breastfeeding success should be documented by a lactation specialist or staff with breastfeeding expertise twice before discharge • Infant has passed at least 1 stool • Weight loss is not greater than 7% of birth weight, or more than 3% per day of age • Total bilirubin concentration has been documented and does not require intervention at the time of discharge • Appropriate follow-up has been arranged • Maternal laboratory studies have been reviewed • Initial hepatitis B vaccine has been administered, or plan for administration has been made • Newborn screening test has been obtained • Car seat study has been passed • Screening hearing test has been performed and appropriate follow-up has been arranged • Family, environmental, and social risk factors have been assessed. • Family education has been completed

Table 9
Indications for births by gestational age

Indications	34–36 wk GA N = 149 (%)	37–38 wk GA N = 100 (%)	39+ wk GA N = 50 (%)
Spontaneous ROM	50	27	18
Spontaneous labor	79	59	48
Spontaneous ROM or labor	93	69	54
Spontaneous ROM and labor	36	17	12
Hypertensive disease	9	11	12
Pregestational diabetes	7	8	2
Nonreassuring FHR	7	10	16
Abruptio placentae	4	0	0
IUGR	3	1	0
Cardiac disease	2	1	0

Abbreviations: FHR, fetal heart rate; GA, gestational age; IUGR, intrauterine growth restriction; N, number; ROM, rupture of membranes.
Data from Lubow JM, How HY, Habli M, et al. Indications for delivery and short-term neonatal outcomes in late preterm as compared with term births. AJOG 2009:e32.

late preterm births in a tertiary care medical center in 2007 and 2008, the indications for delivery included spontaneous preterm birth (36.2%), preterm premature rupture of membranes (17.7%), medically indicated (37.9%), and elective (8.2%).[66] Potentially avoidable deliveries were defined as those in women with stable, but high-risk, indications plus elective deliveries; 17% of late preterm births in this cohort were considered potentially avoidable and possible targets for expectant or innovative management. Stable but high-risk conditions most often included mild preeclampsia (64% of cases), intrauterine growth restriction (17% of cases) or oligohydramnios with reassuring fetal testing, prior classic cesarean delivery, and mild or stable medical conditions. In another cohort of 15,136 singleton late preterm deliveries compared with 170,593 term deliveries, 6.9% of late preterm deliveries were for soft or elective reasons that could be amenable to expectant management.[33]

The percentage of 292,627 singleton late preterm births in the 2001 United States Birth Cohort Linked birth/death files delivered with no recorded indication was 23.2% (**Table 10**).[44] The 4 other categories of indications for delivery accounted for

Table 10
Indications for late preterm delivery and gestational age

GA (wk)	Medical Indication (%)	Obstetric Indication (%)	Congenital Anomaly (%)	Spontaneous Labor (%)	Total with Indications (%)	No Indication (%)
34	15.1	20.6	1.6	45.4	77.9	22.1
35	14.5	16.9	1.3	48.4	77.4	22.6
36	14.1	13.8	1.1	50.3	76.1	23.9
34–36	14.4	15.9	1.3	48.9	76.8	23.2

Abbreviation: GA, gestational age.
Data from Reddy UM, Ko CW, Raju TNK, et al. Delivery indications at late-preterm gestations and infants mortality rates in the United States. Pediatrics 2009;124:237.

76.8% of births, with 45.4% associated with isolated spontaneous labor and 15.9%, 14.4%, and 1.3% associated with obstetric indications, medical indications, and congenital anomalies, respectively. The mothers with no recorded delivery indications were largely characterized as being older; non-Hispanic white race; educated (≥13 years of education); Southern, Midwestern, or Western; multiparous; or having delivered a previous infant with a birth weight greater than or equal to 4000 g. Such characteristics implicate patient-driven factors as important influences on timing of delivery. It is important to confirm this suspicion because infants born with no recorded indication experienced significantly greater neonatal and infant mortality than infants delivered following isolated spontaneous labor (**Table 11**).

In general, avoidance of preterm birth has been a guiding principle for obstetric management of women to avoid morbidity or mortality associated with immaturity.[7,29,67] The exceptions to this principle include situations or illnesses that threaten the life of the mother or fetus. Late preterm and early term infants have only recently been identified as being at risk for morbidity and mortality greater than that for infants born at 39 to 40 weeks' gestation.[2,7,9,14–16,26,29,67] Tocolysis and/or antenatal corticosteroid treatment of women with spontaneous labor between 34 and 39 weeks' gestation have been suggested, but not proven, as potential interventions to improve neonatal outcomes without increasing risk for the women or fetuses.[68–72] Furthermore, expectant management of women with preterm premature rupture of membranes has also been hypothesized to be a care strategy to improve outcomes in affected women, fetuses, and infants.[73–75] Hence, obstetric practices that assumed late preterm and early term infants to have outcomes similar to late term infants may need to be reassessed in large clinical trials to determine whether expectant management, especially beyond the traditional threshold of 34 weeks' gestation, is safe for the fetus, mother, and neonate.[1,2,9,19,20,22,58,67,76]

The optimal balance between risks of late preterm and early term births and risks associated with tocolytic treatment, expectant management of preterm premature rupture of membranes, complications of preeclampsia, and stillbirths is yet to be determined.[58] It is anticipated that improvements in accuracy of fetal assessment of gestational age and surveillance of fetal well-being will better inform clinicians about fetal maturity and status, urgency to deliver, and whether induction of labor or cesarean delivery is indicated. Counseling of women who request delivery before 39 weeks' gestation or cesarean delivery, education of clinicians about the risks of

Table 11
Indications for delivery of late preterm infant, neonatal mortality, and infant mortality

Indication for Delivery of Late Preterm Infants	N	Neonatal Mortality (No. per 1000 Live Births)		Infant Mortality (No. per 1000 Live Births)	
		Rate	RR (95% CI)	Rate	RR (95% CI)
No recorded indication	67909	3.3	Reference	6.8	Reference
Isolated spontaneous labor	143087	1.9	0.6 (0.5–0.7)	4.8	0.7 (0.6–0.8)
Medical	42036	3.8	1.2 (0.9–1.4)	7.0	1.0 (0.9–1.2)
Obstetric	46449	8.8	2.7 (2.3–3.2)	13.3	2.0 (1.7–2.2)
Major anomaly	3697	107.9	33.0 (28.1–38.8)	140.7	20.8 (18.4–23.5)

Abbreviation: N, number.

Data from Reddy UM, Ko CW, Raju TNK, et al. Delivery indications at late-preterm gestations and infants mortality rates in the United States. Pediatrics 2009;124:238.

elective and operative delivery without medical or obstetric indications, and implementation of innovative management guidelines for elective delivery before 39 weeks' gestation or for soft indications hold promise to reduce the number of early term and late preterm births.

SUMMARY

Late preterm and early term infants have significantly greater risks of medical complications and morbidities during the birth hospitalization and during the first weeks after birth than term infants. Neonatal and infant mortality and morbidity rates are largely influenced by gestational age with the lowest rates at 39 to 40 weeks' gestation. Neonatal morbidity and mortality are significantly increased by maternal or fetal illness. Long-term morbidities occur in a small, but significant, percentage of late preterm and early term infants compared with term infants. Academic limitations, social and medical morbidity (such as cerebral palsy and developmental disability), behavioral disorders, and psychiatric illnesses are all more prevalent at lower gestational ages, including those born early term and late preterm.

Most late preterm and early term births are indicated for obstetric and medical reasons. Perhaps as many as 1 in 5 late preterm and early term births can be prevented by implementing management guidelines and new care strategies that limit elective deliveries before 39 weeks' gestation and prove to be safe for mother, fetus, and neonate. Perhaps increased use of antenatal corticosteroids for women with preterm labor at 32 to 34 weeks' gestation could reduce the respiratory complications for those who deliver after 34 weeks. Perhaps corticosteroid administration before elective cesarean delivery will improve neonatal outcomes, or perhaps expectant management of women with preterm premature rupture of membranes at 35 weeks' gestation will reduce neonatal morbidity without an increase in fetal or maternal morbidity. Large randomized trials to test innovative diagnostic and treatment strategies to inform clinicians about optimal management of women at gestations less than 39 weeks are warranted.

REFERENCES

1. Fleischman AR, Oinuma M, Clark SL. Rethinking the definition of "term pregnancy". Obstet Gynecol 2010;116:136–9.
2. Ashton DM. Elective delivery at less than 39 weeks. Curr Opin Obstet Gynecol 2010;22:506–10.
3. Hibbard JU, Wilkins I, Sun L, et al. Consortium on Safe Labor. Respiratory morbidity in late preterm births. JAMA 2010;304:419–25.
4. Dimitriou G, Fouzas S, Georgakis V, et al. Determinants of morbidity in late preterm infants. Early Hum Dev 2010;86:587–91.
5. Young PC, Glasgow TS, Xi L, et al. Mortality of late-preterm (near-term) newborns in Utah. Pediatrics 2007;119:e659–65.
6. Kirby RS, Wingate MS. Late preterm birth and neonatal outcome: is 37 weeks' gestation a threshold level or a road marker on the highway of perinatal risk? Birth 2010;7:169–71.
7. Petrini JR, Dias T, McCormick MC, et al. Increased risk of adverse neurological development of late preterm infants. J Pediatr 2009;154:169–76.
8. Melamed N, Klinger G, Tenenbaum-Gavish K, et al. Short-term neonatal outcome in low-risk, spontaneous, singleton, late preterm deliveries. Obstet Gynecol 2009; 114:253–60.

9. Gouyon JB, Vintejoux A, Sagot P, et al, Burgundy Perinatal Network. Neonatal outcome associated with singleton birth at 34–41 weeks of gestation. Int J Epidemiol 2010;39:769–76.
10. Raju TN, Higgins RD, Stark AR, et al. Optimizing care and outcome for late-preterm (near-term) infants: a summary of the workship sponsored by the National Institute of Child Health and Human Development. Pediatrics 2006;118:1207–14.
11. Hamilton BE, Martin JA, Ventura SJ. Births: preliminary data for 2008. Natl Vital Stat Rep 2010;58(16):1–17.
12. Davidoff MJ, Dias T, Damus K, et al. Changes in the gestational age distribution among U.S. singleton births: impact on rates of late preterm birth, 1992–2002. Semin Perinatol 2006;30:8–15.
13. Martin JA, Hamilton BE, Sutton PD, et al. Births: final data for 2006. Natl Vital Stat Rep 2009;57(7):1–104.
14. Morrison JJ, Rennie JM, Milton PJ. Neonatal respiratory morbidity and mode of delivery after term: influence of timing of elective caesarean section. J Obstet Gynaecol 1995;102(2):101–6.
15. Zenardo V, Simbi AK, Franzoi M, et al. Neonatal respiratory morbidity risk and mode of delivery at term: influence of timing of elective caesarean delivery. Acta Paediatr 2004;93:643–7.
16. Tita A, Landon M, Spong C, et al. Timing of elective repeat cesarean delivery at term and neonatal outcomes. N Engl J Med 2009;360:111–20.
17. American College of Obstetricians and Gynecologists. Fetal lung maturity. Practice Bulletin No. 97. Obstet Gynecol 2008;112:717–26.
18. ACOG Committee on Practice Bulletins – Obstetrics. Induction of labor. Practice Bulletin No. 107. Obstet Gynecol 2009;114:386–97.
19. Oshiro BT, Henry E, Wilson J, et al. Decreasing elective deliveries before 39 weeks of gestation in an integrated health care system. Obstet Gynecol 2009; 113:804–11.
20. Clark SL, Frye DR, Meyers JA, et al. Reduction in elective delivery at <39 weeks of gestation: comparative effectiveness of 3 approaches to change and the impact on neonatal intensive care admission and stillbirth. Am J Obstet Gynecol 2010;203:449, e1–6.
21. Donovan E, Lannon C, Bailit J, et al. A statewide initiative to reduce inappropriate scheduled births at 36(0/7)-3(6/7) weeks' gestation. Am J Obstet Gynecol 2010; 202:243, e1–8.
22. The Joint Commission Introduces Perinatal Care Core Measures. Available at: http://www.jointcommission.org/NewsRoom/NewsReleases/nr_112009.htm. Accessed December 23, 2010.
23. Bastek JA, Sammel MD, Pare E, et al. Adverse neonatal outcomes: examining the risk between preterm, late preterm and term infants. Am J Obstet Gynecol 2008; 199:367.e1–367. e8.
24. Yoder BA, Gordon MC, Barth WH. Late-preterm birth. Does the changing obstetric paradigm alter the epidemiology of respiratory complications? Obstet Gynecol 2009;111:814–22.
25. De Almeida MF, Guinsburg R, da Costa JO, et al. Resuscitative procedures at birth in late preterm infants. J Perinatol 2007;27:761–5.
26. Shapiro-Mendoza CK, Tomashek KM, Kotelchuck M, et al. Effect of late-preterm birth and maternal medical conditions on newborn morbidity risk. Pediatrics 2008;121:e223–32.
27. Wang ML, Dorer DJ, Fleming M, et al. Clinical outcomes of near-term infants. Pediatrics 2004;114:372–6.

28. Engle WA. A recommendation for the definition of "late-preterm" (near-term) and the birth weight-gestational age classification system. Semin Perinatol 2006; 30(1):2–7.
29. Engle WA, Tomashek KM, Wallman C, Committee on Fetus and Newborn. "Late-preterm" infants: a population at risk. A clinical report. Pediatrics 2007;120(6): 1390–401.
30. McIntire DD, Leveno KJ. Neonatal mortality and morbidity rates in late preterm births compared with births at term. Obstet Gynecol 2008;111:35–41.
31. Cheng YW, Nicholson JM, Nakagawa S, et al. Perinatal outcomes in low-risk term pregnancies: do they differ by week of gestation? Am J Obstet Gynecol 2008;47: 330–3.
32. Osrin D. The implications of late-preterm birth for global child survival. Int J Epidemiol 2010;39:645–9.
33. Laughon SK, Reddy UM, Sun L, et al. Precursors for late preterm birth in singleton gestations. Obstet Gynecol 2010;116:1047–55.
34. Khashu M, Narayanan M, Bhargava S, et al. Perinatal outcomes associated with preterm birth at 33 to 36 weeks' gestation: a population-based cohort study. Pediatrics 2009;123:109–13.
35. Pulver LS, Denney JM, Silver RM, et al. Morbidity and discharge timing of late preterm newborns. Clin Pediatr 2010;49:1061–7.
36. Escobar GJ, Greene JD, Hulac P, et al. Rehospitalization after birth hospitalization: patterns among infants of all gestations. Arch Dis Child 2005;90:125–31.
37. Rubaltelli FF, Bonafe L, Tangucci M, et al. Epidemiology of neonatal acute respiratory disorders. Biol Neonate 1998;74:7–15.
38. Gilbert WM, Nesbitt TS, Danielsen B. The cost of prematurity: quantification by gestational age and birth weight. Obstet Gynecol 2003;102:488–92.
39. Jain S, Cheng J. Emergency department visits and rehospitalizations in late preterm infants. Clin Perinatol 2006;33:935–45.
40. Oddie SJ, Hammal D, Richmond S, et al. Early discharge and readmission to hospital in the first month of life in the northern region of the UK during 1998: a case cohort study. Arch Dis Child 2005;90:119–24.
41. Tomashek KM, Shapiro-Mendoza CK, Weiss J, et al. Early discharge among late preterm and term newborns and risk of neonatal mortality. Semin Perinatol 2006; 30:61–8.
42. De Luca R, Boulvain M, Irion O, et al. Incidence of early neonatal mortality and morbidity after late-preterm and term cesarean delivery. Pediatrics 2009;123: e1064–71.
43. Kramer MS, Demissie K, Yand H, et al. The contribution of mild and moderate preterm birth to infant mortality. Fetal and Infant Health Study Group of the Canadian Perinatal Surveillance System. JAMA 2000;284:843–9.
44. Reddy UM, Ko CW, Raju TN, et al. Delivery indications at late-preterm gestations and infant mortality rates in the United States. Pediatrics 2009;124:234–40.
45. Tomashek KM, Shapiro-Mendoza CK, Davidoff MJ, et al. Differences in mortality between late preterm and term singleton infants in the United States, 1995–2002. J Pediatr 2007;151:450–6.
46. Pulver LS, Guest-Warnick G, Stoddard GJ, et al. Weight for gestational age affects the mortality of late preterm infants. Pediatrics 2009;123:e1072–7.
47. Lindstrom K, Lindblad F, Hjern A. Psychiatric morbidity in adolescents and young adults born preterm: a Swedish national cohort study. Pediatrics 2009;123:e47–53.
48. Lindstrom K, Winbladh B, Haglund B, et al. Preterm infants as young adults: a Swedish national cohort study. Pediatrics 2007;120:70–7.

49. Morse SB, Zheng H, Tang Y, et al. Early school-age outcomes of late preterm infants. Pediatrics 2009;123:e622–9.
50. Moster D, Wilcox AJ, Vollset SE, et al. Cerebral palsy among term and postterm births. J Am Med Assoc 2010;304:976–82.
51. Taige NM, Holzman C, Wang J, et al. Late-preterm birth and its association with cognitive and socioemotional outcomes at 6 years of age. Pediatrics 2010;126: 1124–31.
52. Huddy CLJ, Johnson A, Hope PL. Educational and behavioural problems in babies of 32-35 weeks gestation. Arch Dis Child Fetal Neonatal Ed 2001;85:F23–8.
53. Santos IS, Matijasevich A, Domingues MR, et al. Late preterm birth is a risk factor for growth faltering in early childhood: a cohort study. BMC Pediatr 2009;69:71.
54. Linnet KM, Wisborg K, Agerbo E, et al. Gestational age, birth weight, and the risk of hyperkinetic disorder. Arch Dis Child 2008;91:655–60.
55. Moster D, Lie RT, Markestad T. Long-term medical and social consequences of preterm birth. N Engl J Med 2009;359:262–73.
56. Chyi LJ, Lee HC, Hintz SR, et al. School outcomes of late preterm infants: special needs and challenges for infants born at 32 to 36 weeks gestation. J Pediatr 2008;143:25–31.
57. Gurka MJ, LoCasale-Crouch J, Blackman JA. Long-term cognition, achievement, socioemotional, and behavioral development of healthy late-preterm infants. Arch Pediatr Adolesc Med 2010;164:525–32.
58. Loftin RW, Habli M, Snyder CC, et al. Late preterm birth. Rev Obstet Gynecol 2010;3:10–9.
59. Selo-Ojeme DO, Tewari R. Late preterm (32–36 weeks) birth in a North London hospital. J Obstet Gynaecol 2006;26:624–6.
60. American College of Obstetricians and Gynecologists. Late-preterm infants. ACOG Committee Opinion No. 404. Obstet Gynecol 2008;111:1–4.
61. American College of Obstetricians and Gynecologists. Management of preterm labor. ACOG Committee on Practice Bulletins. No. 43. Obstet Gynecol 2003; 101:1039–47.
62. Cedergren MI. Maternal morbid obesity and the risk of adverse pregnancy outcome. Obstet Gynecol 2004;103:219–24.
63. Sibai BM. Preeclampsia as a cause of preterm and late preterm (near-term) births. Semin Perinatol 2006;30:16–9.
64. Merlino A, Ballit J, Mercer BM. Indications for late preterm birth, can obstetricians make a difference? Am J Obstet Gynecol 2008;199(Suppl 6):S234.
65. Lubow JM, How HY, Habli M, et al. Indications for delivery and short-term neonatal outcomes in late preterm as compared with term births. Am J Obstet Gynecol 2009;200:e30–3.
66. Holland MG, Refuerzo JS, Ramin SM, et al. Late preterm birth: how often is it avoidable? Am J Obstet Gynecol 2009;201:404.e1–4.
67. Fuchs K, Gyamfi C. The influence of obstetric practices on late prematurity. Clin Perinatol 2008;35:343–60.
68. Stutchfield P, Whitaker R, Russell I, Antenatal Steroids for Term Elective Caesarean Section (ASTECS) Research Team. Antenatal betamethasone and incidence of neonatal respiratory distress after elective caesarean section: pragmatic randomized trial. BMJ 2005;331(7518):662.
69. Ventolini G, Neiger R, Mathews L, et al. Incidence of respiratory disorders in neonates born between 34 and 36 weeks of gestation following exposure to antenatal corticosteroids between 24 and 34 weeks of gestation. Am J Perinatol 2008; 25:79–83.

70. Roberts D, Dalziel S. Antenatal corticosteroids for accelerating fetal lung matura-tion for women at risk of preterm birth. Cochrane Database Syst Rev 2006;3: CD004454.
71. Joseph KS, Nette F, Scott H, et al. Prenatal corticosteroid prophylaxis for women delivering at late preterm gestation. Pediatrics 2009;124:e835–43.
72. Bastek JA, Sammel MD, Rebele EC, et al. The effects of a preterm labor episode prior to 34 weeks are evident in late preterm outcomes, despite the administration of betamethasone. Am J Obstet Gynecol 2010;203:140,e1–7.
73. Naef RW, Albert JR, Ross EL, et al. Premature rupture of membranes at 34 to 37 weeks' gestation: aggressive versus conservative management. Am J Obstet Gynecol 1998;178:126–30.
74. Mercer BM, Crocker LG, Boe NM, et al. Induction versus expectant management in premature rupture of the membranes with mature amniotic fluid at 32 to 36 weeks: a randomized trial. Am J Obstet Gynecol 1993;169:775–82.
75. Dare MR, Middleton P, Crowther CA, et al. Planned early birth versus expectant management (waiting) for prelabour rupture of membranes at term (37 weeks or more). Cochrane Database Syst Rev 2006;1:CD005302.
76. Dobak WJ, Gardner MO. Later preterm gestation: physiology of labor and impli-cations for delivery. Clin Perinatol 2006;33:765–76.

What We Have Here is a Failure to Communicate: Obstacles to Optimal Care for Preterm Birth

Jay D. Iams, MD[a],*, Edward F. Donovan, MD[b],
Barbara Rose, RN, MPH[c], Mona Prasad, DO, MPH[d]

KEYWORDS

• Communication • Preterm birth • Optimal care • Outcomes

It happened on a Saturday. The man arrived at the hospital the morning after his wife had given birth to their daughter. He had returned early from a business trip after his wife called to say she was about to undergo an urgent cesarean delivery almost 6 weeks before her due date. He had not made it back in time for the birth, arriving several hours later. The nurses on the postpartum unit told him that his wife had finally fallen asleep, and that he should come back after going to see the baby. There he learned that she had been admitted to the neonatal intensive care unit (NICU) because of difficulty breathing. At first he was not worried; this happens sometimes when babies are born early. He knew that doctors and hospitals could do so much for little babies these days, and she weighed almost 4 pounds (1.8 kg). But when he saw her for the first time, he was terrified. All those tubes and wires and flashing monitors, hushed lights and concerned nurses, and 1.8 kg did not look like much in person. Then the doctor, a neonatologist, told him that their little girl was not ready to be born, that babies at 34 weeks' gestation often could not do what full-term babies could

This work was supported in part by grant no. 1U0CMS030227/01 from the Center for Medicare and Medicaid Services, administered by the Ohio Department of Job and Family Services.

[a] Division of Maternal Fetal Medicine, Department of Obstetrics & Gynecology, The Ohio State University Medical Center, 395 West 12th Avenue, Room 554, Columbus, OH 43210-1267, USA
[b] Executive Committee, Ohio Perinatal Quality Collaborative, Cincinnati Children's Hospital Medical Center, 3333 Burnet Avenue, ML 7014, Cincinnati, OH 45229-3039, USA
[c] Ohio Perinatal Quality Collaborative, Cincinnati Children's Hospital Medical Center, 3333 Burnet Avenue, ML 7014, Cincinnati, OH 45229-3039, USA
[d] Division of Maternal Fetal Medicine, The Ohio State University Medical Center, 395 West 12th Avenue, Columbus, OH 43210-1267, USA
* Corresponding author.
E-mail address: jay.iams@osumc.edu

do: breathe easily, stay warm, fight infection, and nourish themselves. The doctor looked tired, and when he commented on it, she said she had been here most of the night since his daughter arrived in the NICU. She was sicker than most, the doctor said, because his wife had not been given a medicine before birth that might have prevented some of the problems the baby was having now. "Why not?", he asked. The doctor said she did not know, that it was customary to give this medicine to women who are ready to deliver early, but his wife did not receive it. The labor and delivery records that accompanied the baby to the NICU said only that his wife had a cesarean birth because of decreased fetal movement, but did not mention steroids, the medicine that could have helped. The man sensed that the doctor and nurses were unhappy that steroids were not given, but he did not pursue it; he wanted to see his wife and let her know about their baby.

When he went back to her room, she was awake and sitting up, clearly exhausted but happy to be a new mother. She told him about how it happened, how she went to a routine obstetrics appointment and told her obstetrician that she had not felt the baby move since the night before. They put her on a monitor for a while and, when the baby's heart tracing was not reassuring, they sent her to the hospital for more tests. There they monitored her again, and then did an ultrasound examination to see whether the baby was breathing and moving and to check the fluid around the baby. A high-risk obstetrician came to see her after that, not her own obstetrician. He explained that the amniotic sac around the baby had very little fluid and some other problems with blood flow she did not understand, and that he would talk to her doctor about it. She was frightened because something similar had happened to her friend Karla in Massachusetts, and her baby had died. Her own obstetrician came in later after finishing in the office. She said the tests showed that the baby was at risk and needed to be delivered, and that inducing labor would take too long, the baby would not tolerate it, and they were going to do a cesarean section, and no, they could not wait for her husband to return. They did not know why this had happened, but it might be related to the itching she had been having recently. They would get some tests. She was scared then, but now relieved and happy. The surgery had been uncomplicated and their daughter weighed almost 4 pounds! When her husband told her that their daughter was in the NICU, attached to wires and tubes, and fighting to breathe, she was shocked and tearful. How could this happen? The obstetrician had said the baby might have a little breathing trouble and maybe some jaundice, but nothing like this! They spent all day Saturday looking for answers, but found only confusion. Her obstetrician said they had saved her baby's life by delivering her now. The NICU nurses were shocked that steroids had not been given, and wondered why she had been delivered early at all. The neonatologist agreed.

On Sunday, the new mother and father were just waking up in the hospital when they heard voices in the hall. One was her obstetrician; the husband recognized the other as the neonatologist he had spoken to the day before. They could not hear what was being said, but it was clear that the doctors were not happy with one another. They heard something about 34 weeks and steroids, and why could they not have waited for a couple days. Her obstetrician had said she was leaving today for some meeting and would not be able to see her on Monday.

In the hall, the neonatologist was disturbed that steroids had not been given, not even 1 dose, to a mother who clearly should have received them at 34 weeks' gestation. The obstetrician was equally firm in her belief that this mother was not a candidate; her dates were confirmed by a first trimester scan. "She was 34 weeks plus 4 days: not a candidate! And besides," she said, "There was no time to wait. The fluid was low, the biophysical profile was 4, and we suspected cholestasis and risked stillbirth." "Even 1 dose would have helped," the neonatologist insisted. "She was being evaluated all afternoon and into the evening: she could have had at least 1 injection an hour or two before delivery. And what's this cholestasis business? Her chart said nothing about that, just decreased fetal movement and low fluid." The obstetrician replied that cholestasis was suspected when the delivery decision was made, but was not confirmed when her laboratory results were returned after the delivery. She said something about The American College of Obstetricians and Gynecologists (ACOG) guidelines and then had to leave to catch her flight. They both walked away annoyed.

This fictional vignette illustrates communication issues about the risks and reasons for late preterm birth, interpretation of literature, and guidelines for antenatal corticosteroids (ANCS) that affect individual patient care. The same suboptimal dialog influences the current national dialog about prematurity. Communication among professional societies, academic disciplines, researchers, funding agencies, and charitable organizations is also affected. Working together in the Ohio Perinatal Quality Collaborative[1] (OPQC), we have discovered that the same is true for perinatal quality improvement collaborations: our different perspectives produce different interpretations of clinical events, vital statistics, research reports, practice guidelines, outcome benchmarks, and the most basic definitions. We think interdisciplinary miscommunication has an adverse effect on our efforts to achieve mutual goals, and that recognizing its existence can improve the health of babies.

HOW DO WE KNOW THAT COMMUNIATION IS NOT OPTIMAL?

The OPQC is a statewide, collaborative quality improvement effort established to promote the reliable use of evidence-based care before and after birth to reduce infant morbidity and mortality.[1] In developing OPQC, we readily agreed on overall goals and pathways, such as optimal use of ANCS, regionalized care for preterm infants, and reduction of inappropriate scheduled births. When we sought specific strategies to reach these goals, we were struck by how often our perspectives differed and began to explore why that was so. Two discussions illustrate these differences:

Optimal Use of ANCS

Despite universal agreement about the neonatal benefits of ANCS given to women who will soon deliver a preterm infant between 24 and 34 weeks' gestation, interdisciplinary discussions about risks, benefits, and optimal strategies of administration have continued for more than 2 decades. First reported in 1972, widespread use of ANCS did not occur in the United States until the National Institute of Child and Human Development (NICHD) held a Consensus Development Conference in 1994 to promote acceptance. The conference was prompted by a Vermont Oxford Network (VON) report[2] that found that fewer than 30% of eligible preterm low birth weight infants were receiving ANCS. Use of ANCS rose significantly after the first consensus conference but, after the high prevalence of repeated courses of ANCS was recognized as an unintended consequence of the conference recommendations, a second consensus conference was convened. Neonatologists were astounded and concerned to learn that repeat courses were deemed necessary because obstetricians could not accurately identify women who would deliver within 1 week. Noting potential growth-related risks of repeated courses, the second consensus conference recommended that ANCS use be limited to a single course.[3] The value of appropriately timed ANCS remains unquestioned, but several unresolved issues still affect practice. What is the shortest interval between administration and delivery that confers benefit? Do fetuses born before 24 or after 34 weeks benefit? Are there long-term risks for infants who received ANCS in utero but delivered at term?

Reported rates of ANCS use vary, from 16% to 61% in the NICHD Neonatal Research Network for infants with birth weights between 401 and 1500 g in 2003,[4] to more than 80% of very low birth weight infants (<1.5 kg) in VON in 2009.[5] Methods to assess appropriate use of ANCS also vary. The California Perinatal Quality Care Collaborative (CPQCC) has set a desired rate of 85%,[6] but notes that rates used by various organizations (eg, the Leapfrog Group, the National Quality Forum, and the Joint Commission) have adopted slightly different criteria for gestational age, birth weight, and denominator populations (either the number of eligible mothers or number of eligible infants who might have received ANCS). These differences between pediatricians and obstetricians about use of ANCS are amplified by separate maternal and neonatal charts. Pediatric charts commonly rely on data abstracted from the obstetric record of the delivery admission. ANCS use is recorded in various locations in the mother's chart, and may or may not include ANCS given during a previous admission, as an outpatient, or in the transferring hospital. Administrative datasets introduce more variables that affect accuracy.[7] The duration of the interval from ANCS administration to birth is another difference. Obstetricians, who interpret the NICHD/ACOG guidelines about not giving ANCS to women whose delivery is imminent to be an exclusion, identify women in whom delivery is expected between 12 and 24 hours and 7 days as candidates; pediatricians tend to advocate ANCS regardless of how short the interval to delivery might be. Regardless of the basis for these divergent opinions, the difference in perspective contributes to miscommunication because neither specialty fully accepts the data supplied by the other. The differences in data collection and interpretation are root causes of continued miscommunication.

Increased Rates of Preterm Birth and Late Preterm Birth

The increase in preterm birth rates after 1990 is explained by obstetricians as resulting from greater use of assisted reproductive techniques, an increase in indicated preterm births initiated by the obstetrician when the health of the mother and/or fetus was deemed to be in jeopardy by prolonging the pregnancy, and the effect of ultrasound on pregnancy dating. Widespread use of ultrasound beginning around 1990 is believed to have shifted the apparent distribution of gestational age at birth to the left as variable intervals of amenorrhea preceding conception were recognized by ultrasound. The effect was to reclassify many apparently postdate pregnancies as term and some that were called term as being preterm. The pediatric interpretation emphasizes the elective delivery of women not in labor, whose medical records often reflect absent or dubious reasons for scheduling the delivery[8] but account for the greatest number of admission to NICUs. Pediatricians also acknowledge the effects of fertility care, but are less aware that ultrasound dating produced a shift in gestational age distribution.

THE ORIGINS OF MISCOMMUNICATION

Our disciplines have always shared the goals of optimal health for the mother, fetus, and newborn. Interdisciplinary communication toward that goal began at a time when obstetrics emphasized protecting maternal health and future reproduction, and pediatrics focused on the newborn. Metrics established in that paradigm, such as the incidence of maternal mortality and low birth weight delivery, were later revised by significant advances in maternal and neonatal care: rates of preterm birth and infant mortality became the primary benchmarks for both specialties. We believe these benchmarks need further revision because of 2 additional advances in care: prenatal ultrasound to determine gestational age and assess fetal health, and improved neonatal care that allows extremely premature infants to survive. These technologies have introduced new information into perinatal decision making that requires revised outcomes and metrics to maintain optimal interdisciplinary communication.

METRICS
We Need to Shift from Weight OR Age OR Maturity to Weight FOR Age AND Maturity

Knowledge deficits about the timing of conception relative to menses and variation in fetal growth explain the adoption of menstrual dating in obstetrics and weight-based data collection in the nursery. When the duration of gestation was unknown or uncertain, birth weight was the only reliable surrogate for fetal age and maturity. In 1972, the differences between preterm and low birth weight were described as: "Infants *who are premature because of curtailed gestation* (gestational age of <37 completed weeks) are designated 'preterm.'. . . Infants *who are premature by virtue of birth weight* (2500 g or less at birth) are designated 'low birth weight' infants."[9] Note the distinction made at that time between age (preterm) and maturity (premature), a subtle difference that has withered over time so that *preterm* has come to mean *not fully mature*, whereas *term* has come to mean *mature*. The conflation of maturity and age was accelerated as ultrasound biometry was integrated with menstrual history to become *best obstetrical dating* in clinical practice, a phenomenon that contributed to an artificial increase in reported preterm births by correcting overestimated gestational age in amenorrheic women previously believed to be postterm women. Ultrasound dating is now accepted by obstetricians, pediatricians, and perinatal epidemiologists as the best method to determine the date of conception,[10] but has not yet been sufficiently integrated into state and national vital statistics so that outcomes from well-dated pregnancies (eg, gestational age confirmed or set by an ultrasound before 20 weeks' gestation) are reported separately from those with uncertain dating (all other methods). This difference is important because the range of possible gestational ages for pregnancies that are not well-dated equals or exceeds 2 weeks on either side of the estimate, a range that affects obstetric management: is the fetus older or younger, or is it symmetrically small or large for its age? When age is uncertain, its relation to maturity becomes more tenuous.

Although we care for the same patient before and after birth and appreciate the importance and consequences of poor growth relative to age, our specialties continue to begin data collection and analysis using our traditional metrics of weight or age. Some progress has been made for very and extremely low birth weight/very preterm infants in presenting outcome data by weight percentiles for gestational age,[11,12] but this practice has not yet been extended to include infants of all gestational ages.

Furthermore, the distinction between maturity and age has not been resurrected, so that gestational age is now used as an accurate surrogate for function, despite evidence and common sense to the contrary. Does anyone really think that all 13 year olds are equally mature? Why should all 34 week olds be expected to be equally mature? The current definition of term is a birth at or after ($37^{0/7th}$ [37 week plus 0 extra days]) weeks' gestation, despite good evidence that many infants at 37 weeks are not fully mature.[13,14] The upper threshold for administration of ANCS is $33^{6/7th}$ weeks' gestation, despite evidence that some infants born after 34 weeks experience morbidity that steroids might have reduced or prevented. These guidelines were adopted when conflation of age and maturity were unavoidable, but that is no longer the case. Gestational age can now be known within 4 to 7 days in most North American women. Assessment of functional maturity has not advanced beyond pulmonary performance. Age should no longer be equated with functional maturity.

OUTCOMES
Clinically Meaningful Data Require Collection Together, Over Time

Preterm birth rate and infant mortality are the outcomes by which our collective efforts are currently judged. Although useful, these rates ignore fetal mortality and offer little information about infant and childhood morbidity. Focusing on the rates of preterm birth and infant mortality ignores the known relationships between stillbirth and preterm birth, and thus promotes the sometimes false assumption that prevention of preterm birth always yields a reduction in infant mortality. A shared perspective on the important outcomes of pregnancy would link fetal, neonatal, and infant metrics to long-term childhood health. The National Center for Health Statistics (NCHS) has moved toward this goal by enhanced reporting of fetal and perinatal mortalities, but this effort is limited by the data provided by the states. Each state defines and collects perinatal data and forwards it to the NCHS, where it is reported by birth weight or by gestational age, and in 1 table by both, but only for the frequency of births in broad categories of weight and age (eg, number of infants born at 28–31 weeks who weighed between 1500 and 1999 g).[15] Because the quality of gestational dating is not often recorded, rates and outcomes cannot be analyzed according to whether gestational dating was or was not optimal (eg, confirmed or set by an ultrasound examination before 20 weeks' gestation).

The Importance of Stillbirth

Obstetric decision making is heavily influenced by weighing the relative risks of fetal death in utero versus the likelihood of neonatal, infant, and childhood morbidity and mortality.[16] Fetal deaths after 28 weeks of pregnancy are more common than neonatal deaths, a fact that dominates obstetric thinking (**Fig. 1**).[17] One question summarizes obstetric thinking: How many days in the NICU equal 1 stillbirth? Fear of stillbirth is appropriate, but estimates of stillbirth risk are uncertain and often overestimated,[18]

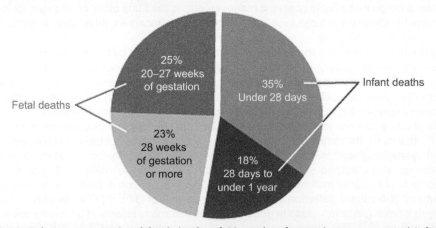

Fig. 1. Relative magnitude of fetal deaths of 20 weeks of gestation or more, and infant deaths: United States, 2005. (*Data from* MacDorman M, Kirmeyer S. The challenge of fetal mortality. NCHS data brief, no 16. Hyattsville (MD): National Center for Health Statistics; 2009.)

whereas the neonatal consequences of late preterm and near-term birth[13,14] are minimized. Obstetricians view the declining fetal mortality as vindication for aggressive obstetrics,[19,20] even as late preterm births increase (**Fig. 2**).[21] Meanwhile, pediatricians whose metrics do not include fetal mortality have seen their intensive care nurseries fill with late preterm and near-term infants whose admission to the NICU often lacks documentation of the reason for early birth,[8] and whose parents were unaware of the risks.[22] Admission to the NICU for near-term infants often occurs hours after the delivery, so that opportunities for direct communication between the obstetrician who made the decision to deliver and the neonatologist caring for the infant in the NICU are delayed or missed entirely.

Resolution or improvement of these contrasting perspectives awaits mutual understanding of the other's viewpoint. In our conversations, obstacles to better understanding seem to be related to specialty-specific measures derived from specialty-specific data. Condition-specific information about the likelihood of stillbirth, coupled with accurate

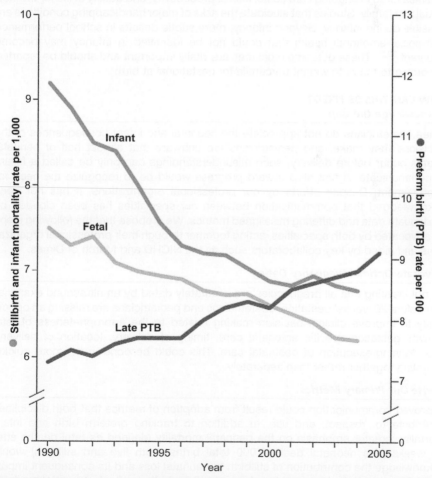

Fig. 2. Stillbirth and infant mortality and preterm birth rates. (*Data from* Ananth CV, Gyamfi C, Jain L. Characterizing risk profiles of infants who are delivered at late preterm gestations: does it matter? Am J Obstet Gynecol 2008;199:329–31.)

information about the age, growth, and maturity of the fetus and its expected short-term and long-term outcomes could inform decision making to reduce perinatal mortality without unnecessarily increasing the rate of preterm birth. Additional studies that simultaneously estimate the risks, at each gestational age, of fetal death and neonatal mortality/morbidity would be helpful.

Long-term Outcomes

Perinatal decision making is also hampered by reliance on intermediate-term or short-term outcomes that are necessary but not sufficient to assess the overall consequences of preterm birth and the effects of prenatal and postnatal care. Short-term survival to 1 month of age or hospital discharge, with or without markers of subsequent neurodevelopmental dysfunction, are inadequate surrogates for infant and childhood mortality and morbidity and lifelong handicap. For example, evaluation of neurodevelopment at age 2 years may identify sensorineural hearing loss. However, the personal and societal consequences of hearing loss are manifest after age 2 years and measured in ongoing care costs, loss of productivity, and quality of life for the individual and family. Studies that elucidate the risks of major handicapping conditions are possible during infancy. Beyond infancy, more subtle deficits in school performance and social-emotional health that could not be identified in infancy may become apparent.[23,24] These outcome measures are vitally important and should be reported according to the birth weight percentile for gestational at birth.

HOW CAN THIS BE FIXED?
Acknowledge the Gap

When obstetricians do not appreciate the neonatal and infant consequences of the decisions they make, and pediatricians are unaware that almost half of perinatal deaths occur before delivery, such misunderstandings can only be called a failure to communicate. A first step toward progress would be to recognize the need for improvement. Despite efforts by our professional organizations, it has not been acknowledged that communication between our specialties has been clouded by inadequate data and differing misaligned metrics. We propose that the following steps be advocated by both specialties, acting together through their professional organizations and aided by key collaborators such as the NICHD and March of Dimes.

Advocate Optimal Pregnancy Dating

By not insisting that all pregnancies are accurately dated by an ultrasound examination before 20 weeks' gestation, obstetricians and pediatricians are missing an opportunity to improve clinical decision making related to the appropriateness of fetal growth, gestation-specific antenatal care, timing of delivery, location of delivery, and planning/execution of postnatal care. This could be done much more quickly by acting together rather than separately.

Revise Our Primary Metrics

Improved communication could result from adoption of metrics that both disciplines contribute to, respect, and use. In addition to tracking preterm birth and infant mortality, greater emphasis on the perinatal mortality (defined as fetal deaths after 20 weeks plus neonatal deaths/1000 total births, both live and stillborn) would acknowledge the contribution of stillbirth to perinatal loss and its consequent importance in prenatal decision making. A composite rate that reflects perinatal mortality and serious morbidity would reflect the efforts of both disciplines, especially if a lower gestational age boundary, such as 22 or 24 weeks, were adopted for this purpose (the lower boundary should reflect the earliest gestational age at which neonatal intervention is common). Similarly, major neonatal, infant, and school-age morbidities are affected by care provided by both disciplines, and should be measured and reported whenever possible through school age. Reporting morbidity data according to gestational age at birth and percentile of growth for age for well-dated pregnancies would establish more accurate expectations to guide care and counseling before and after birth. Because outcomes at each gestational age vary by the adequacy of fetal growth, a perinatal data system that included birth weight, the gestational age at birth, and the method of obstetric dating (eg, good vs all others) would allow fetuses and neonates to receive care appropriate for their percentile of growth for gestational age. Equally important, standardized description of fetuses and newborns by percentiles of weight for gestational age could be an important first step to improved communication between the prenatal and postnatal care givers of the same patient. This approach acknowledges the value of both of the current obstetric (gestational age) and pediatric (birth weight) perspectives. The 2008 Surgeon General's Conference on Prevention of Preterm Birth recommended development of "predictors of perinatal morbidity and mortality that are specific to gestational age and birth weight" with emphasis on "perinatal morbidity and mortality as primary outcome measures" that "consistently integrate gestational age and birth weight in measures" based on "accurate gestational dating (ultrasound in early pregnancy)."[25]

Let's Go Back to Premature!

Update common definitions

The most basic definition, that of preterm birth, has always been artificial, a surrogate for functional maturity that does not track with age before or after birth. The current definition is no longer relevant to what is known about fetal growth and development.[26] The most common boundaries of preterm birth ($20^{0/7th}$ and $36^{6/7th}$ weeks of gestation)[27] are supported more by tradition than cause or outcomes. Rates of short-term and long-term morbidity and mortality are higher in infants born between $36^{0/7th}$ and $38^{6/7th}$ weeks' gestation than at 39 and 40 weeks' gestation,[28] attesting to the artificiality of $37^{0/7th}$ weeks as being term. The lower boundary is similarly flawed. Births at 17, 18, and 19 weeks confer an increased risk of subsequent births between 20 and 36 weeks,[29,30] but are still reported together with all other losses in the first half of pregnancy, where outcomes are not well described.[31] Pediatricians and obstetricians should ask that perinatal epidemiologists and professional organizations adopt a definition of full term that reflects these data. The Institute of Medicine's Committee on Preterm Birth (composed of pediatricians, obstetricians, and perinatal epidemiologists) recommended exactly this step in 2006,[32] as did the Surgeon General's Conference on Preterm Birth in 2008.[25] To date, neither the American Academy of Pediatrics nor ACOG has petitioned Congress or the NCHS to make these changes. We believe that current evidence indicates that maturity is achieved at $39^{0/7th}$ weeks. Infants born before $39^{0/7th}$ weeks' gestation should be recognized as having some risk of being less than fully mature. A return to the use of the word premature would emphasize this possibility for all infants born before $39^{0/7th}$ weeks of gestation.

Promote Clinical Research Collaboration

Specialty-specific research should be supported, but research proposals that feature integrated interdisciplinary collaboration throughout pregnancy, birth, and childhood should receive priority funding. Prospective determination of gestational age and hypothesis-driven collection of biospecimens during pregnancy are particularly important.

Promote Interdisciplinary Communication in Fellowship

Unlike residency training, fellowship training in neonatology and maternal fetal medicine allows adequate time to foster collaborative education, research, and patient care. Evidence of interdisciplinary collaboration throughout fellowship should become a standard feature of fellowship certification in both disciplines.

Collaborative Quality Improvement Efforts

Quality improvement projects offer an opportunity to work together toward mutual goals outside traditional academic and hospital specialty boundaries. Funding agencies should give preference to truly collaborative projects where the success of prenatal and intrapartum interventions are measured by infant and childhood outcomes.

Collaborative Clinical Care

Timing and location of delivery affect antenatal and postnatal care of the mother, fetus, and newborn. Decisions about perinatal care require collaboration and consultation. Similarly, but less apparent, perinatal decisions to withhold or withdraw intensive care also are better made collaboratively to assure optimal continuity of care and communication between the family and their caregivers. We recognize that these recommendations will require rethinking many current practices, and believe that to be an appropriate step toward improved communication.

REFERENCES

1. Ohio Perinatal Quality Collaborative Writing Committee. A statewide initiative to reduce inappropriate scheduled births at 36(0/7)-38(6/7) weeks' gestation [Erratum appears in Am J Obstet Gynecol 2010;202(6):603]. Am J Obstet Gynecol 2010;202(3):243, e1–8.
2. Investigators of the Vermont-Oxford Trials Network Database Project. The Vermont-Oxford Trials Network: very low birth weight outcomes for 1990. Pediatrics 1993;91:540–5.
3. Goldenberg RL, Wright LL. Repeated courses of antenatal steroids. Obstet Gynecol 2001;97:316–7.
4. Vohr BR, Wright LL, Dusick AM, et al. Center differences and outcomes of extremely low birth weight infants. Pediatrics 2004;113:781–9.
5. Vermont Oxford Network member website. Available at: https://nightingale.vtoxford.org/. Accessed February 13, 2011.
6. California Perinatal Quality Care Collaborative. Available at: http://www.cpqcc.org/quality_improvement/qi_toolkits/antenatal_corticosteroid_therapy_rev_october_2009/toolkit_revision_summary. Accessed February 13, 2011.
7. Leapfrog Group. Available at: http://www.leapfroggroup.org/news/leapfrog_news/4788210. Accessed February 13, 2011.
8. Reddy UM, Ko CW, Raju TN, et al. Delivery indications at late-preterm gestations and infant mortality rates in the United States. Pediatrics 2009;124:234–40.
9. Chase HC, Byrnes ME. Trends in "prematurity": United States: 1950–67. Rockville (MD): US Department of Health, Education, and Welfare, Public Health Service, Health Services and Mental Health Administration, NCHS, 1972; DHEW publication no. (HSM)72-1030. Vital and health statistics; series 3, no. 15, from Blackmore CA, Rowley DL, Kiely JL. Birth Outcomes. Available at: http://www.cdc.gov/Reproductivehealth/ProductsPubs/DatatoAction/birout2.pdf. Accessed February 13, 2011.

10. Taipale P, Hiilesmaa V. Predicting delivery date by ultrasound and last menstrual period in early gestation. Obstet Gynecol 2001;97:189–94.

11. Tyson JE, Parikh NA, Langer J, et al. Intensive care for extreme prematurity—moving beyond gestational age. N Engl J Med 2008;358:1672–81.

12. Stoll BJ, Hansen NI, Bell EF, et al. Neonatal outcomes of extremely preterm infants from the NICHD Neonatal Research Network. Pediatrics 2010;126(3):443–56.

13. McIntire DD, Leveno KJ. Neonatal mortality and morbidity rates in late preterm births compared with births at term. Obstet Gynecol 2008;111:35–41.

14. Clark SL, Miller DD, Belfort MA, et al. Neonatal and maternal outcomes associated with elective term delivery. Am J Obstet Gynecol 2009;200:156, e1–4.

15. Martin JA, Hamilton BE, Sutton PD, et al. no 1. Births: final data for 2008. National vital statistics reports, vol. 59. Hyattsville (MD): National Center for Health Statistics; 2010.

16. Joseph KS. Theory of obstetrics: an epidemiologic framework for justifying medically indicated early delivery. BMC Pregnancy Childbirth 2007;7:4.

17. MacDorman M, Kirmeyer S. The challenge of fetal mortality. NCHS data brief, no 16. Hyattsville (MD): National Center for Health Statistics; 2009.

18. Reddy UM, Laughon SK, Sun L, et al. Prepregnancy risk factors for antepartum stillbirth in the United States. Obstet Gynecol 2010;116(5):1119–26.

19. MacDorman MF, Kirmeyer S. Fetal and perinatal mortality, United States, 2005. Natl Vital Stat Rep 2009;57(8):1–19.

20. MacDorman MF, Declercq E, Zhang J. Obstetrical intervention and the singleton preterm birth rate in the United States from 1991–2006. Am J Public Health 2010; 100(11):2241–7.

21. Ananth CV, Gyamfi C, Jain L. Characterizing risk profiles of infants who are delivered at late preterm gestations: does it matter? Am J Obstet Gynecol 2008;199: 329–31.

22. Goldenberg RL, McClure EM, Bhattacharya A, et al. Women's perceptions regarding the safety of births at various gestational ages. Obstet Gynecol 2009;114:1254–8.

23. Talge NM, Holzman C, Wang J, et al. Late preterm birth and its association with cognitive and socioemotional outcomes at 6 years of age. Pediatrics 2010;126: 1124–31.

24. Lipkind HS, Slopen ME, Pfeiffer MR, et al. School age outcomes of late preterm infants. Am J Obstet Gynecol 2011;204:S37, SMFM Abstr 64.

25. Ashton DM, Lawrence HC 3rd, Adams NL 3rd, et al. Surgeon general's conference on the prevention of preterm birth. Obstet Gynecol 2009;113(4):925–30.

26. Fleischman AR, Oinuma M, Clark SL. Rethinking the definition of "term pregnancy". Obstet Gynecol 2010;116:136–9.

27. Creasy RK, Resnik R, Iams JD, et al, editors. Creasy and Resnik's maternal-fetal medicine: principles and practice. 6th edition. Philadelphia: Saunders Elsevier; 2008.

28. Raju TN. Late-preterm births: challenges and opportunities. Pediatrics 2008;121: 402–3.

29. Edlow AG, Srinivas SK, Elovitz M. Second-trimester loss and subsequent pregnancy outcomes: what is the real risk? Am J Obstet Gynecol 2007;197(6):581, e1–6.

30. McManemy J, Cooke E, Amon E, et al. Recurrence risk for preterm delivery. Am J Obstet Gynecol 2007;196:576, e1–6.

31. Creinin MD, Simhan H. Can we communicate gravidity and parity better? Obstet Gynecol 2009;113(3):709–11.

32. Behrman RE, Butler AS, editors. Preterm birth: causes, consequences, and prevention. Institute of Medicine (US) committee on understanding premature birth and assuring healthy outcomes. Washington, DC: National Academies Press (US); 2007.

Controversy: Antenatal Steroids

Ronald Wapner, MD[a], Alan H. Jobe, MD, PhD[b],*

KEYWORDS

- Prematurity • Respiratory distress syndrome • Corticosteroids
- Neurodevelopmental outcomes

There is no controversy about the core conclusion that women at risk of preterm delivery before 32 to 34 weeks' gestational age should be treated with antenatal steroids. This practice is supported by the initial comprehensive meta-analysis of Crowley, Chambers, and Keirse in 1990,[1] the National Institutes of Health Consensus Development Conference in 1994,[2] the second Consensus Conference to evaluate repeated courses of antenatal steroids in 2000,[3] and the practice recommendations of obstetric societies worldwide. Three recent meta-analyses by the Cochrane Collaboration on the benefits of antenatal steroids,[4] the choice of steroid and dosing,[5] and repeat doses of corticosteroids[6] comprehensively summarize the available clinical information to about 2007. However, there are many unanswered questions about which steroid and dose to use and about their use in selected populations. This review focuses on those areas of uncertainty.

CURRENT STATE OF ANTENATAL STEROID USE
Current Practice

This therapy is based on the initial Liggins and Howie[7] trial (1972) that used betamethasone as a 1:1 mixture of betamethasone phosphate and betamethasone acetate. The choice of the corticosteroid was empiric and based on Liggins research with fetal sheep, the available information about maternal to fetal transfer of fluorinated corticosteroids, and preparations available at that time for clinical use. Most clinical trials of a single course of corticosteroids and virtually all trials of repeated treatments have used the betamethasone acetate plus phosphate formulation available as Celestone.[4,6] The other corticosteroid that has been tested in clinical trials is dexamethasone phosphate.[5] As with any drug therapy, optimization of treatments requires

Disclosure: Some off-label products are mentioned in the article.
a Department of Obstetrics and Gynecology, Columbia University Medical Center, New York, NY, USA
b Division of Pulmonary Biology, Cincinnati Children's Hospital Medical Center, The University of Cincinnati, 3333 Burnet Avenue, Cincinnati, OH 45229-3039, USA
* Corresponding author.
E-mail address: alan.jobe@chmcc.org

Clin Perinatol 38 (2011) 529–545
doi:10.1016/j.clp.2011.06.013
0095-5108/11/$ – see front matter © 2011 Elsevier Inc. All rights reserved.

perinatology.theclinics.com

information about the drugs, the dose, the treatment intervals, and potential toxicity. There is minimal information for antenatal corticosteroids because the therapy was developed and tested by investigators without industry support and without the intent to have the treatment licensed. Despite a clear consensus that the use of antenatal corticosteroids is standard of care, there has been no review or approval by the Federal Drug Agency in the United States. Although clinical trials have included more than 6000 patients, multiple questions remain about all facets of the pharmacology of corticosteroids for this unique strategy to treat the pregnant woman to benefit the fetus.

Differences Between Betamethasone and Dexamethasone

The drugs are similar fluorinated corticosteroids with primarily glucocorticoid and minimal mineralicorticoid effects. The only structural difference is the isomeric position of a methyl group on position 16 of the ring structure. However, these drugs do have distinct activities. Betamethasone and dexamethasone have comparable potencies that are 25 times greater than cortisol for genomic effects because they have similar high affinities for the glucocorticoid receptor that regulates gene expression.[8] However, nongenomic effects on ion channels for example are about 6-fold higher for dexamethasone than for betamethasone.[9] The few direct comparisons of dexamethasone with betamethasone in developing annals also show differences in the drugs. For example, Ozdenir and colleagues,[10] reported that betamethasone promoted more lung maturation with less growth restriction in fetal mice than did dexamethasone. Pregnant sheep developed labor more consistently with fetal infusions with betamethasone than with dexamethasone, and the fetal betamethasone treatment decreased maternal progesterone more than dexamethasone.[11] Subtle differences in fetal responses to maternal treatments may also occur in humans. There are reports that betamethasone decreased fetal heart rate variability and changed fetal behavior more than did dexamethasone,[12,13] although Subtil and colleagues[14] did not detect differences in fetal heart rate responses to the 2 drugs. Independent of the formulations, betamethasone and dexamethasone are not equivalent drugs.

Dose and Route

The initial 2-dose 12-mg betamethasone treatment given at a 24-hour interval used by Liggins and Howie[7] has been accepted as the standard in almost all trials that have used betamethasone acetate plus phosphate.[4] The dexamethasone 4-dose 6-mg treatment at 12-hour intervals was modeled to achieve similar receptor occupancy.[15] The Liggins and Howie trial continued beyond the initial publication with randomization to evaluate twice the dose of betamethasone, with no apparent added benefit.[16] The dose and intervals for treatment have not been systematically evaluated in the human.

The pharmacokinetics of these drugs are complex. These corticosteroids are prodrugs in that soluble betamethasone phosphate and dexamethasone phosphate are dephosphorylated rapidly (half-life <1 hour) by phosphatases to the active drugs.[17] The terminal half-life for the free corticosteroids in plasma is about 4 hours, but receptor occupancy should persist for considerably longer.[18] After an initial high plasma level in the mother, fetal plasma levels of betamethasone or dexamethasone are about 30% of maternal levels in both humans and sheep.[15,19] In contrast, betamethasone acetate as a milled particle of 4 to 12 μm in the betamethasone acetate plus phosphate preparation is relatively insoluble. The free betamethasone enters the plasma slowly after deacetylation and has a terminal half-life of about 14 hours.[18] Plasma free betamethasone levels in the pregnant ewe peak within minutes of injection with betamethasone phosphate and then decrease rapidly. In contrast, betamethasone acetate yields peak betamethasone levels that are about one-tenth that achieved with betamethasone phosphate in the plasma of the ewe. Betamethasone levels are virtually undetectable in fetal blood after maternal treatment with betamethasone acetate.[17]

Recent experiments in sheep models show how little is known about how these treatments modulate fetal maturation. In fetal sheep models, lower maternal doses of betamethasone phosphate were as effective as the clinical dose for lung maturation with fewer effects on fetal growth.[20,21] Single intramuscular (IM) doses of cortisol (fetal), dexamethasone (fetal), or betamethasone phosphate (maternal) do not induce lung maturation in sheep.[17,22,23] In contrast, 4 doses of cortisol given to the fetus at 4-hour intervals or 4 doses of betamethasone phosphate given to the ewe do induce lung maturation.[22] These results show the need for a sustained fetal exposure for the maturational response.

The assumption has been that the benefits and risks of antenatal corticosteroid therapy result from direct fetal exposures to the agent. The rationale for including the betamethasone acetate in the treatment was that prolonged fetal exposure would be achieved. However, both maternal and fetal plasma free betamethasone levels are low after maternal treatment with betamethasone acetate.[17] A single maternal dose of betamethasone acetate is as effective for fetal lung maturation as is the standard 2-dose betamethasone acetate plus phosphate treatment in fetal sheep (**Fig. 1**). Therefore, very low fetal exposures to betamethasone can induce lung maturation. The implication is that betamethasone acetate alone might achieve the clinical goals with minimal fetal exposure to a corticosteroid. A preparation of betamethasone acetate is not available for clinical use.

Another twist to the relationships between fetal plasma levels of betamethasone and fetal effects is shown in **Fig. 2**. A fetal IM injection with betamethasone acetate plus phosphate (0.5 mg/kg fetal weight) results in higher fetal plasma betamethasone levels for 3 hours than does a maternal injection of 0.5 mg/kg maternal weight.[19]

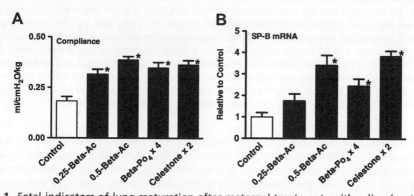

Fig. 1. Fetal indicators of lung maturation after maternal treatments with saline (control), 1 dose of 0.25 mg/kg betamethasone acetate (0.25, Beta-Ac), 1 dose of 0.5 mg/kg Beta-Ac, 4 doses of 0.25 mg/kg betaphosphate (Beta-PO₄) given at 12-hour intervals, or 2 doses of Celestone (0.5 mg/kg of a 1:1 mixture of Beta-Ac and Beta-PO₄ given at a 24-hour interval). All fetuses were delivered prematurely 48 hours after the initial treatment. (*A*) Lung compliance measured by the lung gas volume at 40 cm H_2O pressure increased for all treated groups relative to controls. (*B*) The mRNA for the surfactant protein (SP)-B also increased in the fetal lungs. *$P<.05$ versus controls. (*Data from* Jobe AH, et al. Betamethasone dose and formulation for induced lung maturation in fetal sheep. Am J Obstet Gynecol 2009; 201(6):611,e1–7.)

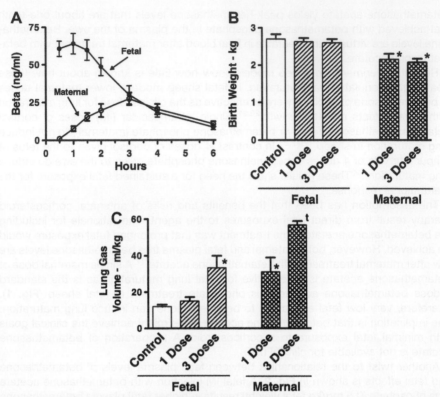

Fig. 2. Plasma levels of betamethasone (Beta), birth weights, and lung gas volumes. (*A*) Beta levels in fetal plasma after maternal treatments with 0.5 mg/kg beta-acetate plus phosphate (maternal) or after fetal treatment with the same dose based on estimated fetal weight (fetal). (*B*) One or 3 weekly fetal treatments with this dose did not decrease birth weight, whereas maternal treatments decreased birth weight. (*C*) Lung gas volume measured at 40 cm H_2O pressure as a measure of lung maturation increased more with maternal than fetal treatments. *$P<.05$ versus control, $^tP<.05$, 3 doses maternal versus 3 doses fetal. ([*A*] *Data from* Berry LM, Polk DH, Ikegami M, et al. Preterm newborn lamb renal and cardiovascular responses after fetal or maternal antenatal betamethasone. Am J Physiol 1997;272(6 Pt 2): R1972–9; and [*B, C*] Jobe AH, Newnham J, Willet K, et al. Fetal versus maternal and gestational age effects of repetitive antenatal glucocorticoids. Pediatrics 1998;102:1116–25.)

Nevertheless, the maternal treatment induces more fetal lung maturation than is achieved with the fetal treatment.[24] Furthermore, the higher direct fetal exposure to betamethasone does not cause fetal growth restriction, whereas the maternal treatment does. These results show that lung maturation is not optimally induced by high fetal plasma levels of betamethasone. Maternal treatment resulting in lower fetal exposure to the corticosteroid induces more lung maturation.

A clinical trial also has identified another quirk of corticosteroid dosing for fetal lung maturation. Betamethasone and dexamethasone can be given orally. Egerman and colleagues[25] randomized women to IM or oral dexamethasone at equivalent effective doses to test the hypothesis that oral treatment would be effective. The trial was stopped because of adverse outcomes in the oral dexamethasone arm of the trial (**Table 1**). The oral treatment was associated with large increases in newborn sepsis and intraventricular hemorrhage (IVH) with no indication of added benefit for

Table 1
A comparison of outcomes for women randomized to 6 mg dexamethasone every 12 hours ×
4 IM or 8 mg dexamethasone every 12 hours × 4

	Oral	IM	P
Number	99	84	—
RDS (%)	34.3	29.8	.53
Newborn sepsis (%)	10.1	1.2	.01
IVH	10.1	2.4	.04
Necrotizing enterocolitis	1.2	5.1	.13
Neonatal death	7.1	4.8	.55

Data from Egerman RS, Mercer BM, Doss JL, et al. A randomized, controlled trial of oral and intramuscular dexamethasone in the prevention of neonatal respiratory distress syndrome. Am J Obstet Gynecol 1998;179:1120–3.

respiratory distress syndrome (RDS) or death outcomes. There is no good explanation for these adverse outcomes after oral treatment.

The experimental literature does not support the currently used corticosteroids and treatment schedules as optimal for the indication of fetal maturation. The results in animal models suggest that prolonged, but very low fetal exposures to maternal corticosteroids should be evaluated to minimize fetal risks. Furthermore, fetal exposure to the corticosteroid may not be necessary. Perhaps placental responses to the corticosteroids signal the desired fetal effects.

Clinical Outcomes with Betamethasone versus Dexamethasone

Nevertheless, the clinician must treat with an available drug. Based on the earlier discussion, comparisons of the 2-dose betamethasone acetate plus phosphate treatment with the 4-dose dexamethasone phosphate treatment are not comparisons of equivalent fetal exposures to the same drug. There are 2 approaches to evaluating the relative benefits or risks of these drug treatments: a direct analysis of trials that randomized women to betamethasone or dexamethasone, or an indirect analysis of the trials that compared each drug with placebo and then a comparison of the outcomes relative to the placebo controls (**Table 2**).[5] The placebo-controlled trials were performed before 1990 and included primarily more mature infants, whereas the dexamethasone to betamethasone comparison trials were more recent. The indirect comparison identified less RDS with betamethasone as the only significant difference. The direct comparison qualitatively favors dexamethasone for the outcome of severe IVH primarily because of the recent trial reported by Elimian and colleagues.[26]

Table 2
Dexamethasone versus betamethasone risk ratio (95% CI)

Outcomes	Direct Comparison[a]	Indirect Comparison[b]
RDS	1.06 (0.88–1.28)	1.44 (1.14–1.78)
Severe IVH	0.40 (0.13–1.24)	0.47 (0.09–2.33)
Fetal/neonatal death	1.28 (0.46–3.52)	0.96 (0.71–1.30)

[a] *Data from* Brownfoot FC, Crowther CA, Middleton P. Different corticosteroids and regimens for accelerating fetal lung maturation for women at risk of preterm birth. Cochrane Database Syst Rev 2008;4:CD006764.
[b] *Data from* Roberts D, Dalziel S. Antenatal corticosteroids for accelerating fetal lung maturation for women at risk of preterm birth. Cochrane Database Syst Rev 2006;3:CD004454.

There has been a concern that maternal dexamethasone phosphate treatments may increase periventricular leukomalacia in newborns because of sulfites used for preservative.[27] We believe this situation is unlikely given the sulfite dose and volume of distribution in the mother. Infants are exposed to higher amounts of sulfite from hyperalimentation and other drugs that they receive. The clinical experience of the National Institute of Child Health and Human Development (NICHD) neonatal research network for more than 300 infants was an increase in death with antenatal dexamethasone treatment relative to betamethasone (odds ratio [OR] 1.66; confidence interval [CI] 1.07–2.57).[28] Another large recent series reported significantly less RDS and bronchopulmonary dysplasia for betamethasone-exposed than dexamethasone-exposed infants.[29] Data for the generally favorable long-term outcomes are available only for betamethasone-exposed infants.[4] Despite the multiple trials, no definitive recommendation can be made in favor of 1 drug treatment over the other.

CLINICAL QUESTIONS
Efficacy at Very Early Gestational Ages

Although treatment guidelines advise the use of antenatal corticosteroid for pregnancies at risk of preterm delivery from 24 weeks' to 32 to 34 weeks' gestation, there are minimal data from randomized trials for treatments with deliveries before 28 weeks' gestational age.[4] The irony is that preterm infants delivered at these very early gestational ages are most likely to benefit from the corticosteroid effects to decrease RDS, IVH, and death. These infants also are of most interest for contemporary perinatal care. The lack of information is historical in origin because the placebo-controlled trials performed before 1990 enrolled few pregnancies with deliveries at less than 28 weeks. A recent meta-analysis and systemic review of corticosteroid use before 26 weeks' gestation reported no benefits.[30] The investigators acknowledged that the trials and the meta-analysis were underpowered. We also suggest that there are other difficulties with accessing outcomes in these very early gestation outcomes. For diseases like RDS, the incidence is high and the corticosteroid treatment may not prevent RDS. For example, Garite and colleagues[31] found no decrease in RDS, but a significant decrease in the severity of RDS. The care strategies and clinical outcomes also have changed since these trials were performed. New randomized placebo trials are unlikely to be performed to resolve this question.

The biology of corticosteroid effects on the developing fetus and recent clinical experiences are 2 avenues to the evaluation of the usefulness of antenatal corticosteroids for very preterm deliveries. Lung tissue from 12-week to 24-week human fetuses in explant culture responds to corticosteroids, with an increase in epithelial maturation and the appearance of lamellar bodies, the storage organelles for surfactant.[32] Fetal monkeys at early gestations respond to maternal corticosteroid treatments with lung maturation.[33] Thus, there is no biologic reason to believe that the fetal human lung would not respond to antenatal corticosteroids at even previable gestational ages.

Clinical experiences are prone to bias based on the decision to treat with corticosteroids. Nevertheless, the information does represent current practice and outcomes for these high-risk pregnancies. The outcomes for all infants born with gestational ages less than 26 weeks in the United Kingdom and Ireland in 1995 were reported by Costeloe and colleagues.[34] Antenatal corticosteroids were given to 65% of the women, and the exposed newborns had decreased death (OR 0.57, CI 0.37–0.85), and decreased severe IVH (OR 0.39, CI 0.22–0.77), but not a decrease in RDS. For a more recent cohort of 181 infants born at 23 weeks' gestation, the 25% who received a complete course of antenatal corticosteroids had an OR for death of

0.18 and a CI 0.06 to 0.54, relative to unexposed infants, although overall morbidity and mortality were high.[35] A recent series from Japan also reported a decrease in RDS and IVH for infants exposed to antenatal corticosteroids who were delivered at 24 to 25 weeks. Death was decreased for infants delivered at 22 to 23 weeks and at 24 to 25 weeks relative to infants not exposed to antenatal corticosteroids.[36] Given the probable benefits, if the expectation is to care for a very preterm infant, then a single course of antenatal corticosteroids is indicated.

Use in the Late Preterm Period

Most studies have evaluated antenatal steroid use only up to 34 weeks' gestation. This upper gestational limit is arbitrary and was chosen to include the sickest neonates in whom prematurity-associated lung disease was life threatening. Recently, it has been realized that there is a significant disease burden that continues beyond this gestational period, because 3 of every 4 preterm births occur between 34 and 37 weeks' gestation.[37–46] It is estimated that more than 250,000 infants born at 34 weeks or later are admitted to the neonatal intensive care unit (NICU) each year, many of these for respiratory distress. At 34 weeks nearly 50% of infants require intensive care, and this drops to 15% at 35 weeks and is still 8% at 36 weeks.[47,48]

In understanding the potential benefit of antenatal steroid treatment in the late preterm period it should be remembered that not all respiratory distress is caused by surfactant deficiency and that antenatal steroids have multiple effects. One of the important steps in lung transition to air breathing is the removal of lung fluid. Through much of gestation, fetal lung development requires the active secretion of fluid into the alveolar spaces, which occurs via a chloride secretory mechanism.[49,50] As term approaches, lung fluid begins to be transferred from the lumen, across the apical membrane into the interstitium. This process occurs through passive movement of Na from the lumen into the interstitium through Na-permeable ion channels followed by active extrusion of Na from the cell across the basolateral membrane into the serosal space.[51] ENaC regulate the passive transfer of Na and are rate limiting in this process, which is maximally timed to occur in late gestation. Steroids play a key role in ENaC changes and thus in the absorption of fetal lung fluid.[52,53]

Preliminary data suggest that corticosteroids have an effect on reducing respiratory morbidity in this population by both enhancing borderline surfactant production and by initiating lung fluid removal. In a retrospective cohort analysis, Ventolini and colleagues[54] reported that infants born in the late preterm period who had previously received antenatal corticosteroids (from 24 to 34 weeks) had significantly reduced rates of overall respiratory distress (24.4% vs 81.3%) as well as a reduced rate of RDS (surfactant deficiency) (7.5% vs 35.5%).

Although the individual risk of a late preterm neonate requiring significant respiratory support is small, as a group it becomes substantial.[37–46,55] In addition, the accrued medical costs and parental anxiety of mild respiratory difficulties, including transient tachypnea, cannot be ignored. To address this question, the members of the Maternal Fetal Medicine Units Network in collaboration with the National Heart, Lung, and Blood Institute have initiated a prospective randomized trial of antenatal steroids for pregnant women likely to deliver in this window and who have not received steroid treatment earlier. The trial will recruit approximately 2800 singleton and twin gestations and should be completed in 2014.

Repeated or Rescue Courses

Although treatment with a single course of antenatal corticosteroids has been clearly integrated into clinical care, controversy exists as to whether the beneficial effects are time limited and whether retreatment is required. It is clear from animal and human studies that some of the effects of treatment such as surfactant production are reversible[56] after approximately 7 to 10 days, but the impact of time on other beneficial effects as well as the overall clinical impact are less well described.[57] Until recently, most clinical studies have suggested that the maximal effect of treatment does diminish over time, but all of these observational evaluations have been limited by multiple confounding factors.[57–60]

Over the last decade several multicentered, prospective, randomized trials have been performed comparing a single course of treatment with retreatment at various intervals ranging from 1 to 2 weeks. These results have been summarized in a Cochrane review[6] that includes results for more than 2000 women. In this analysis, treatment with repeat courses of corticosteroids is associated with a reduction in the overall occurrence of respiratory distress (relative risk [RR] 0.82, CI 0.72–0.93) and in the frequency of severe neonatal lung disease (RR 0.60, CI 0.48–0.75). In addition, repeat doses reduced overall serious infant morbidity (RR 0.79, CI 0.67–0.93). No significant differences were seen in other outcomes assessed, including chronic lung disease, perinatal mortality, IVH, periventricular leukomalacia, and maternal infection. The investigators conclude that the acute short-term pulmonary benefits for neonates support the use of repeat doses of antenatal corticosteroids.

Although repeat courses of antenatal corticosteroids may improve neonatal pulmonary status, there are concerns that repetitive retreatment may be harmful. Although the Cochrane review showed no overall reduction in birth weight of infants exposed to repeat steroids, most fetuses had only 1 or 2 subsequent courses of treatment. However, in the US NICHD trial[61] in which undelivered pregnancies were all retreated weekly until 34 weeks' gestation, 64% of infants had 4 or more repeat courses. In this subgroup receiving multiple exposures, there was a significant reduction in birth weight and an increase in small-for-gestational-age infants.[62] Placental size in the repeat group was also smaller.[63]

The ultimate evaluation of the efficacy and safety of repeat courses of antenatal steroids is the impact of treatment on the long-term health of the infant. The 3 largest multicentered national trials have now published their 2-year to 3-year follow-up.[62,64,65] The results of these studies are reassuring, with no difference in weight, neurodevelopment outcome or other health parameters in the group receiving multiple courses. In the US study in particular, in which a large number of infants were exposed to more than 4 courses, there was no difference in any anthropometric or developmental parameters by 2 years of age. However, of some concern was the finding of cerebral palsy in 6 infants in the repeat corticosteroid group. All received 4 or more courses of corticosteroids, none had any perinatal complications, and 5 were born at 34 weeks or later in gestation. Only 1 child in the placebo group was diagnosed with cerebral palsy. Overall the number of cases of cerebral palsy was small, and these results did not reach statistical significance (RR 5.7, CI 0.7–46.7). However, the predominance of this finding in infants exposed to 4 or more courses suggests that caution should be advised in exposing the fetus to multiple courses of steroids and that routine prophylactic retreatment is inadvisable.

Ideally, antenatal steroid treatment should be given so that birth occurs more than 24 hours after the initial course and within 7 days. Obstetricians are limited in their ability to predict preterm delivery with such accuracy, with approximately 50% of patients given an initial course of antenatal corticosteroids remaining undelivered 7 to 10 days later.[66] Women treated before 28 weeks' gestation seem more likely to give birth more than 7 days later than those treated after 28 weeks.[67]

To maximize the likelihood that every neonate has been treated during their ideal therapeutic window without requiring routine repetitive dosing, a rescue approach has been suggested in which initial treatment is given when a substantial risk of preterm birth is suspected, and if delivery does not occur within 7 to 14 days, a single retreatment (rescue) course is administered when preterm birth seems imminent. The efficacy of this approach has recently been reported by Garite and colleagues,[68] who randomized patients who remained at risk for preterm delivery 2 weeks or longer after their initial treatment to receive either a repeat course of betamethasone or a placebo when preterm delivery was highly likely. The group receiving an active drug rescue course had reduced composite morbidity (OR 0.65 [0.44–0.97]), a lower frequency of RDS (OR 0.64 [0.43–0.95]), and less need for postnatal surfactant treatment (OR 0.65 [0.43–0.98]). There was no reduction in bronchopulmonary dysplasia or the need for ventilator support. Birth weights and the frequency of intrauterine growth restriction were similar in both groups.

A few other observations from this study that may be of guidance to the clinician are noteworthy. In evaluating the timing and duration of the rescue effect, these investigators showed that the largest and most significant improvement in composite morbidity was seen in infants delivering between 2 and 7 days from the first dose of the rescue course. Although not a predesignated analysis, the investigators examined in which gestational ages the greatest efficacy of rescue treatment was seen. The reduction in composite morbidity was limited to babies born at less than 33 weeks, with no difference in outcome thereafter.

There is no consistent agreement among experts on the need and appropriateness of repeat administration of antenatal steroids. To address this inconsistency, a group of investigators representing each of the major trials of repeat and rescue dosing have recently been funded to perform an individual patient data meta-analysis to determine the efficacy and safety of various repeat dosing approaches. Led by Caroline Crowther of the University of Adelaide, this study should answer many of the remaining questions. In the meantime, it seems safe to administer a single rescue course if preterm birth at less than 33 weeks seems likely. The dose should be timed in an attempt to have delivery within 2 to 7 days from the first dose of the rescue course. Retreatment of infants beyond 33 weeks seems not to be effective or necessary.

Twins

The efficacy of antenatal corticosteroid use in twin gestations remains uncertain. The impact of antenatal corticosteroids in this clinical subcategory has never been evaluated in prospective trials of treated and untreated twins, so information is available only from cohort studies with multiple potential confounders or from subgroups of twins included within larger prospective trials of mostly singletons. This lack of information is unfortunate because twins and higher-order multiple gestations are an increasingly important contributor to preterm birth. The rate of twin births has increased 65% over the last 30 years and triplet gestations have increased more than 400%. Almost 60% of twins deliver at less than 37 completed weeks of gestation and more than 10% before 32 weeks.[69]

Most studies have shown no significant benefit to antenatal corticosteroid administration in twins or if one is shown it seems to be less than that seen with singletons.[70,71] A recent Cochrane meta-analysis performed by Roberts and Dalziel[4] showed a nonsignificant reduction in the rate of RDS in twins after the administration of steroids (OR 0.85, 95% CI 0.60–1.20). Similarly, in one of the largest population based studies evaluating the impact of steroids in twins, Blickstein and colleagues[71] reported that a complete course has a similar 40% to 50% reduction in RDS compared with no steroid treatment of both singletons and twins but that the effect is plurality dependent. Compared with treated singletons the OR for RDS in twins was 1.4 and in triplets it was 1.8.

There are several reasons that steroid treatment has not been confirmed to reduce RDS in twins. Initially it was speculated that the larger volume of distribution of women carrying twins and the larger fetal volume may result in reduced steroid exposure of the fetus. It has been shown that compared with women carrying a singleton, the half-life of betamethasone is shorter and the clearance greater in women carrying twins.[72] However, most recently, Gyamfi and colleagues[73] have measured both maternal and fetal (cord) betamethasone levels in both singleton and twin gestations and reported no difference. The cord betamethasone levels were higher in twins.

The most likely reason that twins have shows improvement after steroids is related to the small sample size of most studies, giving them insufficient power to confirm a difference. For example, the Cochrane analysis is based on only 4 studies with 167 twins and 157 controls. Confirming the 0.85 OR seen in this analysis would take a sample size of almost 4000 twin gestations.

From a practice standpoint it seems reasonable to treat women with twins who are at risk for preterm birth with a single course of antenatal steroids using the same dosing regimen as with singletons. One problem with this approach is predicting when to treat so that the maximum numbers of preterm infants are exposed and so that unnecessary treatment is minimized. To evaluate this approach, Murphy and colleagues[74] compared 2 twin cohorts at risk for preterm birth. One group received prophylactic steroids every 2 weeks starting at 24 weeks, whereas the other group received a rescue course if preterm delivery appeared imminent. In this comparison, there was no significant benefit to routine treatment, with more than a 7.5-fold greater risk of unnecessary exposure. However, in the rescue group almost one-third of infants delivering preterm did not receive a complete course of treatment.

Maternal Obesity

Obesity is known to alter the maternal volume of distribution, raising the question of whether the dosing of antenatal steroids should be adjusted based on maternal body weight. Although obesity does not seem to alter drug absorption, tissue distribution and drug elimination may be changed.

Gyamfi and colleagues[73] recently evaluated the impact of maternal obesity on both maternal and cord betamethasone levels. After controlling for the number of days since steroid treatment, number of courses, plurality, and gestational age there was no significant difference in maternal or cord betamethasone levels in obese patients.

Elective Cesarean Section

Delivery by cesarean section in the near-term period without preceding labor increases the occurrence of fetal respiratory morbidity.[39,75] Compared with infants delivered vaginally those delivered by prelabor cesarean section have a 2.3-fold to 6.8-fold increased risk of respiratory morbidities, including transient tachypnea, surfactant deficiency, and pulmonary hypertension. The risk of an NICU admission is doubled.[49,76,77] Even after 37 weeks' gestation, the risk of morbidity is inversely related to gestational age. In a large series of women delivering by repeat cesarean delivery, births at 37 weeks and at 38 weeks were associated with an increased risk of adverse respiratory outcomes compared with deliveries in the 39th week.[78] Mechanical ventilation, newborn sepsis, hypoglycemia, admission to the NICU, and hospitalization for 5 days or more were increased by a factor of 1.8 to 4.2 for births at 37 weeks and 1.3 to 2.1 for births at 38 weeks. The risk of any adverse outcome decreased from 15.3% to 8% from 37 to 39 completed weeks; the risk of RDS decreased from 3.7% to 0.9%, and transient tachypnea decreased from 4.8% to 2.7%.

Ideally, all prelabor cesarean deliveries would occur only after 39 completed weeks of gestation but this is not always possible because obstetric conditions of the mother or child may make a near-term delivery necessary. Whether administration of steroids in these cases is appropriate is uncertain, but a recent study suggests that it may be helpful. The Antenatal Steroids for Term Cesarean Section (ASTECS)[79] trial addressed the value of antenatal corticosteroids in patients undergoing elective cesarean section at term. Candidates were randomized to a course of antenatal betamethasone or no treatment. The study enrolled 998 women, 503 of whom received active treatment. Corticosteroids significantly decreased the rate of admission to the special care nursery for respiratory distress (RR 0.46, CI 0.23–0.93), with nonsignificant reductions in all respiratory morbidities. Although suggestive, the study was not blinded and did not use a placebo. In addition, respiratory distress was unconventionally defined as tachypnea (rate >60 breaths per minute) with grunting, recession, or nasal flaring. The investigators hypothesized that corticosteroid treatment decreased respiratory complications by increasing epithelial Na channel (ENaC) expression and function, thus allowing the lung to convert from active fluid secretion to sodium and fluid absorption. Because term infants, even after elective cesarean delivery, have a low incidence of respiratory morbidity, the number needed to treat to prevent 1 case of RDS is between 80 and 100 compared with 20 and 30 in the late preterm period and approximately 5 for infants at less than 32 weeks.[80]

Inflammation and Corticosteroids

There is not much controversy about corticosteroid treatment of women at risk of preterm delivery with ruptured membranes, although membrane rupture is a strong surrogate indicator for clinically silent chorioamnionitis. Clinical experience and a meta-analysis of the trial data support the benefits of antenatal corticoid treatments despite preterm rupture of membranes or a retrospective diagnosis of histologic chorioamnionitis.[81,82] A problem for the analysis of current clinical series is that most women have received antenatal corticosteroids. For example, 87% of women from a consecutive series of 457 deliveries at less than 32 weeks' gestation received corticosteroids, and the women not treated differed in the incidence of preeclampsia and type of preterm birth.[83] Decisions about which women may benefit from antenatal corticosteroids in the future may depend on new information about how infection/inflammation affects the pregnancy and outcomes. For example, new information that much of the histologic chorioamnionitis is associated with nonculturable organisms detected by polymerase chain reaction analyses will change how the perinatal community thinks about and diagnoses antenatal infections.[84] In experimental models with live *Ureaplasma*, the organism most frequently associated with histologic chorioamnionitis, the maturational effects on the fetal lung depend on the amount of inflammation and the chronicity of the infection, variables that are not considered clinically.[85] Further, fetal inflammatory and immune modulatory responses to the combined exposures of antenatal corticosteroids and fetal inflammation are complex and depend on the timing and the order of the exposures.[86] We know little about how the interactions of these responses may benefit or harm the fetus.

AN INTERNATIONAL PERSPECTIVE

Although antenatal corticosteroids are standard of care for pregnancies at risk of preterm delivery before 32 to 34 weeks worldwide, the use of antenatal corticosteroids in resource-poor environments is estimated to be only about 10% for women at risk.[87] This low use has been recognized as a target to improve outcomes by the World Health

Organization. However, there are multiple unanswered questions about how to best improve outcomes for the approximately 30% of newborn deaths within the first month of life attributed to prematurity.[88] The drug-related issues are substantial. Betamethasone acetate plus phosphate may be the drug of choice for the developed world, but the stability of this preparation has been poorly studied. The need to give repeated timed injections in low-resource environments is also a challenge. However, the largest challenge is the identification of the deliveries at risk in populations with no or minimal antenatal care or gestational dating and with a high incidence of fetal growth restriction. Furthermore, these populations with significant incidences of malaria, tuberculosis, and human immunodeficiency virus may be at risk if treated with corticosteroids. Even if treatments can be given effectively for home and low-level clinic deliveries, there is no benefit unless the care for the preterm infant is improved. Antenatal corticosteroids should be targeted for pregnancies at risk of delivering infants with birth weights of perhaps more than 1500 g, because the very preterm infants will likely not survive in these environments without risk of significant handicaps. However, the attack rates for antenatal corticosteroid responsive problems in these later gestational age infants remain essentially unstudied even in the developed world.[89] The NICHD has started a trial to evaluate if antenatal corticosteroids can benefit these late-preterm deliveries. The use of antenatal corticosteroids in resource-poor environments is challenging and may not be effective or free from risk.

REFERENCES

1. Crowley P, Chalmers I, Keirse MJ. The effects of corticosteroid administration before preterm delivery: an overview of the evidence from controlled trials. Br J Obstet Gynaecol 1990;97(1):11–25.
2. NIH, Consensus development panel on the effect of corticosteroids for fetal maturation on perinatal outcomes. Effect of corticosteroids for fetal maturation on perinatal outcomes. JAMA 1995;273(5):413–8.
3. Antenatal corticosteroids revisited: repeat courses. NIH Consens Statement 2000;17(2):1–10.
4. Roberts D, Dalziel S. Antenatal corticosteroids for accelerating fetal lung maturation for women at risk of preterm birth. Cochrane Database Syst Rev 2006;3: CD004454.
5. Brownfoot FC, Crowther CA, Middleton P. Different corticosteroids and regimens for accelerating fetal lung maturation for women at risk of preterm birth. Cochrane Database Syst Rev 2008;4:CD006764.
6. Crowther CA, Harding JE. Repeat doses of prenatal corticosteroids for women at risk of preterm birth for preventing neonatal respiratory disease. Cochrane Database Syst Rev 2007;3:CD003935.
7. Liggins GC, Howie RN. A controlled trial of antepartum glucocorticoid treatment for prevention of RDS in premature infants. Pediatrics 1972;50(4):515–25.
8. Lipworth BJ. Therapeutic implications of non-genomic glucocorticoid activity. Lancet 2000;356(9224):87–9.
9. Buttgereit F, Brand MD, Burmester GR. Equivalent doses and relative drug potencies for non-genomic glucocorticoid effects: a novel glucocorticoid hierarchy. Biochem Pharmacol 1999;58(2):363–8.
10. Ozdemir H, Guvenal T, Cetin M, et al. A placebo-controlled comparison of effects of repetitive doses of betamethasone and dexamethasone on lung maturation and lung, liver, and body weights of mouse pups. Pediatr Res 2003;53(1):98–103.

11. Derks JB, Giussani DA, Van Dam LM, et al. Differential effects of betamethasone and dexamethasone fetal administration of parturition in sheep. J Soc Gynecol Investig 1996;3(6):336–41.

12. Senat MV, Minoui S, Multon O, et al. Effect of dexamethasone and betamethasone on fetal heart rate variability in preterm labour: a randomised study. Br J Obstet Gynaecol 1998;105(7):749–55.

13. Rotmensch S, Liberati M, Vishne TH, et al. The effect of betamethasone and dexamethasone on fetal heart rate patterns and biophysical activities. A prospective randomized trial. Acta Obstet Gynecol Scand 1999;78(6):493–500.

14. Subtil D, Tiberghien P, Devos P, et al. Immediate and delayed effects of antenatal corticosteroids on fetal heart rate: a randomized trial that compares betamethasone acetate and phosphate, betamethasone phosphate, and dexamethasone. Am J Obstet Gynecol 2003;188(2):524–31.

15. Ballard PL, Ballard RA. Scientific basis and therapeutic regimens for use of antenatal glucocorticoids. Am J Obstet Gynecol 1995;173(1):254–62.

16. Liggins GC, Howie RN. Prevention of respiratory distress syndrome by maternal steroid therapy. In: Gluck L, editor. Modern perinatal medicine. Chicago: Year-book Publishers; 1974. p. 415–24.

17. Jobe AH, Nitsos I, Pillow JJ, et al. Betamethasone dose and formulation for induced lung maturation in fetal sheep. Am J Obstet Gynecol 2009;201(6): 611,e1–7.

18. Samtani MN, Lohle M, Grant A, et al. Betamethasone pharmacokinetics after two prodrug formulations in sheep: implications for antenatal corticosteroid use. Drug Metab Dispos 2005;33(8):1124–30.

19. Berry LM, Polk DH, Ikegami M, et al. Preterm newborn lamb renal and cardiovascular responses after fetal or maternal antenatal betamethasone. Am J Physiol 1997;272(6 Pt 2):R1972–9.

20. Loehle M, Schwab M, Kadner S, et al. Dose-response effects of betamethasone on maturation of the fetal sheep lung. Am J Obstet Gynecol 2010;202(2):186,e1–7.

21. Kutzler MA, Ruane EK, Coksaygan T, et al. Effects of three courses of maternally administered dexamethasone at 0.7, 0.75, and 0.8 of gestation on prenatal and postnatal growth in sheep. Pediatrics 2004;113(2):313–9.

22. Jobe AH, Newnham JP, Moss TJ, et al. Differential effects of maternal betamethasone and cortisol on lung maturation and growth in fetal sheep. Am J Obstet Gynecol 2003;188:22–8.

23. Jobe AH, Moss TJ, Nitsos I, et al. Betamethasone for lung maturation: testing dose and formulation in fetal sheep. Am J Obstet Gynecol 2007;97(5):523–6.

24. Jobe AH, Newnham J, Willet K, et al. Fetal versus maternal and gestational age effects of repetitive antenatal glucocorticoids. Pediatrics 1998;102:1116–25.

25. Egerman RS, Mercer BM, Doss JL, et al. A randomized, controlled trial of oral and intramuscular dexamethasone in the prevention of neonatal respiratory distress syndrome. Am J Obstet Gynecol 1998;179:1120–3.

26. Elimian A, Garry D, Figueroa R, et al. Antenatal betamethasone compared with dexamethasone (betacode trial): a randomized controlled trial. Obstet Gynecol 2007;110(1):26–30.

27. Baud O, Foix-L'Helias L, Kaminski M, et al. Antenatal glucocorticoid treatment and cystic periventricular leukomalacia in very premature infants. N Engl J Med 1999;341(16):1190–6.

28. Lee BH, Stoll BJ, McDonald SA, et al. Adverse neonatal outcomes associated with antenatal dexamethasone versus antenatal betamethasone. Pediatrics 2006;117(5):1503–10.

29. Feldman DM, Carbone J, Belden L, et al. Betamethasone vs dexamethasone for the prevention of morbidity in very-low-birthweight neonates. Am J Obstet Gynecol 2007;197(3):284,e1–4.

30. Onland W, de Laat MW, Mol BW, et al. Effects of antenatal corticosteroids given prior to 26 weeks' gestation: a systematic review of randomized controlled trials. Am J Perinatol 2011;28(1):33–44.

31. Garite TJ, Rumney PJ, Briggs GG, et al. A randomized, placebo-controlled trial of betamethasone for the prevention of respiratory distress syndrome at 24 to 28 weeks' gestation. Am J Obstet Gynecol 1992;166(2):646–51.

32. Gonzales LW, Ballard PL, Ertsey R, et al. Glucocorticoids and thyroid hormones stimulate biochemical and morphological differentiation of human fetal lung in organ culture. J Clin Endocrinol Metab 1986;62(4):678–91.

33. Bunton TE, Plopper CG. Triamcinolone-induced structural alterations in the development of the lung of the fetal rhesus macaque. Am J Obstet Gynecol 1984; 148(2):203–15.

34. Costeloe K, Hennessy E, Gibson AT, et al. The EPICure study: outcomes to discharge from hospital for infants born at the threshold of viability. Pediatrics 2000;106(4):659–71.

35. Hayes EJ, Paul DA, Stahl GE, et al. Effect of antenatal corticosteroids on survival for neonates born at 23 weeks of gestation. Obstet Gynecol 2008;111(4):921–6.

36. Mori R, Kusuda S, Fujimura M. Antenatal corticosteroids promote survival of extremely preterm infants born at 22–23 weeks of gestation. J Pediatr 2011; 159(1):110–4,e1.

37. Davidoff MJ, Dias T, Damus K, et al. Changes in the gestational age distribution among U.S. singleton births: impact on rates of late preterm birth, 1992 to 2002. Semin Perinatol 2006;30(1):8–15.

38. Hibbard JU, Wilkins I, Sun L, et al. Respiratory morbidity in late preterm births. JAMA 2010;304(4):419–25.

39. Yoder BA, Gordon MC, Barth WH Jr. Late-preterm birth: does the changing obstetric paradigm alter the epidemiology of respiratory complications? Obstet Gynecol 2008;111(4):814–22.

40. Hjalmarson O. Epidemiology and classification of acute, neonatal respiratory disorders. A prospective study. Acta Paediatr Scand 1981;70(6):773–83.

41. Krantz ME, Wennergren M, Bengtson LG, et al. Epidemiological analysis of the increased risk of disturbed neonatal respiratory adaptation after caesarean section. Acta Paediatr Scand 1986;75(5):832–9.

42. Wennergen M, Krantz M, Hjalmarson O, et al. Low Apgar score as a risk factor for respiratory disturbances in the newborn infant. J Perinat Med 1987;15(2): 153–60.

43. Dani C, Reali MF, Bertini G, et al. Risk factors for the development of respiratory distress syndrome and transient tachypnoea in newborn infants. Italian Group of Neonatal Pneumology. Eur Respir J 1999;14(1):155–9.

44. Rubaltelli FF, Dani C, Reali MF, et al. Acute neonatal respiratory distress in Italy: a one-year prospective study. Italian Group of Neonatal Pneumology. Acta Paediatr 1998;87(12):1261–8.

45. Clark RH. The epidemiology of respiratory failure in neonates born at an estimated gestational age of 34 weeks or more. J Perinatol 2005;25(4):251–7.

46. Wang ML, Dorer DJ, Fleming MP, et al. Clinical outcomes of near-term infants. Pediatrics 2004;114(2):372–6.

47. Dudell GG, Jain L. Hypoxic respiratory failure in the late preterm infant. Clin Perinatol 2006;33(4):803–30 [abstract: viii–ix].

48. Angus DC, Linde-Zwirble WT, Clermont G, et al. Epidemiology of neonatal respiratory failure in the United States: projections from California and New York. Am J Respir Crit Care Med 2001;164(7):1154-60.
49. Jain L, Eaton DC. Physiology of fetal lung fluid clearance and the effect of labor. Semin Perinatol 2006;30(1):34-43.
50. Bland RD. Lung epithelial ion transport and fluid movement during the perinatal period. Am J Physiol 1990;259(2 Pt 1):L30-7.
51. Jain L. Alveolar fluid clearance in developing lungs and its role in neonatal transition. Clin Perinatol 1999;26(3):585-99.
52. Jain L, Chen XJ, Ramosevac S, et al. Expression of highly selective sodium channels in alveolar type II cells is determined by culture conditions. Am J Physiol Lung Cell Mol Physiol 2001;280(4):L646-58.
53. Venkatesh VC, Katzberg HD. Glucocorticoid regulation of epithelial sodium channel genes in human fetal lung. Am J Physiol 1997;273(1 Pt 1):L227-33.
54. Ventolini G, Neiger R, Mathews L, et al. Incidence of respiratory disorders in neonates born between 34 and 36 weeks of gestation following exposure to antenatal corticosteroids between 24 and 34 weeks of gestation. Am J Perinatol 2008; 25(2):79-83.
55. Escobar GJ, Greene JD, Hulac P, et al. Rehospitalisation after birth hospitalisation: patterns among infants of all gestations. Arch Dis Child 2005;90(2):125-31.
56. Vidaeff AC, Ramin SM, Gilstrap LC 3rd, et al. Characterization of corticosteroid redosing in an in vitro cell line model. Am J Obstet Gynecol 2004;191(4):1403-8.
57. Vermillion ST, Soper DE, Newman RB. Is betamethasone effective longer than 7 days after treatment? Obstet Gynecol 2001;97(4):491-3.
58. Sehdev HM, Abbasi S, Robertson P, et al. The effects of the time interval from antenatal corticosteroid exposure to delivery on neonatal outcome of very low birth weight infants. Am J Obstet Gynecol 2004;191(4):1409-13.
59. Ring AM, Garland JS, Stafeil BR, et al. The effect of a prolonged time interval between antenatal corticosteroid administration and delivery on outcomes in preterm neonates: a cohort study. Am J Obstet Gynecol 2007;196(5):457,e1-6.
60. National Institutes of Health Consensus Development Panel. Antenatal corticosteroids revisited: repeat courses-National Institutes of Health Consensus Development Conference Statement, August 17-18, 2000. Obstet Gynecol 2001;98(1): 144-50.
61. Wapner RJ, Sorokin Y, Thom EA, et al. Single versus weekly courses of antenatal corticosteroids: evaluation of safety and efficacy. Am J Obstet Gynecol 2006; 195(3):633-42.
62. Wapner RJ, Sorokin Y, Mele L, et al. Long-term outcomes after repeat doses of antenatal corticosteroids. N Engl J Med 2007;357(12):1190-8.
63. Sawady J, Mercer BM, Wapner RJ, et al. The National Institute of Child Health and Human Development Maternal-Fetal Medicine Units Network Beneficial Effects of Antenatal Repeated Steroids study: impact of repeated doses of antenatal corticosteroids on placental growth and histologic findings. Am J Obstet Gynecol 2007;197(3):281,e1-8.
64. Crowther CA, Doyle LW, Haslam RR, et al. Outcomes at 2 years of age after repeat doses of antenatal corticosteroids. N Engl J Med 2007;357(12):1179-89.
65. Murphy KE, Hannah ME, Willan AR, et al. Multiple courses of antenatal corticosteroids for preterm birth (MACS): a randomised controlled trial. Lancet 2008; 372(9656):2143-51.
66. Modi N, Lewis H, Al-Naqeeb N, et al. The effects of repeated antenatal glucocorticoid therapy on the developing brain. Pediatr Res 2001;50(5):581-5.

67. McLaughlin KJ, Crowther CA, Vigneswaran P, et al. Who remains undelivered more than seven days after a single course of prenatal corticosteroids and gives birth at less than 34 weeks? Aust N Z J Obstet Gynaecol 2002;42(4):353–7.
68. Garite TJ, Kurtzman J, Maurel K, et al. Impact of a 'rescue course' of antenatal corticosteroids: a multicenter randomized placebo-controlled trial. Am J Obstet Gynecol 2009;200(3):248,e1–9.
69. Martin JA, Hamilton BE, Sutton PD, et al. Births: final data for 2002. Natl Vital Stat Rep 2003;52(10):1–113.
70. Choi SJ, Song SE, Seo ES, et al. The effect of single or multiple courses of antenatal corticosteroid therapy on neonatal respiratory distress syndrome in singleton versus twin pregnancies. Aust N Z J Obstet Gynaecol 2009;49(2): 173–9.
71. Blickstein I, Shinwell ES, Lusky A, et al. Plurality-dependent risk of respiratory distress syndrome among very-low-birth-weight infants and antepartum corticosteroid treatment. Am J Obstet Gynecol 2005;192(2):360–4.
72. Ballabh P, Lo ES, Kumari J, et al. Pharmacokinetics of betamethasone in twin and singleton pregnancy. Clin Pharmacol Ther 2002;71(1):39–45.
73. Gyamfi C, Mele L, Wapner RJ, et al. The effect of plurality and obesity on betamethasone concentrations in women at risk for preterm delivery. Am J Obstet Gynecol 2010;203(3):219,e1–5.
74. Murphy DJ, Caukwell S, Joels LA, et al. Cohort study of the neonatal outcome of twin pregnancies that were treated with prophylactic or rescue antenatal corticosteroids. Am J Obstet Gynecol 2002;187(2):483–8.
75. Hansen AK, Wisborg K, Uldbjerg N, et al. Risk of respiratory morbidity in term infants delivered by elective caesarean section: cohort study. BMJ 2008; 336(7635):85–7.
76. Hansen AK, Wisborg K, Uldbjerg N, et al. Elective caesarean section and respiratory morbidity in the term and near-term neonate. Acta Obstet Gynecol Scand 2007;86(4):389–94.
77. Kolas T, Saugstad OD, Daltveit AK, et al. Planned cesarean versus planned vaginal delivery at term: comparison of newborn infant outcomes. Am J Obstet Gynecol 2006;195(6):1538–43.
78. Tita AT, Landon MB, Spong CY, et al. Timing of elective repeat cesarean delivery at term and neonatal outcomes. N Engl J Med 2009;360(2):111–20.
79. Stutchfield P, Whitaker R, Russell I. Antenatal betamethasone and incidence of neonatal respiratory distress after elective caesarean section: pragmatic randomised trial. BMJ 2005;331(7518):662.
80. Sinclair JC. Meta-analysis of randomized controlled trials of antenatal corticosteroid for the prevention of respiratory distress syndrome: discussion. Am J Obstet Gynecol 1995;173(1):335–44.
81. Harding JE, Pang J, Knight DB, et al. Do antenatal corticosteroids help in the setting of preterm rupture of membranes? Am J Obstet Gynecol 2001;184(2):131–9.
82. Elimian A, Verma U, Beneck D, et al. Histologic chorioamnionitis, antenatal steroids, and perinatal outcomes. Obstet Gynecol 2000;96(3):333–6.
83. Goldenberg RL, Andrews WW, Faye-Petersen OM, et al. The Alabama preterm birth study: corticosteroids and neonatal outcomes in 23- to 32-week newborns with various markers of intrauterine infection. Am J Obstet Gynecol 2006; 195(4):1020–4.
84. DiGiulio DB, Romero R, Amogan HP, et al. Microbial prevalence, diversity and abundance in amniotic fluid during preterm labor: a molecular and culture-based investigation. PLoS One 2008;3(8):e3056.

85. Knox CL, Dando SJ, Nitsos I, et al. The severity of chorioamnionitis in pregnant sheep is associated with in vivo variation of the surface-exposed multiple-banded antigen/gene of *Ureaplasma parvum*. Biol Reprod 2010;83(3):415–26.
86. Kallapur SG, Kramer BW, Moss TJ, et al. Maternal glucocorticoids increase endotoxin-induced lung inflammation in preterm lambs. Am J Physiol Lung Cell Mol Physiol 2003;284(4):L633–42.
87. Darmstadt GL, Bhutta ZA, Cousens S, et al. Evidence-based, cost-effective interventions: how many newborn babies can we save? Lancet 2005;365(9463): 977–88.
88. Bassani DG, Kumar R, Awasthi S, Million Death Study Collaborators. Causes of neonatal and child mortality in India: a nationally representative mortality survey. Lancet 2010;376:1853–60.
89. Bastek JA, Sammel MD, Rebele EC, et al. The effects of a preterm labor episode prior to 34 weeks are evident in late preterm outcomes, despite the administration of betamethasone. Am J Obstet Gynecol 2010;203(2):140,e1–7.

Late Preterm Birth: Preventable Prematurity?

Sowmya S. Mohan, MD, Lucky Jain, MD, MBA*

KEYWORDS

• Late preterm birth • Prematurity • Infant mortality
• Infant morbidity

Prematurity is one of the leading causes of infant morbidity and mortality globally. Over the years, however, advances in medicine and technology have enhanced the ability to care for babies at very early gestations. There has also been a shift in the distribution of births away from term/post-term gestations and toward earlier gestational ages.[1] These changes have added to the burden of premature births, which reached an all-time high of 12.7% of live births in 2007.[2] Premature infants (born at <37 completed weeks' gestation or <260 days, counting from the first day of the last menstrual period[3]) can be categorized into subgroups of very preterm (gestation of <32 weeks), moderately preterm (between $32^{0/7}$ and $33^{6/7}$ weeks' gestation), and late preterm infants (born between $34^{0/7}$ and $36^{6/7}$ weeks' gestation) (**Fig. 1**).[4] The gestational age limits defining each subgroup of premature infants were established in 2005 by a panel of experts from the National Institutes of Health and the National Institute of Child Health and Human Development.[5] While developing these criteria, the group took into account many factors, including the obstetric guidelines that consider 34 weeks a maturational milestone in the developing fetus. Current obstetric guidelines recommend that antenatal steroids not be offered to mothers with anticipated delivery at gestational ages beyond 34 weeks because surfactant is generally considered adequate at this point in development.[5] The problem lies in the belief that late preterm infants are mature (due to their larger size) and behave more like term babies instead of smaller, more typical premature infants. The assumption that late preterm infants are capable of a smooth transition to extrauterine life has led to more lenient criteria for the earlier delivery of these babies—often without clear medical indication or a clear understanding of the consequences of such a decision. In reality, late preterm infants behave more like their smaller premature counterparts in that they have a higher incidence of transient tachypnea of the newborn,[6,7] respiratory distress syndrome,[7,8] persistent pulmonary hypertension of the newborn,[9] respiratory failure, prolonged

Department of Pediatrics, Emory University School of Medicine, 2015 Uppergate Drive, Atlanta, GA 30322, USA
* Corresponding author.
E-mail address: ljain@emory.edu

Clin Perinatol 38 (2011) 547–555
doi:10.1016/j.clp.2011.06.005   **perinatology.theclinics.com**

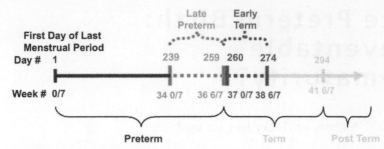

Fig. 1. Definition of late preterm and early term. (*From* Engle WA, Kominiarek MA. Late preterm infants, early term infants, and timing of elective deliveries. Clin Perinatol 2008;35:325; with permission.)

physiologic jaundice, late neonatal sepsis,[3] thermoregulation issues, feeding difficulties, and a host of other problems that affect them during the neonatal period and have potential long-term consequences.

There is another side to this story, however, a belief that the same obstetric practices that have increased early term and late preterm births have led to a greater than 50% rise in cesarean section rates in the past decade alone and have helped drive down stillbirths to an all-time low (**Fig. 2**).[10] It is also not clear whether a late preterm pregnant woman threatened by preterm labor, preterm rupture of membranes, or a host of medical conditions should be expeditiously delivered or managed expectantly. Although the past 5 years have led to a new focus on late preterm births and yielded new information, there are many unknowns that need to be addressed (**Box 1**). The focus of this article is to present both sides of the story,

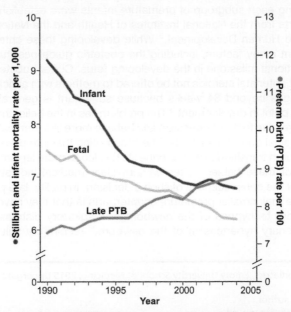

Fig. 2. Stillbirth and infant mortality rates in comparison with late preterm births, 1990–2005. (*Reprinted from* Ananth C, Gyamfi C, Jain L. Characterizing risk profiles of infants who are delivered at late preterm gestations: does it matter? Am J Obstet Gynecol 2008;199:329–31; with permission.)

Box 1
Late preterm infants: the knowns and the unknowns

1. What's known
   a. Mortality rises with each week lost in gestation below 39 weeks.
   b. Excess morbidity, mostly transient, is related to global immaturity.
   c. Birth at earlier gestations has an impact on health and mortality beyond the neonatal period.
   d. Long-term neurologic outcomes are a cause of concern.

2. What's unknown
   a. Are adverse outcomes due to early delivery or due to the events preceding late preterm birth?
   b. Are outcomes after preterm labor, preterm rupture of membranes, or medically indicated late preterm birth different?
   c. Can late preterm births and iatrogenic prematurity be safely reduced?
   d. Can interventions, such as antenatal steroids, improve outcomes?

---

one that highlights the many problems and morbidities faced by this subgroup of premature infants and the other that justifies their early delivery.

THE LATE PRETERM INFANT

Although not as underdeveloped as their more premature counterparts, late preterm infants are at a considerably higher risk for complications after birth. Due to their near-term gestation and size, they are often not monitored closely in mother and baby units and can spiral down quickly due to a delay in identifying their problems. In recent years, there has been an increasing awareness of their unique set of complications, such as delayed neonatal transition, wet lung syndrome, hypothermia, hypoglycemia, and hyperbilirubinemia.[11] As detailed in **Box 2**, the problems facing late preterm infants are not unique to this group of newborns but these complications have distinct differences in their manifestations and management.

With statistics showing that as many as 75% of preterm births are classified as late preterm,[12] up to one-third of all neonatal ICU (NICU) admissions in the United States

---

Box 2
Morbidities late preterm infants are at greatest risk for due to their physiologic immaturity and limited compensatory responses to the extrauterine environment compared with term infants

Late preterm infants are at greater risk (compared with term babies) for morbidities, such as

1. Temperature instability
2. Hypoglycemia
3. Respiratory distress
4. Apnea
5. Jaundice

Data from Engle WA, Tomashek KM, Wallman C. "Late preterm" infants: a population at risk. Pediatrics 2007;120:1390–401.

---

are attributed to late preterm infants.[13] The reasons for admission to the NICU in this cohort of premature infants, range from short stays for problems, such as transient tachypnea of the newborn, to more complicated and extended stays for problems, such as persistent pulmonary hypertension of the newborn. In addition to the social and emotional impacts on parents of a sick late preterm newborn in an NICU, the cost of NICU care (up to $3500/day) can have a significant economic impact. This has prompted many studies and debate over the allocation of medical resources. One study done in the State of California, showed that in 1996 alone, the State could have saved $49.9 million in health care costs by preventing nonmedically indicated deliveries between 34 and 37 weeks of gestation.[14]

In addition to these sobering statistics, the higher risk of complications associated with late preterm infants often continues after the initial hospitalization. For example, late preterm infants have an increased incidence of hospital readmissions and sick visits compared with full-term infants. In a 2007 study by Tomashek and colleagues,[15] late preterm infants who were discharged home early (<2 days after birth) from the hospital had a 4.3% rate of readmission to the hospital (compared with 2.7% of term infants). Another study reported that for late preterm infants reporting to an emergency department after initial discharge from the birthing hospital, their primary diagnosis was an extension of their initial prematurity.[16] Given all this and the disproportionately high number of late preterm infants delivered, the overall socioeconomic impact of late preterm births can be significant.[16] Strategies are needed to reduce the preventable fraction of late preterm births that have been occurring with increasing frequency in the past few years.

ETIOLOGY OF LATE PRETERM BIRTHS

The rate of preterm births in the United States is much higher than in other developed nations.[17] Because late preterm births are the fastest growing subset from this high risk group, it is important to have a better understanding of the etiology of prematurity and late preterm births so that the modifiable factors leading to the high rate of late preterm births in the United States are addressed.

From 1990 to 2006, the rate of late preterm births rose 20% from 6.8 to 8.1. In other words, 1 of every 15 babies born in 1990 was a late preterm infant in comparison statistics from 2006 showing that the problem had worsened and as many as 1 in every 12 births was classified as late preterm.[18] When looking at the issue of late preterm births, it is customary to divide the births into 2 groups. The first group is spontaneous late preterm births (ie, premature labor with intact membranes or premature rupture of membranes with subsequent concern for infection, inflammation, and so forth) where there is limited control on preventing the birth and the focus lies in a better understanding of the management of the neonate during the perinatal period. The second group includes premature babies born after the induction of labor or performance of a cesarean section for maternal or fetal indications (ie, preeclampsia, eclampsia, or intrauterine growth retardation) or for other reasons (ie, convenience) (**Fig. 3**). Given these 2 categories, a high number of late preterm births can be attributed to multiple factors (including higher rates of induced deliveries and cesarean sections, efforts to reduce stillbirths, greater maternal age, increased use of artificial reproductive technology [which raises the risk of multiple births], and the false belief that neonatal outcomes will be good after 34 weeks' gestation [leading to a lower threshold for intervention during the late preterm period]),[17,18] which potentially may be able to be influenced and, therefore, outcomes improved.

PTD Subtypes

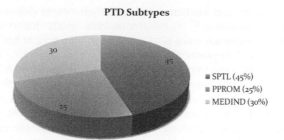

- SPTL (45%)
- PPROM (25%)
- MEDIND (30%)

Fig. 3. Etiology of late preterm births. (*Data from* Martin JA, Kirmeyer S, Osterman M, et al. Born a bit too early: recent trends in late preterm births. NCHS Data Brief 2009;24:1–8.)

One of the factors affecting the rate of late preterm births occurring in the United States is the change that has taken place in the management of labor and delivery in the past 20 years. Specifically, there has been a marked increase in the number of inductions of labor and cesarean sections performed[18] at 34 to 36 weeks' gestation, which has influenced the upswing in the late preterm birth rate.[19,20] As seen in **Fig. 4**, vaginal births of late preterm infants for which labor was induced more than doubled (from 7.5% to 17.3%) between 1990 and 2006. In addition, there was a 46% increase in the percentage of late preterm births delivered by cesarean section during that same time period.[18,21] Inappropriate interventions may be a substantial factor in the increase in late preterm births in the United States.[17] Researchers have showed that some physicians are pursuing early delivery for a range of indications even when there is little evidence supporting such action. In a retrospective chart review study led by Kuehn and colleagues in 2010,[17] the investigatorsinvesin found that one-fifth of late preterm births had documented reason for medically indicated late preterm delivery that was not a generally accepted medical indication (based on guidelines set forth from the American College of Obstetricians and Gynecologists and consensus expert opinion). This lack of stringent criteria for early delivery can translate into poorer outcomes for neonates, such as those seen in late preterm infants.[17] Researchers found that infants who were delivered between 34 and 36 weeks without a medical indication were more likely to need ventilator support and were at higher risk of major neonatal morbidity (intraventricular hemorrhage,

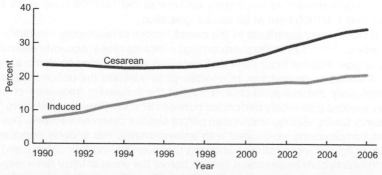

Fig. 4. Induction of labor and cesarean delivery rates among late preterm births: United States, 1990–2006. (*Data from* Martin JA, Kirmeyer S, Osterman M, et al. Born a bit too early: recent trends in late preterm births. NCHS Data Brief 2009;24:1–8.)

necrotizing enterocolitis, and ventilator support) than infants delivered early due to accepted medical indications.[17] Furthermore, this study found that physician-initiated late preterm deliveries were also associated with poorer neonatal outcomes than were spontaneous late preterm births.[17]

It has been argued that the trend of increasing late preterm births is in part due to a drive to decrease stillbirths (some data suggest that in certain circumstances, early delivery may prevent stillbirth). An analysis of the available US data shows, however, that the drop in stillbirth rate shows little temporal relationship to stillbirth rates. Noting the increasing number of late preterm deliveries and the complications associated with it, however, researchers concede that physicians may be overreacting and delivering many neonates too early.[17] Although the decrease in stillbirths during the same time period as the increase in late preterm deliveries can be seen in **Fig. 2**, the increase in perinatal infant morbidity and long-term consequences of premature birth need to be considered and the decision to deliver at an earlier gestation should be based on medical indications for delivery and not on associating gestational age (such as 34 weeks) as a marker for perceived improved outcomes.[10]

RISKS OF LATE PRETERM BIRTHS

The risks associated with late preterm births are many and may be avoidable, if a pregnancy is allowed to progress (assuming there are no medical indications for early delivery).

Respiratory

Several studies have consistently shown that the late preterm infants have higher respiratory morbidity and mortality compared with full-term infants. Many late preterm infants develop respiratory distress soon after birth (sustained distress for more than 2 hours after birth accompanied by grunting, flaring, tachypnea, retractions, or supplemental oxygen requirement), which studies show occurs more often in late preterm infants than in term newborns (28.9% vs 4.2%, respectively).[7] In addition, within the early term and late preterm groups, babies with a gestational age of 37 weeks are 5 times as likely, and babies born at 35 weeks were 9 times as likely, to have respiratory distress compared with babies born at 38 to 40 weeks.[22] For each gestational age week, infants delivered by elective cesarean section tend to do more poorly. Madar and colleagues[23] found that the incidence of respiratory distress was significantly increased with every week of gestation below 39 weeks: 30/1000 infants born at 34 weeks' gestation developed respiratory distress as did 14/1000 born at 35 weeks' gestation, and 7.1/1000 born at 36 weeks' gestation.

Several factors may contribute to the overall burden of respiratory morbidity in late preterm infants.[9,24–28] Given the shortcomings clinicians face in accurate estimation of gestational age, elective inductions and cesarean sections may have increased the burden of iatrogenic prematurity. In an attempt to minimize the occurrence of iatrogenic respiratory distress syndrome in light of the increasing frequency of elective cesarean sections (commonly performed between 37 and 40 weeks' gestation),[29] fetal lung maturity testing was recommended before elective cesarean sections. Due to the risks and complications associated with amniocentesis, this is done infrequently,[30] especially in light of recent studies showing that even late preterm infants and some early term infants born by cesarean section before the onset of labor have respiratory distress despite having mature surfactant profiles. This prompted the American College of Obstetricians and Gynecologists to recommend scheduling elective cesarean section at 39 weeks or later or waiting for the onset of spontaneous labor[31] but, unfortunately, factors related to the convenience of scheduled elective cesarean section deliveries for both families and providers have continued to influence the timing of elective cesarean section.[30]

Mortality

Perhaps one of the most disturbing aspects of late preterm births is the high infant mortality rate in comparison with other groups of infants. Birth/infant death files from 1995 to 2002 in the United States showed that despite significant declines in mortality rates for late preterm and term infants since 1995, the infant mortality rate in 2002 was 3 times higher in late preterm infants than term infants (7.9 vs 2.4 deaths/1000 live births).[15] In addition, a large study involving 133,022 infants born at 34 to 40 weeks' gestation found that neonatal mortality rates were significantly higher for the late preterm infants (1.1, 1.5, and 0.5 per 1000 live births at 34, 35, and 36 weeks, respectively—compared with 0.2 per 1000 live births at 39 weeks' gestation [$P<.001$]).[6] Therefore, it is not surprising that the relative risk of death increased for every decreasing week in gestational age less than 40 weeks.[32] In addition to mortality, this group of late preterm infants adds a substantial burden to the neurocognitive and pulmonary morbidity rates in premature infants.[33]

PREVENTION OF LATE PRETERM BIRTHS

Awareness of complications associated with late preterm infants has had a remarkable effect; 2008 was the second straight year that the United States that preterm rate declined—this was the first 2- year decline in nearly 3 decades.[34] The late preterm rate had risen 25% between 1990 and 2006 (from 7.3% to 9.1%), so it was encouraging to see the 0.3% decline from 2006 to 2008 (9.1% down to 8.8%, respectively).[34] A part of this decline is attributed to a 4% decrease in preterm cesarean sections and a decrease (from 7.7% to 7.2%) of induced preterm vaginal births. In addition, noninduced vaginal births also decreased during this time period and there was no change in the proportions of multiple births (multiples are at greater risk than singletons of preterm delivery and, therefore, a change in the number of multiple pregnancies/deliveries can potentially confound systematic problems with medical practices that can affect the number of late preterm infants born each year).[34] Even though this shift in trends is encouraging, the US preterm birth rate remains high and there are changes that need to be made to continue to decrease the number of late preterm births in the United States.

One of the changes that could affect the number of late preterm deliveries is halting the practice of performing cesarean deliveries that are scheduled for the convenience of patients and physicians.[21] Other factors contributing to the high late preterm birth rate (and overall preterm birth rate) are public health issues, such as educating pregnant women about smoking cessation and expanded access to health care coverage for women of childbearing age. In addition, improved adherence to practice guidelines (ie, regarding fertility treatments and early cesarean sections and inductions and progesterone supplementation during pregnancy) can have a significant impact on the number of preterm/late preterm births each year.[21]

Another factor that could prevent late preterm deliveries is educating health care providers who make the decision to medically intervene at an earlier gestational age despite a lack of clear indication and parents who are often not aware of the potential complications associated with late preterm births.[35,36]

These issues notwithstanding, efforts to reduce prematurity are a shining example of a collaborative effort between obstetricians and neonatologists to decrease preventable morbidity. Resigning to the notion that preterm labor and delivery have a multifactorial etiology allows accepting that there are risk factors, such as genetics, predisposition to preterm labor, and environmental/socioeconomic factors, that may not be modifiable. The recent success with reducing late preterm births suggests otherwise.

REFERENCES

1. Davidoff MJ, Dias T, Damus K, et al. Changes in the gestational age distribution among U.S. singleton births: impact on rates of late preterm birth, 1992 to 2002. Semin Perinatol 2006;30(1):8–15.
2. Martin JA, Hamilton BE, Sutton PD, et al. National vital statistics reports: from the Centers for Disease Control and Prevention, National Center for Health Statistics, National Vital Statistics System. Births: final data for 2005. Natl Vital Stat Rep 2007;56(6):1–103.
3. Raju TN. Epidemiology of late preterm (near-term) births. Clin Perinatol 2006; 33(4):751–63.
4. Engle WA, Kominiarek MA. Late preterm infants, early term infants, and timing of elective deliveries. Clin Perinatol. 2008 Jun DTBS- Local Disk MEDLINE 2008; 35(2):325–41, vi.
5. Raju TN, Higgins RD, Stark AR, et al. Optimizing care and outcome for late-preterm (near-term) infants: a summary of the workshop sponsored by the National Institute of Child Health and Human Development. Pediatrics 2006; 118(3):1207–14.
6. McIntire DD, Leveno KJ. Neonatal mortality and morbidity rates in late preterm births compared with births at term. Obstet Gynecol 2008;111(1):35–41.
7. Wang ML, Dorer DJ, Fleming MP, et al. Clinical outcomes of near-term infants. Pediatrics 2004;114(2):372–6.
8. Clark RH. The epidemiology of respiratory failure in neonates born at an estimated gestational age of 34 weeks or more. J Perinatol 2005;25(4):251–7.
9. Roth-Kleiner M, Wagner BP, Bachmann D, et al. Respiratory distress syndrome in near-term babies after caesarean section. Swiss Med Wkly 2003;133(19/20):283–8.
10. Ananth CV, Gyamfi C, Jain L. Characterizing risk profiles of infants who are delivered at late preterm gestations: does it matter? Am J Obstet Gynecol 2008;199: 329–31.
11. Engle WA, Tomashek KM, Wallman C. "Late-preterm" infants: a population at risk. Pediatrics 2007;120(6):1390–401.
12. Adamkin D. Late Preterm Infants: severe hyperbilirubinemia and postnatal glucose homeostasis. J Perinatol 2009;29:S12–7.
13. Angus DC, Linde-Zwirble WT, Clermont G, et al. Epidemiology of neonatal respiratory failure in the United States: projections from California and New York. Am J Respir Crit Care Med 2001;164(7):1154–60.
14. Gilbert WM, Nesbitt TS, Danielsen B. The cost of prematurity: quantification by gestational age and birth weight. Obstet Gynecol 2003;102(3):488–92.
15. Tomashek KM, Shapiro-Mendoza CK, Davidoff MJ, et al. Differences in mortality between late-preterm and term singleton infants in the United States, 1995–2002. J Pediatr 2007;151(5):450–6, 456,e451.
16. Jain S, Cheng J. Emergency department visits and rehospitalizations in late preterm infants. Clin Perinatol 2006;33(4):935–45 [abstract xi].
17. Kuehn BM. Scientists probe the role of clinicians in rising rates of late preterm birth. JAMA 2010;303(12):1129–30.

18. Martin JA, Kirmeyer S, Osterman M, et al. Born a bit too early: recent trends in late preterm births. NCHS Data Brief 2009;24:1–8.

19. Fuchs K, Wapner R. Elective cesarean section and induction and their impact on late preterm births. Clin Perinatol 2006;33(4):793–801.

20. Bettegowda VR, Dias T, Davidoff MJ, et al. The relationship between cesarean delivery and gestational age among US singleton births. Clin Perinatol 2008; 35(2):309–23.

21. Voelker R. US Preterm Births: "D" is for Dismal. JAMA 2010;303(2):116–7.

22. Escobar GJ, Clark RH, Greene JD. Short-term outcomes of infants born at 35 and 36 weeks gestation: we need to ask more questions. Semin Perinatol 2006;30(1): 28–33.

23. Madar J, Richmond S, Hey E. Surfactant-deficient respiratory distress after elective delivery at 'term'. Acta Paediatr 1999;88(11):1244–8.

24. Hansen AK, Wisborg K, Uldbjerg N, et al. Risk of respiratory morbidity in term infants delivered by elective caesarean section: cohort study. BMJ 2008;336(7635):85–7.

25. Kolas T, Saugstad OD, Daltveit AK, et al. Planned cesarean versus planned vaginal delivery at term: comparison of newborn infant outcomes. Am J Obstet Gynecol 2006;195(6):1538–43.

26. Levine EM, Ghai V, Barton JJ, et al. Mode of delivery and risk of respiratory diseases in newborns. Obstet Gynecol 2001;97(3):439–42.

27. Morrison JJ, Rennie JM, Milton PJ. Neonatal respiratory morbidity and mode of delivery at term: influence of timing of elective caesarean section. Br J Obstet Gynaecol 1995;102(2):101–6.

28. Villar J, Carroli G, Zavaleta N, et al. Maternal and neonatal individual risks and benefits associated with caesarean delivery: multicentre prospective study. BMJ 2007;335(7628):1025.

29. Hales KA, Morgan MA, Thurnau GR. Influence of labor and route of delivery on the frequency of respiratory morbidity in term neonates. Int J Gynaecol Obstet 1993;43(1):35–40.

30. Dudell GG, Jain L. Hypoxic respiratory failure in the late preterm infant. Clin Perinatol 2006;33(4):803–30.

31. Aap, Acog. Guidelines for perinatal care. 6th edition. ELK Grove Village (IL): American Academy of Pediatrics; 2002.

32. Young PC, Glasgow TS, Li X, et al. Mortality of late-preterm (near-term) newborns in Utah. Pediatrics 2007;119(3):e659–65.

33. Kramer MS, Demissie K, Yang H, et al. The contribution of mild and moderate preterm birth to infant mortality. Fetal and Infant Health Study Group of the Canadian Perinatal Surveillance System. JAMA 2000;284(7):843–9.

34. Martin JA, Osterman MJ, Sutton PD. Are preterm births on the decline in the United States? Recent data from the National Vital Statistics System. NCHS Data Brief 2010;39:1–8.

35. Kuehn BM. Groups take aim at US preterm birth rate. JAMA 2006;296(24): 2907–8.

36. Greene MF. Making small risks even smaller. N Engl J Med 2009;360(2):183–4.

Term Pregnancy: Time for a Redefinition

Steven L. Clark, MD[a,*], Alan R. Fleischman, MD[b]

KEYWORDS

• Term pregnancy • Stillbirths • Preterm birth • Infants

Historically, term pregnancy has been defined as one in which 260 to 294 days have elapsed since the first day of the last menstrual period.[1–3] Infants born before this interval (<37 completed weeks of gestation) have traditionally been classified as preterm infants, whereas those delivered beyond this interval (42 weeks and beyond) are designated as postterm infants. However, these definitions are largely arbitrary. Furthermore, although the potential hazards of both preterm birth and postterm pregnancy have been long recognized, little attention has, until recently, been given to the differential morbidity experienced by neonates born at different times within the 5-week interval classically considered term gestation.[3] There is a growing body of evidence demonstrating the existence of significant differences both in the antenatal risks faced by such fetuses and in their outcomes as infants. Because the designation term pregnancy and the distinction between term, preterm, and postterm pregnancy carry with them significant clinical implications with respect to the management of pregnancy complications, the timing of both elective and indicated delivery, and the oversight of postterm pregnancy, a reevaluation of the concept of term pregnancy in light of current data is needed.

HISTORICAL PERSPECTIVES

"We possess no reliable means of estimating the exact date (of confinement) but are obliged to content ourselves with the method proposed by Naegele, which is based upon the belief that labor occurs two hundred eighty days from the beginning of the last menstrual period." So wrote Williams[4] over a century ago in the first edition of what was to become the classic text, *Williams Obstetrics*. Under these circumstances, it is not surprising that Williams was vague in his definition of both preterm and post-term birth, although clearly recognizing even then the dangers of both. It was not until half a century later, in 1948, that the World Health Assembly proposed an international definition of a premature infant as one with a birth weight of less than 2500 g and/or

[a] Women's and Children's Clinical Services Group, Hospital Corporation of America, 217 Melrose Road, PO Box 404, Twin Bridges, MT 59754, USA
[b] March of Dimes, Albert Einstein College of Medicine, 1275 Mamaroneck Avenue White Plains, NY 10605, USA
* Corresponding author.
E-mail address: steven.clark1@hcahealthcare.com

Clin Perinatol 38 (2011) 557–564
doi:10.1016/j.clp.2011.06.014
0095-5108/11/$ – see front matter © 2011 Elsevier Inc. All rights reserved.

a gestational age of less than 38 completed weeks.[3-6] In 1961, a report by the Expert Committee on Maternal and Child Health of the World Health Organization first recognized a distinction between premature and low-birth-weight infants.[3-6] In 1970, the Second European Congress of Perinatal Medicine somewhat arbitrarily changed the boundary between preterm and term infants to 37 weeks' rather than 38 weeks' gestation.[3,7] Accepted by the US National Center for Health Statistics in 1972, this recommendation seems to be the basis for the current definition of prematurity recognized by both the American College of Obstetricians and Gynecologists and the American Academy of Pediatrics.[3]

In contrast, the precise origins of the traditional definition of postterm pregnancy as one exceeding 42 completed weeks' gestation are somewhat more obscure but seem to have originated in a report from Sweden in 1956 demonstrating a dramatic increase in perinatal mortality seen beyond this time during the years 1943 to 1952.[3,8]

Thus, current definitions of both preterm and postterm pregnancy are either completely arbitrary or based primarily on data collected 40 to 50 years ago and then perpetuated to the point of canonization without serious reassessment of the validity of such distinctions.[9-11] Considering that ultrasonographic dating of pregnancy was then virtually unknown, current techniques for monitoring high-risk pregnancies were nonexistent, newborn intensive care was primitive by current standards, and perinatal outcomes were primarily based on crude assessments of mortality rather than more subtle indices of long-term morbidity, these definitions would seem to have limited relevance to the practice of twenty-first century medicine. Indeed, a serious examination of available data suggests that perpetuation of these antiquated definitions may result in significant harm.[3]

PRETERM BIRTH

The short-term and long-term implications of preterm birth before 37 completed weeks' gestation are well recognized. The recent examination of the outcomes of larger preterm infants born between 34 weeks and 36 weeks 6 days reveals that even these infants suffer significantly increased mortality and morbidity compared with term infants.[12-15] The complications include an increased incidence of transient tachypnea of the newborn, respiratory distress syndrome, pulmonary hypertension, apnea, temperature instability, jaundice, and poor feeding.[16-18] Perhaps more troubling has been the recent recognition that such infants are also prone to poorer long-term neurologic performance, including cerebral palsy, lower reading and math scores, and higher participation in special education during early grades.[19-25] This problem is of special concern given the relatively large percentage of preterm infants born beyond 34 weeks' gestation. Indeed, one recent report demonstrated that infants born between 34 and 37 weeks' gestation accounted for 75% of all preterm deliveries in the United States.[21] Such abnormal developmental findings should not come as a surprise because there is an increase of 35% in brain size and a 5-fold increase in white matter volume during the last 6 to 8 weeks of pregnancy.[24] This recognition of morbidity has led to the general acceptance of a new gestational subclass within the definition of preterm, the late preterm infant, defined as a child born between 34 weeks 0 days and 36 weeks 6 days of gestation.[20,22] Making this distinction allows more careful analysis of this significant group of premature infants.

EARLY TERM BIRTH

Most studies examining long-term neurologic outcomes of preterm infants published before the last several years did not include infants born after 37 weeks' gestation, apparently out of deference to the traditional definition of prematurity. However, recent reports focusing on differential outcomes of term infants have demonstrated significant short-term morbidity, including respiratory distress and need for mechanical ventilation as well as increased neonatal intensive care admission rates, for infants born before 39 completed weeks compared with those born beyond this point **(Fig. 1)**.[26–32] Because these results were remarkably consistent in a series of unselected (indicated and elective) repeat cesarean deliveries and a series of purely elective deliveries, it seems that these adverse outcomes are primarily related to gestational age per se, rather than the indication for delivery before 39 weeks.[30,31] In addition, an analysis of US singleton live births at term between 1995 and 2001 found that the mortality rate decreased with increasing gestational age from 0.66 per 1000 live births at 37 weeks to 0.33 per 1000 live births at 39 weeks and remained stable from 39 to 40 weeks.[27] The rates for neonatal infection and sudden infant death syndrome also decreased with increasing gestational age. A subsequent analysis of the 2001 National Center for Health Statistics birth cohort of singleton gestations also found increased neonatal and infant mortality rates for births at 37 and 38 weeks' gestation compared with 39 weeks' gestation.[26] Thus, the current data are unequivocal in documenting increased morbidity and mortality among infants born at term between 37 and 38 weeks' gestation compared with those born at or beyond 39 completed weeks.

Long-term studies of neurologic function in infants born between 37 and 38 weeks compared with those born at 39 to 40 weeks modeled after studies recently conducted in late preterm infants are lacking at present. However, the biologic continuum evident in early human brain growth suggests that findings similar to those observed in late preterm infants might be expected among term infants born before 39 weeks' gestation. Although the frequency of such long-term learning disabilities are expected to be lower in the 37- to 38-week age groups, the fact that purely elective delivery before 39 weeks' gestation may involve 10% to 15% of all children born in the United States makes these observations of particular potential relevance for the 4 million

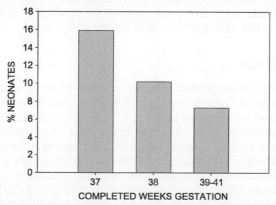

Fig. 1. Adverse neonatal outcomes and newborn intensive care admissions for early term deliveries compared with neonates delivered between 39 and 41 completed weeks' gestation. (*Data from* Clark SL, Miller DD, Belfort MA, et al. Neonatal and maternal outcomes associated with elective term delivery. Am J Obstet Gynecol 2009;200:156,e1–4; and Tita AT, Landon MB, Spong CY, et al. Timing of elective repeat cesarean delivery at term and neonatal outcomes. N Engl J Med 2009;360:111–20.)

children currently born annually in the United States.[30] At present, the risk of long-term intellectual impairment in infants born between 37 and 38 weeks remains biologically plausible but speculative. However, the clear presence of short-term morbidity and mortality among such infants, as well as the increased risk of cesarean delivery associated with induction of labor should be sufficient to interdict the practice of elective delivery before 39 weeks' gestation.[30,33,34] Changing such a well-established but misguided practice is difficult and seems to be best accomplished using an approach that includes both physician and patient education and hospital oversight.[35,36] Elective delivery before 39 weeks' gestation has been recently adopted as a national quality metric by both the National Quality Forum and the Joint Commission.[37,38]

An additional concern is the inaccuracy of gestational dating associated with those pregnancies that do not have the benefit of early ultrasonographic confirmation. Because the estimated date of delivery can vary as much as 2 weeks based on history alone or ultrasonographic values late in pregnancy, elective delivery at 37 or 38 weeks can inadvertently result in a preterm birth at 35 to 36 weeks' gestation.

Concerns have been expressed regarding a possible adverse effect of delayed delivery beyond 37 weeks on the rate of stillbirths.[39] No evidence exists to support such a hypothesis. Because delivery at any gestational age by definition eliminates the possibility of stillbirth beyond that point, some cases of stillbirth must occur at 37 to 39 weeks' gestation that would have been avoided with earlier delivery.[35] However, this number is sufficiently small to be statistically undetectable in a recent series of almost half a million deliveries.[35] In addition, recent data have demonstrated that the small number of unexpected stillbirths occurring between 37 and 39 weeks' gestation (0.8/1000 births) is counterbalanced by an excess number of cases of infant death, including sudden infant death syndrome (2.7–4.1/1000) occurring in infants born within this 2-week interval.[26,40]

In terms of both neonatal morbidity and mortality, a 37-week threshold for the definition of term pregnancy has no biologic basis; rather, there seems to be a clear and continuous relationship between gestational age and both neonatal morbidity and mortality from early pregnancy onward, with a nadir at about 39 weeks' gestation.[40,41] Based on such considerations, the authors strongly support the use of early term to describe gestations between 37 weeks 0 days and 38 weeks 6 days to avoid the inaccurate and potentially detrimental connotation of equality of outcomes beyond 37 weeks implicit in the traditional definition of term pregnancy.[3]

POSTTERM PREGNANCY

Postterm pregnancy is associated with an increase in antepartum and neonatal death, intrauterine growth restriction, oligohydramnios, meconium aspiration, macrosomia, and the need for cesarean delivery.[42–47] Such clinical morbidity has pathophysiologic underpinnings in an increased prevalence of placental apoptosis and higher umbilical cord erythropoietin levels in pregnancies extending beyond 41 weeks. Newer techniques for monitoring prolonged pregnancies and an increased willingness to intervene with delivery have reduced absolute perinatal morbidity and mortality in these infants. However, relative morbidity and mortality associated with pregnancies that extend beyond 40 and 41 weeks' gestation continue to be represented by an increasing biologic continuum with no clear clinical threshold.[40,41] As elegantly demonstrated by Smith, even the actual risks of pregnancy extending beyond 40 to 41 weeks may currently be muted by the common practice of delivery before this time, a practice so prevalent that the mean gestational age of infants born in the United States has now been reduced from 40 to 39 weeks' gestation

(Fig. 2).[10,40] Thus, the arbitrary use of 42 weeks and 0 days to define a biologic threshold for risk of morbidity or death is not supported by the available literature; most recent data support a significantly increased risk of adverse perinatal outcomes beginning by 41 weeks' gestation.

WHAT'S IN A NAME

Despite the biologic continuity of risk associated with gestational age, some categorical delineation of gestational age is necessary both for the collection and comparison of perinatal outcomes data and to guide clinical practice. However, the available data suggest that the use of 37 and 42 weeks as bookends defining a normal duration of pregnancy is really no longer scientifically supportable. The use of term to describe all pregnancies in this 5-week range has several potential hazards that are seen regularly in clinical practice and take the form of both overintervention and underintervention. At one end of the spectrum, many women are delivered electively once the biologically nonexistent 37-week threshold has been attained, a practice encouraged by the normalization of deviance relating to an anecdotal preponderance of good short-term outcomes seen with this practice.[30,35] Similarly, well-meaning clinicians may inappropriately delay delivery of a subset of pregnancies complicated by fetal growth restriction or maternal preeclampsia waiting for the magical 37-week line to be crossed. At the other end of the spectrum, physicians may fail to realize the reality of the risk associated with pregnancies continuing beyond 41 weeks because the fetus is, technically, not postterm. Patients may also be inappropriately influenced in their decisions and the pressures they bring to bear on their health care providers by a mistaken belief that the 37- to 42-week interval has some rational physiologic basis.[36]

The available data suggest that the present definition of term pregnancy requires subclassification based on the epidemiologic and biologic evidence (**Table 1**). Such a modification of terminology does not imply any immediate change in clinical management of pregnancies between 37 and 42 weeks' gestation beyond that justified by appropriately conducted gestational age–specific clinical trials. However, such

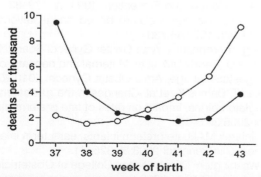

Fig. 2. Perinatal mortality and gestational age. Open circles represent the cumulative probability of perinatal death × 1000. Closed circles represent perinatal mortality rate per 1000 births. (*From* Smith GC. Life table analysis of the risk of perinatal death at term and postterm in singleton pregnancies. Am J Obstet Gynecol 2001;184:489; with permission.)

Table 1
Proposed definitions

Description	Gestational Age
Preterm	<36 wk and 6 d
Late preterm	34 wk and 0 d to 36 wk and 6 d
Term	37 wk and 0 d to 40 wk and 6 d
Early term	37 wk and 0 d to 38 wk and 6 d
Postterm	>41 wk

a change would serve to bring the description of gestational age in line with biologic reality and would enhance both research and clinical practice to the betterment of the fetus/infants.

REFERENCES

1. World Health Organization (WHO). International statistical classification of diseases and related health problems (rev. 10, vols. 1 and 2, ICD-10). Geneva (Switzerland): WHO; 1992.
2. American Academy of Pediatrics/American College of Obstetricians and Gynecologists. Appendix D: standard terminology for reporting of reproductive health statistics in the United States. In: Guidelines for perinatal care. 6th edition. Elk Grove (IL): American Academy of Pediatrics/American College of Obstetricians and Gynecologists; 2007. p. 389–404.
3. Fleishman AR, Oinuma M, Clark SL. Rethinking the definition of term pregnancy. Obstet Gynecol 2010;116:136–9.
4. Williams JW. Williams obstetrics. London. 1st edition. New York: D. Appleton and Company; 1903.
5. Drillien CM. Chapter 4: the low-birth weight infant. In: Cockburn F, Drillien CM, editors. Neonatal medicine. Osney Mead (United Kingdom): Blackwell Scientific Publications; 1974. p. 51–61.
6. Blackmore CA, Rowley DL, Kiely JL. Preterm birth. In: From data to action: CDC's Public health surveillance for women, infants and children. Atlanta (GA): The Centers for Disease Control and Prevention; 1994. p. 179–83.
7. Working party to discuss nomenclature based on gestational age and birthweight. Arch Dis Child 1970;45:730.
8. Lindell A. Prolonged pregnancy. Acta Obstet Gynecol Scand 1956;35:136–63.
9. Bailit JL, Gregory KD, Reddy UM, et al. Maternal and neonatal outcomes by labor onset type and gestational age. Am J Obstet Gynecol 2010;202:245,e1–12.
10. Davidoff MJ, Dias T, Damus K, et al. Changes in the gestational age distribution among U.S. singleton births: impact on rates of late preterm birth, 1992 to 2002. Semin Perinatol 2006;30:8–15.
11. Engle WA, Kominiarek MA. Late preterm infants, early term infants, and timing of elective deliveries. Clin Perinatol 2008;35:325–41.
12. Preterm labor. Washington, DC: American College of Obstetricians and Gynecologists; 1995. Technical Bulletin #206.
13. Tomashek KM, Shapiro-Mendoza CK, Davidoff MJ, et al. Differences in mortality between late-preterm and term singleton infants in the United States, 1995–2002. J Pediatr 2007;151(5):450–6.

14. Engle WA. A recommendation for the definition of "late preterm" (near-term) and the birth weight-gestational age classification system. Semin Perinatol 2006;30:2–7.

15. Raju TN, Higgins RD, Stark AR, et al. Optimizing care and outcome for late-preterm (near-term) infants: a summary of the workshop sponsored by the National Institute of Child Health and Human Development. Pediatrics 2006;118:1207–14.

16. McIntire DD, Leveno KJ. Neonatal mortality and morbidity rates in late preterm births compared with births at term. Obstet Gynecol 2008;111:35–41.

17. Hibbard JU, Wilkins I, Sun L, et al. Consortium on Safe Labor. Respiratory morbidity in late preterm infants. JAMA 2010;304:419–25.

18. Colin AA, McEvoyu C, Castile RG. Respiratory morbidity and lung function in preterm infants of 32–36 weeks gestational age. Pediatrics 2010;126:115–28.

19. Gurka MJ, LoCasale-Crouch J, Blackman JA. Long term cognitive, achievement, socioemotional and behavioral development of healthy late preterm infants. Arch Pediatr Adolesc Med 2010;114:525–32.

20. Morse SB, Zheng H, Tany Y, et al. Early school-age outcomes of late preterm infants. Pediatrics 2009;123:e622–9.

21. Melamed N, Klinger G, Tenenbaum-Gavish K, et al. Short term neonatal outcome in low risk spontaneous, singleton, late preterm deliveries. Obstet Gynecol 2009; 114:253–60.

22. Engle WA, Tomushek KM, Walman C. "Late preterm" infants: a population at risk. Pediatrics 2007;120:1398–401.

23. Chyi LJ, Lee HC, Hintz SR, et al. School outcomes of late preterm infants: special needs and challenges for infants born at 32–36 weeks gestation. J Pediatr 2008; 153:25.

24. Jain L. School outcomes in late preterm infants: a cause for concern. J Pediatr 2008;153:5–6.

25. Petrini JR, Dias T, McCormick MC, et al. Increased risk of adverse neurological development for late preterm infants. J Pediatr 2009;154(2):169–76.

26. Reddy UM, Ko CW, Willinger M. "Early" term births (37–38 weeks) are associated with increased mortality. Am J Obstet Gynecol 2006;195:S202.

27. Zhang X, Kramer MS. Variations in mortality and morbidity by gestational age among infants born at term. J Pediatr 2009;154:358–62, 362,e1.

28. Hansen AK, Wisborg K, Uldbjerg N, et al. Elective caesarean section and respiratory morbidity in the term and near-term neonate. Acta Obstet Gynecol Scand 2007;86:389–94.

29. Morrison JJ, Rennie JM, Milton PJ. Neonatal respiratory morbidity and mode of delivery at term: influence of timing of elective caesarean section. Br J Obstet Gynaecol 1995;102:101–6.

30. Clark SL, Miller DD, Belfort MA, et al. Neonatal and maternal outcomes associated with elective term delivery. Am J Obstet Gynecol 2009;200:156,e1–4.

31. Tita AT, Landon MB, Spong CY, et al. Timing of elective repeat cesarean delivery at term and neonatal outcomes. N Engl J Med 2009;360:111–20.

32. Wilmink FA, Hukkelhoven CW, Lunshof S, et al. Neonatal outcome following elective cesarean section beyond 37 weeks of gestation: a 7-year retrospective analysis of a national registry. Am J Obstet Gynecol 2010;202:250,e1–8.

33. ACOG Committee on Practice Bulletins—Obstetrics. ACOG practice bulletin. No. 107, August 2009. Induction of labor. Obstet Gynecol 2009;114:386–97.

34. Glantz JC. Term labor induction compared with expectant management. Obstet Gynecol 2010;115:70–6.

35. Clark SL, Frye DR, Meyers JA, et al. Reduction in elective delivery prior to 39 weeks gestation—comparative effectiveness of 3 approaches to change

and the impact on neonatal outcome and stillbirth. Am J Obstet Gynecol 2010; 203:449,e1–6.

36. Goldenberg RL, McClure EM, Bhattacharya A, et al. Women's perceptions regarding the safety of births at various gestational ages. Obstet Gynecol 2009;114:1254–8.

37. The National Quality Forum. NQF #0469. Elective delivery prior to 39 completed weeks gestation. Endorsed on: October 28, 2008. Available at: http://qualityforum. org/Measures_List.aspx. Accessed January 20, 2009.

38. The Joint Commission. Specifications manual for Joint Commission National Quality Core Measures (2010A1). Available at: http://www.jointcommission.org/ PerformanceMeasurement/PerformanceMeasurement/Perinatal+Care+Core+ Measure+Set.htm. Accessed January 20, 2009.

39. Greene MF. Making small risks even smaller. N Engl J Med 2009;360:183–4.

40. Smith GC. Life table analysis of the risk of perinatal death at term and post term in singleton pregnancies. Am J Obstet Gynecol 2001;184:489.

41. Heimstad R, Romundstad PR, Eik-Nes SH, et al. Outcome of pregnancies beyond 37 weeks of gestation. Obstet Gynecol 2006;108:500–8.

42. Caughey AB, Musci TJ. Complications of term pregnancies beyond 37 weeks of gestation. Obstet Gynecol 2004;103:57.

43. Clausson B, Cnattingus S, Axelsson O. Outcomes of post-term births: the role of fetal growth restriction and malformations. Obstet Gynecol 1999;94:758.

44. Hilder L, Costeloe K, Thilaganathan B. Prolonged pregnancy: evaluating gestation-specific risks of fetal and infant mortality. Br J Obstet Gynaecol 1998;105:169–73.

45. Alexander JM, McIntire DD, Levino KJ. Forty weeks and beyond: pregnancy outcomes by week of gestation. Obstet Gynecol 2000;96:291.

46. Nakling J, Backe B. Pregnancy risk increases from 41 weeks of gestation. Acta Obstet Gynecol Scand 2006;85:663–8.

47. Olesen AW, Westergaard JG, Olsen J. Perinatal and maternal complications related to post-term delivery: a national register based study, 1978–1993. Am J Obstet Gynecol 2003;189:222–7.

Quality Improvement Opportunities to Prevent Preterm Births

Bryan T. Oshiro, MD[a],*, Scott D. Berns, MD, MPH[b,c]

KEYWORDS

• Prematurity • Preterm • Quality improvement

Prematurity (or preterm birth) continues to be one of the most common complications plaguing obstetrics, and is the leading cause of perinatal morbidity and mortality in the United States. The financial impact of preterm birth is also enormous. The Institute of Medicine estimated the annual societal cost to be at least $26.2 billion.[1] In recent years there has been a great deal of research improving our ability to understand the various causes of preterm labor and premature rupture of the membranes, and improving our predictive and diagnostic abilities. Although there has been a great deal of effort, attention, and importance placed on trying to prevent preterm deliveries through research and by organizations such as the Institute of Medicine, the March of Dimes, and the National Institute of Child Health and Human Development to name but a few, there had been very little progress in decreasing the overall preterm birth rate in the United States until 2006 when preterm birth rates began to fall slightly. Between 2006 and 2009 the preterm birth rates in the United States decreased annually and went from 12.8% to 12.2%.[2] Even though randomized prospective trials using 17-hydroxyprogesterone caproate (17-P) in patients with prior spontaneous labor showed a significant decrease in recurrent preterm birth, this has not been universally implemented 8 years after the first trial was published.[3] Indeed, it has been estimated that the routine use of 17-P could reduce the preterm birth rate by 2% and prevent as many as 10,000 preterm births annually in the United States.[4] Thus, widespread use of 17-P could help to achieve the Healthy People 2020 objective of a national preterm birth rate of 11.4%.[5]

However, preventing preterm birth is a complex problem that cannot be addressed by a single approach such as giving progesterone; as progesterone has not been

The authors have nothing to disclose.

[a] Department of Obstetrics and Gynecology, Loma Linda University School of Medicine, 11234 Anderson Street, Suite 3400, Loma Linda, CA 92354, USA

[b] March of Dimes National Office, 1275 Mamaroneck Avenue, White Plains, NY 20605, USA

[c] Department Pediatrics, Warren Alpert Medical School of Brown University, 593 Eddy Street, Providence, RI, USA

* Corresponding author.

E-mail address: boshiro@llu.edu

Clin Perinatol 38 (2011) 565–578

doi:10.1016/j.clp.2011.06.010

0095-5108/11/$ – see front matter © 2011 Elsevier Inc. All rights reserved.

perinatology.theclinics.com

shown to be efficacious in all cases, such as in patients with a twin gestation.[6] Even evaluating who is at risk and diagnosing preterm labor can be challenging.

Quality improvement measures have been developed and employed in many areas of medicine with great success, such as in preventing line sepsis or ventilator-associated pneumonias in intensive care units.[7,8] However, few quality improvement projects have been implemented in preventing prematurity. Quality improvement projects are designed to improve the performance of a system, and work well when there is little controversy and operate according to existing knowledge. Therefore, the goal of quality improvement in terms of preventing premature delivery rests on taking the existing scientific knowledge and applying it systematically to reduce premature deliveries and, conversely, to eliminate practices that are harmful or ineffective. Due to the complex nature of the causes of prematurity, developing and instituting a quality improvement program to prevent preterm births can be challenging. However, using quality improvement principles and techniques learned from patient safety may prove invaluable in rapidly implementing and translating evidence-based preterm birth prevention methodologies onto the front line of routine patient care.

DEFINING QUALITY IMPROVEMENT

In striving to identify quality improvement strategies to prevent preterm birth, it is important to first define "quality" and subsequently "quality improvement." *Quality* has been defined by the Institute of Medicine (IOM) as "the degree to which health services for individuals and populations increase the likelihood of desired health outcomes and are consistent with current professional knowledge."[9] In addition, the IOM states that safety is "freedom from accidental injury" and not freedom from errors.[10] Quality encompasses doing the *right thing* (the needed health services), at the *right time* (when needed), and in the *right way* (appropriate interventions), to achieve the best possible results. Patient safety involves identifying adverse events, analyzing why these events occur, and putting mechanisms in place to prevent these adverse events.

Early efforts to improve the quality of care in health care focused primarily on evaluating errors and in identifying and eliminating substandard practices, commonly known as *quality assurance*. This model was the first to be adopted by the Joint Commission in the 1950s. The focus therefore was on eliminating outlier events, and often involved trying to determine who was at fault after something went wrong. These efforts did not make systematic improvements in the overall quality of care. James Reason, a clinical psychologist, theorized that these traditional efforts to decrease errors by solely focusing on individuals and individual efforts would not be effective, as humans are fallible. People eventually will make a mistake. Therefore he reasoned that systems need to be created to decrease unwanted variability and increase the reliability in the system in which we deliver care.[11] The IOM reported in *Crossing the Quality Chasm* that "If we want safer, higher-quality care, we will need to have redesigned systems of care."[12]

In 1966 Avedis Donabedian described a model of quality improvement, which consisted of 3 components that would enable global change in improving quality. As Donabedian explained, structure, process, and outcomes define the system of care, and all play a role in measuring and evaluating quality.[13] *Structure* assesses who is providing care, in what capacity, and where; *Process* identifies how the care is being provided and may assess the interactions between patients and providers; while *Outcomes* evaluate the impact on care through measurement of a patient or group of patients' health status. This concept comprised one of the first efforts at improving care across the system.

Fundamental to improving health care delivery is to realize that a problem exists. Thus, *quality improvement* is about understanding what the problems are, knowing what the goal is, addressing and improving system performance, then measuring the outcome of the performance improvement plan. At the core of improving system performance and systems change is reducing variability. These tenets were born from the work of Shewhart, Deming, and Juran in the early part of the twentieth century, with their focus on increasing the efficiency of American industry.[14] These investigators identified the need to minimize the opportunity for human error by standardizing and streamlining production processes, which led to decreased variability and overall system improvement.[15] In *Crossing the Quality Chasm*, the IOM made it clear that the health care system needs to be better designed to maximize safety, essentially making it "harder for people to do something wrong and easier for them to do it right."[12]

Furthermore, the IOM committee proposed 6 aims to improve health care delivery for the twenty-first century, stating that health care should be:

1. Safe—avoiding injuries to patients from the care that is intended to help them
2. Effective—providing services based on scientific knowledge to all who could benefit and refraining from providing services to those not likely to benefit (avoiding underuse and overuse, respectively)
3. Patient-centered—providing care that is respectful of and responsive to individual patient preferences, needs, and values, and ensuring that patient values guide all clinical decisions
4. Timely—reducing waits and sometimes harmful delays for both those who receive and those who give care
5. Efficient—avoiding waste, including waste of equipment, supplies, ideas, and energy
6. Equitable—providing care that does not vary in quality because of personal characteristics such as gender, ethnicity, geographic location, and socioeconomic status.

A health care system that could improve in these 6 dimensions would provide a safer environment to provide care. To achieve such a system, the IOM committee also proposed the following rules to redesign and improve care for patients[12]:

1. *Care should be based on continuous healing relationships.* Patients should receive care whenever they need it and in many forms, not just face-to-face visits. Health care should be available at all times, every day or night.
2. *Care should be customized according to patients' needs and values.* The system should be designed to meet the most common types of needs, but should be able to respond to individual patient choices and preferences.
3. *The patient is the source of control.* Patients should be given the necessary information and the opportunity to exercise the degree of control they choose over health care decisions that affect them.
4. *Shared knowledge and the free flow of information.* Patients should have unfettered access to their own medical information and to clinical knowledge. Clinicians and patients should communicate effectively and share information.
5. *Care should be evidence-based.* Patients should receive care based on the best available scientific knowledge. It should not vary illogically from clinician to clinician or from place to place.
6. *Ensure safety as a system priority.* Patients should be safe from injury caused by the health care system.
7. *Assure transparency to assist with informed decisions.* The system should make information available to patients and their families that allows them to make

informed decisions when selecting a health plan, hospital, or clinical practice, or when choosing among alternative treatments.

8. *Patient needs should be anticipated.* The system should anticipate the needs of the patient rather than reacting to them.

9. *Continuous decreased waste of resources.* The system should not waste resources or patients' time.

10. *Collaboration and cooperation should occur among clinicians and institutions.* Clinicians and institutions should actively collaborate and communicate to ensure an appropriate exchange of information and coordination of care.

However, these changes must be accepted and implemented by fallible human beings. Physicians, nurses, and other health care providers are highly trained and many times are indoctrinated with a sense that errors can be avoided by individual effort.[16] In running complex operations such as in operating nuclear-powered warships, the inevitability of failure has been anticipated and safeguards to avoid catastrophic failures have been built in. To date, the navy has not had a single disaster involving a nuclear reactor. Organizations that operate under such hazardous conditions without or lower than expected errors are known as high-reliability organizations (HROs). According to the Agency for Healthcare Research and Quality, the common features of HROs are[17]:

- Preoccupation with failure: the acknowledgment of the high-risk, error-prone nature of an organization's activities and the determination to achieve and deliver safe care
- Commitment to resilience: the development of capacities to detect unexpected threats and contain them before they cause harm, or bounce back when they do
- Sensitivity to operations: HROs are mindful of the complexity of the systems in which they work and strive to quickly identify abnormalities and problems in the system to reduce or eliminate errors
- A culture of safety: members are free to draw attention to potential hazards or from actual failures without fear of censure from management
- Reluctance to simplify: HROs refuse to simplify or ignore the explanations for difficulties and problems that they face.

If we are to overcome the challenges of managing a complicated problem such as decreasing preterm births, we must become an HRO. What are the steps then needed to implement quality initiatives and move us in this direction? Leape[16] suggests the following:

- Reduce reliance on memory: by using checklists, protocols, and computerized decision aids
- Improve information access: information should be displayed where and when it is needed in a form that is easy to access
- Error proofing: critical tasks should be structured so errors cannot be made
- Standardization: increases both the efficiency and the reliability of delivering quality care
- Training: instruction of health care workers in procedures or problem solving should include greater emphasis on possible errors and how to prevent them.

However, the most important and fundamental change that is needed if there is to be meaningful progress in providing safe and consistent care is a cultural one. Health care providers need to accept that medical errors are inevitable and cannot be avoided by being more diligent or making more of an effort. Errors must be accepted as evidence of system flaws.[16] Strong leadership is important in implementing quality changes. It is necessary to remove obstacles, energize constituents, create a vision, and implement quality standards and guidelines.

Finally, to actualize and institute quality improvement projects, certain quality improvement approaches and tools can be used. Ellsbury and Ursprung[18] have suggested the following "seven questions to consider when designing a quality initiative":

1. What problem should one select?
2. Who will be on the project team?
3. What is the goal?
4. What will one measure?
5. How will one analyze the measurements?
6. What changes will one make to create an improvement?
7. How will one test the changes?

Next, in implementing change, an efficient "trial-and-learning" or "cycles of testing" methodology is employed. One such example is the PDSA (Plan-Do-Study-Act) tool or paradigm. This concept was originally described by Walter Shewhart of Bell Laboratories in the 1930s and was later refined by W. Edward Deming. This model was used effectively by Toyota, and is summarized in **Box 1**.[19]

Keeping these principles and questions in mind, in creating a quality improvement initiative, goal(s) need to be clearly elucidated. Measurement is the key to assessing change and improving performance, including decreased variability. The ultimate goal of quality improvement in health care, including reducing preterm births, is to improve the consistent delivery of evidence-based care and providing it at the right time, in the right place, and in the right manner. A detailed example of this

---

Box 1
PDSA summary

Plan

- State the objectives of the cycle
- Make predictions about what will happen next and why
- Develop a plan to carry out the changes (Who? What? Where? What data needs to be collected?)

Do

- Introduce the change(s)
- Collect data
- Document problems and unexpected observations
- Begin analysis of the data

Study

- Complete the analysis of the data
- Summarize what was learned

Act

- What modifications should be made?
- What will happen in the next cycle?

methodology to decrease elective deliveries before 39 weeks' gestational age is provided in Appendix A.

IDENTIFYING QUALITY IMPROVEMENT OPPORTUNITIES TO PREVENT PRETERM BIRTHS

The overarching goal of prematurity prevention is to decrease perinatal morbidity and mortality. To do this we must understand and manage the process. Because the current process for prematurity prevention is ambiguous and inconsistent, it becomes a challenge to measure. Thus an important step would be to apply what is known to be effective or beneficial and to eliminate that which is shown to be ineffective. As these can be very complex, involving various aspects of health care delivery, the application of the quality improvement process should target various segments at various entry points into the health care system. These include prenatal care office visits and management in labor and delivery—at postpartum both immediately and in the office, and at preconception or interconception time periods. Care should be standardized as much as possible to reduce variation. Once variation is reduced, performance can then be measured. Quality improvement opportunities to prevent preterm births[14] are listed in **Box 2**.

FRAMEWORK FOR QUALITY IMPROVEMENT TO PREVENT PRETERM BIRTHS
Describe the System

Describing the system can be done through a variety of methods that may include flowcharts, optimal attributes (eg, care that is effective, efficient, equitable, family-centered, safe, and timely), or key attributes. The description of the system is always in the context of the aim of the quality improvement initiative. For example, the flow-chart shown in **Fig. 1**, in the form of a "fishbone" diagram, illustrates the components of a system to eliminate nonmedically indicated (elective) deliveries before 39 weeks' gestational age.[20]

This system can also be described through a listing of key attributes in approaching this quality improvement initiative:

- Clinician education: provide clinicians with data about patient complications
- Patient education: provide women with educational materials that define "full term"
- Public awareness campaign: use public service announcements and social marketing to educate the public
- Elective delivery hospital policy: establish clear policies around indications for deliveries before 39 weeks of completed gestation
- Use standard forms for scheduling elective induction or cesarean section: consistently provide guidance on indications for deliveries before 39 weeks of completed gestation
- Physician leadership: hospital leader(s) clearly identified, specifically those who can approve "exceptions" to the policy
- Data collection forms and trend charts: collect process and outcome data over time and share with clinicians and staff.

Determine the Performance of the System Over Time to Reduce Preterm Births

A set of measures that balances clinical outcomes should be developed. In a quality improvement effort to reduce preterm births, a balanced set of measures may include:

- Percent reduction in preterm birth
- Percent of eligible women receiving the quality improvement clinical intervention

- Patient and/or family satisfaction with the intervention
- Staff productivity and/or efficiency
- Staff satisfaction with the preterm birth reduction initiative, including their role in the intervention
- The quality improvement initiative's impact on cost (to patient, provider/hospital, and/or insurer).

Box 2
Quality improvement opportunities to prevent preterm births

- Optimizing preconception, interconception, and prenatal health
  - Identify risk factors for preterm birth (eg, previous preterm birth)
  - Proper pregnancy spacing
  - Smoking cessation
  - Teen pregnancy prevention
  - Screening for illicit substances
- Access
  - Insurance coverage for everyone
  - Provider availability
  - Early entry into prenatal care
- Standardizing assessments
  - Early ultrasound dating
  - Standardized assessments incorporated into prenatal and antepartum care (eg, decreasing elective deliveries before 39 weeks)
- Increased use of fetal fibronectin testing and vaginal ultrasound to measure cervical length for patients presenting with symptoms of preterm labor
- Increased use of 17α-hydroxyprogesterone caproate administration
- Cerclage placements in appropriate candidates
- Tightened guidelines in assisted reproductive technologies
- Appropriate use of tocolytics
- Therapies to optimize the neonate
  - Antenatal steroids
  - Group B *Streptococcus* screening and prophylaxis
  - Antibiotics for preterm premature rupture of membranes
  - Magnesium sulfate for neuroprotection
  - Maternal transfer to a tertiary care hospital capable of taking care of the neonate
- Eliminating ineffective treatments
  - Hydration
  - Bed rest
  - Prolonged tocolytic use

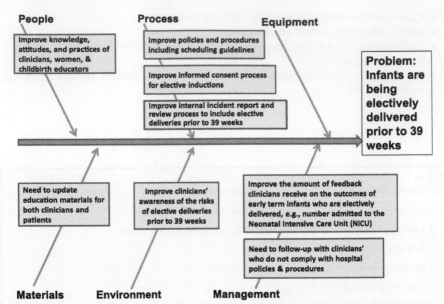

Fig. 1. Fishbone diagram. (*From* Main E, Oshiro B, Chagolla B, et al. Elimination of non-medically indicated (elective) deliveries before 39 weeks gestational age. A California tool-kit to transform maternity care. Available at: www.marchofdimes.com/professionals/medicalresources_39weeks.html; with permission.)

Determine Whether Changes in the System Result in Improvement Over Time

The example in **Fig. 2** shows the impact over time of a quality improvement initiative, beginning in January 2001, at Intermountain Healthcare hospitals to reduce elective deliveries before 39 weeks' gestation.[21]

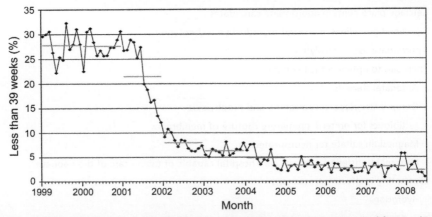

Fig. 2. Decreasing elective deliveries before 39 weeks. Intermountain Healthcare. (*Data from* Oshiro BT, Henry E, Wilson J. Decreasing elective deliveries before 39 weeks of gestation in an integrated health care system. Obstet Gynecol 2009;113:804–11.)

Aim to Understand What Changes Along the Time Series Continuum Actually Improved Performance and Affected Outcomes

In the example shown in **Table 1** from Magee Women's Hospital, in their efforts to eliminate elective inductions prior to 39 weeks, the investigators were able to show over time that a formal approach to scheduling inductions made the most significant impact on the outcome measure of interest, elective inductions prior to 39 weeks' gestation.[22]

Aggregate the Learning Across a Variety of Sites

The Intermountain Healthcare example (see **Fig. 2**) to reduce elective deliveries before 39 weeks' gestation illustrates this aggregation of learning across multiple hospital sites. Other examples include similar initiatives done at Hospital Corporation of America hospitals as well as the Ohio Perinatal Quality Collaborative. Both show similarly impactful results on outcome measures.[23,24]

The criteria for a rigorous and potentially impactful quality improvement initiative that catalyzes systems change, including those to reduce preterm births, are[25]:

- Aim of the project is focused on performance improvement
- Performance measures are balanced and clearly related to the aim
- Whether through flowchart, key attributes, or other method, the description of the redesigned system is clear
- In moving to the new system, the key learning that occurred is well documented
- Measures across the time series can be linked with system changes that have been made
- Sustainability is shown by continuing to measure, long after the changes have been made.

Table 1
Reduction of induction risks: a departmental quality improvement project, Magee Women's Hospital

	3 Mo 2004	3 Mo 2005	14 Mo 2006–2007
Quality improvement approach	Baseline	Education and voluntary guidelines	Formal approval needed to schedule outside guidelines
Deliveries (N)	2139	2260	10895
Elective inductions <39 wk (N)	23	21	30
Total elective inductions (rate, %)	11.8	10.0	4.3 (P<.001)
Elective nulliparous inductions (N)	29	33	87
Elective nulliparous inductions → cesarean section (N)	10	5	12
Elective nulliparous inductions → cesarean section (rate, %)	35.7	15.2	13.8 (P<.01)
Total induction rate (%)	24.9	20.1	16.6

Data from Fisch JM, English D, Pedaline S, et al. Labor induction process improvement: a patient quality-of-care initiative. Obstet Gynecol 2009;113:797–803.

SUMMARY

Although premature delivery rates have begun to decline recently, prematurity still remains a cause of significant morbidity for newborns as well as being the leading cause of neonatal mortality. Expertise and consistency in health care delivery must be fostered in order to put into clinical practice those effective discoveries made by basic and clinical researchers. Women and their babies are not benefiting from available preterm birth prevention and treatment modalities, due to diagnostic errors, inconsistent care, failures in communication, and not being administered proven therapies in a timely manner. For example, in one study only 13.2% of preterm labor patients received optimal group B streptococcal chemoprophylaxis before delivery.[26] In addition, whereas the administration of antenatal steroids to women delivering prematurely has been paramount in improving the outcome of neonates delivered prematurely, the consistent administration of antenatal steroids to all at-risk mothers has been problematic. It was reported in one study that only 80% of eligible patients received the recommended course of antenatal steroids before delivery.[27] Although programs have been instituted to increase the appropriate administration of antenatal steroids in the past, they have not been uniformly successful.[28] Because of these continued inconsistencies and failures, the Joint Commission has added antenatal steroid administration as one of the 5 perinatal care core measures,[29] and hospitals have begun to institute programs to comply with this and other perinatal care core measures.

There have been only a few large-scale quality improvement projects or systems initiatives that have addressed prematurity directly. Several have been sponsored by the March of Dimes. One such project was introduced in 2005 by the California Chapter of the March of Dimes. This organization spearheaded the development and introduction of a preterm labor assessment toolkit,[30] and have been promoting its use in hospitals across the state as well as across the United States. This toolkit promotes a standardized process of preterm labor assessment when patients present to labor and delivery with signs and symptoms of preterm labor. Implementation of this toolkit, including a standardized protocol for preterm labor assessment, has been shown to reduce the rate of unnecessary hospital admissions with concomitant reductions in health care costs.[31]

Given the limited evidence-based opportunities to prevent preterm birth, implementing a quality improvement initiative to prevent preterm birth is a challenging undertaking. To optimize the prospects for the success of such an initiative, one must clearly identify the intervention, describe the system for change, measure the performance of the system over time, and determine whether changes in the system actually result in improvement. Institutional will and commitment to patient safety, being a high-reliability organization combined with provider leadership, and patient engagement in quality improvement are paramount. With these components in place, one becomes well positioned to institute a quality improvement initiative to prevent preterm birth.

APPENDIX A

The Plan-Do-Study-Act (PDSA) methodology or cycle can be applied to simple or more complex processes with the goal of making the processes more reliable. An approach to decreasing elective deliveries before 39 weeks' gestational age using the PDSA approach is shown here.[20]

Action Items	Details
PLAN	
Convene multidisciplinary quality improvement team of key stakeholders	• Key stakeholders may include: physicians/nurses/clerical staff; risk/quality management
Determine outcome measure(s) and data collection process	• Neonatal intensive care unit (NICU) admissions for babies delivered <39 weeks • Identify morbidities measures: neonatal and maternal • Electronic records, chart reviews, logs • Outline monitoring and ongoing evaluation of morbidities associated with <39-week deliveries
Determine process measure(s) and data collection process	• Scheduling process, including documentation to identify gestational age, indication for elective delivery • Process of oversight, guidelines enforcement and communication chain that prohibit elective deliveries <39 weeks
Align scheduling process with process to identify whether elective deliveries are appropriate and can be scheduled	• Step 1: Check that gestational age and medical indication are documented in scheduling form • Step 2: If criteria are missing or do not match specific guidelines (outlined in a checklist, for example), first level of communication is triggered (eg, call to Obstetrics Provider to request information) • Step 3: Additional chains of communication are triggered so that scheduling criteria are met and resolved
Develop or adopt scheduling form(s)	Identify who fills out forms and who reviews forms for required elements for scheduling
Aim for consensus on key concepts	• What is the "appeal process" for cases not covered by the guidelines? • Outline consequences if a provider refuses to follow the guidelines
Develop departmental policy	Policy reflects scheduling and documentation process, oversight and enforcement process to reduce or eliminate elective inductions and cesarean sections prior to 39 weeks' gestation that are not medically indicated
Collect baseline outcome and process measure data to identify areas in need of attention; data collected before implementation allows specific analysis of change after implementation	• Conduct chart reviews of scheduled inductions and cesarean deliveries for a minimum of 2 months before implementation • Assess the level of understanding of the issues by providers and patients • Assess barriers to change
Conduct educational presentations and Grand Rounds for key stakeholders	• Neonatal risks of Early Term Birth • Successful quality improvement projects that reduced elective Early Term Births
Develop a plan and timeline for implementation	First implementation plan runs for 1–2 months; first evaluation ("Study") is completed within 1–2 months
	(continued on next page)

Action Items	Details
DO	
Communicate new departmental policy	Identify point person to communicate policy with each group; eg, Department Chair, Quality Improvement Committee Chair or MD Project Lead communicates with Obstetrics Providers; Nursing Director communicates with Nursing Staff
Implement use of new processes and forms for a predetermined pilot period of time	Implement new processes and forms for 1–2 months; evaluate within 1–2-month time period
STUDY	
After predetermined pilot period, review and assess effectiveness of policy and forms implementation; analyze impact on obstetric service, process and patient outcomes	Depending on the intent and resources of the department, this action item can be conducted as in-depth analysis or a less intensive overview of trends of process and outcome measures including: • Review of elective procedures • Indications • Neonatal outcomes
ACT	
Reconvene quality improvement team to identify additional changes to continue improvement process	• Edit scheduling forms, guidelines • Clarify implementation plan • Provide additional guidance to providers about department policy, scheduling and documentation requirements
Inform staff of changes	Process measures may require additional change over time; process measures can change during the implementation process, but outcome measures remain more constant
Obtain ongoing feedback on strengths and areas for improvement	Feedback reminds everyone about the importance of the project, fosters teamwork, and gives everyone a voice. Providing feedback can be as simple as posting monthly data in prominent spots on Labor & Delivery; data can include process and outcome measures, ie, number of elective births and number of NICU admissions in that population

REFERENCES

1. Behrman RE, Butler AS, editors. Preterm birth: causes, consequences, and prevention. Washington, DC: National Academies Press; 2007.
2. Hamilton BE, Martin JA, Ventura SJ. 3. Births: preliminary data for 2009. National Vital Statistics Reports, 59. Hyattsville (MD): National Center for Health Statistics; 2010.
3. Meis PJ, Klebanoff M, Thom T, et al. Prevention of recurrent preterm delivery by 17 alpha-hydroxyprogesterone caproate. N Engl J Med 2003;348:2379–85.
4. Petrini JN, Callaghan WM, Klebanoff M. Estimated effect of 17 alpha-hydroxyprogesterone caproate on preterm birth in the United States. Obstet Gynecol 2005; 105:267–72.

5. Healthy People.gov/2020 topics and objectives: maternal, infant and child health. Available at: http://www.healthypeople.gov/2020/topicsobjectives2020/objectiveslist. aspx?topicid=2. Accessed May 2, 2011.

6. Rouse DJ, Caritis SN, Peaceman AM, et al. A trial of 17 alpha-hydroxyprogesterone caproate to prevent prematurity in twins. N Engl J Med 2007;357:454–61.

7. Pronovost P, Needham D, Berenholtz S, et al. An intervention to decrease catheter-related bloodstream infections in the ICU. N Engl J Med 2006;355: 2725–32.

8. Resar R, Pronovost P, Haraden C, et al. Using a bundle approach to improve ventilator care processes and reduce ventilator-associated pneumonia. Jt Comm J Qual Patient Saf 2005;31:243–8.

9. Lohr KN, editor. Medicare: a strategy for quality assurance. Washington, DC: National Academies Press; 1990.

10. Kohn KT, Corrigan JM, Donaldson MS, editors. To err is human: building a safer health care system. Washington, DC: National Academies Press; 1999.

11. Reason J. Human error: models and management. BMJ 2000;320:768–70.

12. Institute of Medicine. Crossing the quality chasm: a new health system for the 21st century. Washington, DC: National Academies Press; 2001.

13. Donabedian A. Evaluating the quality of medical care. Milbank Mem Fund Q 1966;44(Suppl):166–206.

14. Berns SD, editor. Toward improving the outcome of pregnancy III. Enhancing perinatal health through quality, safety and performance initiatives. White Plains (NY): March of Dimes; 2010.

15. Luce JM, Bindman AB, Lee PR. A brief history of health care quality assessment and improvement in the United States. West J Med 1994;160:263–8.

16. Leape LL. Error in medicine. JAMA 1994;272:1851–7.

17. U.S. Dept. of Health and Human Services Agency on Healthcare Research and Quality: transforming hospitals into high reliability organizations. Available at: http://www.ahrq.gov/qual/hroadvice/hroadvice1.htm#fig6. Accessed May 2, 2011.

18. Ellsbury DL, Ursprung R. A primer on quality improvement methodology in neonatology. Clin Perinatol 2010;37:87–99.

19. Speroff T, O'Connor GT. Study designs for PDSA quality improvement research. Qual Manag Health Care 2004;13:17–32.

20. Main E, Oshiro B, Chagolla B, et al. Elimination of non-medically indicated (elective) deliveries before 39 weeks gestational age. A California toolkit to transform maternity care. Available at: www.marchofdimes.com/professionals/medicalresources_ 39weeks.html. Accessed May 2, 2011.

21. Oshiro BT, Henry E, Wilson J. Decreasing elective deliveries before 39 weeks of gestation in an integrated health care system. Obstet Gynecol 2009;113:804–11.

22. Fisch JM, English D, Pedaline S, et al. Labor induction process improvement: a patient quality-of-care initiative. Obstet Gynecol 2009;113:797–803.

23. Clark SL, Frye DR, Meyers JA, et al. Reduction in elective delivery at <39 weeks of gestation: comparative effectiveness of 3 approaches to change and the impact on neonatal intensive care admission and stillbirth. Am J Obstet Gynecol 2010;203:449.e1–6.

24. Donovan EF, Lannon C, Bailit J, et al. A statewide initiative to reduce inappropriate scheduled births at 36(07)-38(6/7) weeks' gestation. Am J Obstet Gynecol 2010;202:243.e1–8.

25. Nolan T. System changes to improve patient safety. BMJ 2000;320:771–3.

26. Goins WP, Talbot TR, Schaffner W, et al. Adherence to perinatal group B streptococcal prevention guidelines. Obstet Gynecol 2010;115:1217–24.

27. Howell EA, Stone J, Kleinman LG, et al. Approaching NIH guideline recommended care for maternal-infant health: clinical failures to use recommended antenatal steroids. Matern Child Health J 2010;14:430–6.
28. Wirtschafter DD, Danielsen BH, Main EK. Promoting antenatal steroid use for fetal maturation: results from the California perinatal quality care collaborative. J Pediatr 2006;148:606–12.
29. Specifications manual for Joint Commission National Quality Core Measures: perinatal core measure PC-03. Available at: http://manual.jointcommission.org/releases/TJC2011A/PerinatalCare.html. Accessed May 2, 2011.
30. Preterm labor assessment toolkit. Available at: www.marchofdimes.com/professionals/medicalresourcespretermlabor.html. Accessed May 2, 2011.
31. Rose CH, McWeeney DT, Brost BC, et al. Cost-effective standardization of preterm labor evaluation. Am J Obstet Gynecol 2010;203:250,e1–5.

Index

Note: Page numbers of article titles are in **boldface** type.

A

Abruption. *See* Placental abruption.
Academic problems, 447
Agency for Healthcare Research and Quality, 568
Alloimmunization, delivery indicated for, 426–427
Anemia, fetal, delivery indicated for, 426–427
Animal models
    for inflammation and infection, 391–396
    for maternal stress, 365–366
Antibiotics, for infections, 388–389
Arithmetic disability, 447
Asphyxia
    cerebral palsy risk in, 457
    neuroprotection for, 460–463
Assent, versus consent, in decision-making, 481–482
Asthma, delivery indicated for, 426
Attention-deficit disorders, 447–448, 503–506

B

Bacteremia, fetal, 389
Behavioral outcomes, of preterm infants, 447–448
    early term, 503–506
    extremely preterm, 477
    late preterm, 503–506
"Best Interests" Standard, 479
Betamethasone, antenatal
    current practice using, 529–530
    dose for, 530–533
    outcomes of, 533–534
    versus dexamethasone, 530, 533–534
Biomarkers, for inflammation
    in animal models, 392–396
    in humans, 390–391
Birth asphyxia
    cerebral palsy risk in, 457
    neuroprotection for, 460–463
Birth weight, versus gestational age, in decision-making, 472
Brain injury, 443–444, 460–463

Clin Perinatol 38 (2011) 579–589
doi:10.1016/S0095-5108(11)00076-5
0095-5108/11/$ – see front matter © 2011 Elsevier Inc. All rights reserved.

perinatology.theclinics.com

Moving?

Make sure your subscription moves with you!

To notify us of your new address, find your **Clinics Account Number** (located on your mailing label above your name), and contact customer service at:

Email: journalscustomerservice-usa@elsevier.com

800-654-2452 (subscribers in the U.S. & Canada)
314-447-8871 (subscribers outside of the U.S. & Canada)

Fax number: 314-447-8029

Elsevier Health Sciences Division
Subscription Customer Service
3251 Riverport Lane
Maryland Heights, MO 63043

*To ensure uninterrupted delivery of your subscription, please notify us at least 4 weeks in advance of move.

Moving?

Make sure your subscription moves with you!

To notify us of your new address, find your Clinics Account Number (located on your mailing label above your name), and contact customer service at:

Email journalscustomerservice-usa@elsevier.com

800-654-2452 (subscribers in the U.S. & Canada)
314-447-8871 (subscribers outside of the U.S. & Canada)

Fax number: 314-447-8029

Elsevier Health Sciences Division
Subscription Customer Service
3251 Riverport Lane
Maryland Heights, MO 63043

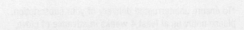

Printed and bound by CPI Group (UK) Ltd, Croydon, CR0 4YY

03/10/2024

01040452-0011